THE BIG BOOK OF

# ENDURANCE TRAINING
# AND
# RACING

# THE BIG BOOK OF

# ENDURANCE TRAINING AND RACING

## Dr. Philip Maffetone

FOREWORD BY
**Mark Allen**

Skyhorse Publishing

Skyhorse Publishing books may be purchased in bulk at special discounts for sales promotion, corporate gifts, fund-raising, or educational purposes. Special editions can also be created to specifications. For details, contact the Special Sales Department, Skyhorse Publishing, 555 Eighth Avenue, Suite 903, New York, NY 10018 or info@skyhorsepublishing.com.

www.skyhorsepublishing.com

10 9 8 7 6 5 4 3 2 1

Library of Congress Cataloging-in-Publication Data

Maffetone, Philip.
 The big book of endurance training and racing / Philip Maffetone ; foreword by Mark Allen.
    p. cm.
  Includes index. 4452 3842 12/10
  ISBN 978-1-61608-065-5 (pbk. : alk. paper)
 1. Physical education and training. 2. Physical fitness--Physiological aspects. 3. Muscle strength. 4. Running--Training. I. Allen, Mark, 1958- II. Title.
  GV711.5.M35 2010
  613.7'1--dc22

                    2010017692

Printed in Canada

# CONTENTS

## SECTION II
### Diet and Nutrition

## SECTION III
### The Importance of Self-Care and Injury Prevention

MARK ALLEN

# FOREWORD

**W**elcome to *The Big Book of Endurance Training and Racing*. Hopefully, the information you find in these pages will change your life. It did for me when I began training under the guidance of Dr. Phil Maffetone.

My athletic career started in 1968 when I answered an ad in the local paper announcing swim-team tryouts. At the time I literally couldn't swim more than the length of a twenty-five-yard pool without having to stop and catch my breath. In the nearly thirty years since, I have tried almost every training theory and coaching style in the pursuit of personal athletic excellence. The evolution to my present program was not easy. The years of regimented swim coaching had ingrained in me a very narrow-minded training philosophy, which was to do things faster. If I could just train with more yardage, and train faster, then I would most certainly race faster. Or so I thought.

My race results from this type of program were mediocre at best. "Do more, faster" really only works for those so talented that their genetics override the lunacy of their training and take them to greatness anyway. I ended my twelve-year swimming career completely burned out, physically and mentally. I also ended it feeling like I just hadn't reached my potential. But at the time, I couldn't put my finger on why.

Fortunately, I was given a second chance to explore the limits of my athletic abilities. In 1982, I embarked on what has been a dream trip through the world of the triathlon. It wasn't always smooth, though. My initiation years mirrored my swimming career. Due specifically to the swimming mentality, "Do more, faster," a few great results were separated by injuries and sporadic improvement. But unlike swimming, which is not an impact sport, the price of unwise training in triathlons is not only mental decay, but physical as well. Something needed to change.

Just about this time, I was introduced to Dr. Phil Maffetone, who had enjoyed a good deal of success training triathletes. I was warned that his methods were probably going to sound crazy at first, but assured that they really worked. That was 1984. And, yes, at the time his philosophy on training was almost completely opposite to my "do more, faster" approach. Now it's a new millennium, and his training techniques that once seemed crazy are almost universally accepted as the only method that will allow you to reach your peak performance year after year. Using Phil's training program and consulting with him over the years, I have been able to rack up a long list of international triathlon victories, including six Ironman Hawaii titles, the last of which came at age thirty-seven!

In *The Big Book of Endurance Training and Racing,* Dr. Maffetone details the training philosophy that I have used throughout my triathlon career. If you have used these tools and techniques, you know they work. If you haven't, welcome to what will undoubtedly be a whole new level of athletic performance. Take the time to follow his program. Leave your ego at the door, because in the short term it might seem like you aren't going anywhere. But long term, I guarantee you will see the results you know your body is capable of.

*Mark Allen is a six-time Ironman Hawaii champion and was named by* Outside *magazine the fittest man in the world.*

# PREFACE

The Big Book of Endurance Training and Racing is for triathletes, runners, cyclists, swimmers, cross-country skiers, and other athletes seeking greater endurance. You will learn about the many important tools that help you achieve optimal athletic potential—and keep you healthy and injury-free for many productive years.

Commitment and dedication to your sport cannot be accomplished without careful planning. I want to assist you in getting even more from your body. The successful road to training and racing is relatively simple. It includes having a clear strategy with short- and long-term goals, monitoring progress to assure your plan is working and to prevent overtraining, and, of course, proper nutrition.

This book gives you a fresh look at successful endurance training and competition. My system offers a truly "individualized" approach, which I have continually updated and refined over three decades of training and treating athletes, who range from world champions to weekend warriors.

My general philosophy regarding endurance contains four key points:

1. **Build a great aerobic base.** This essential physical and metabolic foundation helps accomplish several important tasks: it prevents injury and maintains a balanced physical body; it increases fat burning for improved stamina, weight loss, and sustained energy; and it improves overall health in the immune and hormonal systems, the intestines and liver, and throughout the body.

2.  **Eat well.** Specific foods influence the developing aerobic system, especially the foods consumed in the course of a typical day. Overall, diet can significantly influence your body's physical, chemical, and mental state of fitness and health.

3.  **Reduce stress.** Training and competition, combined with other lifestyle factors, can be stressful and adversely affect performance, cause injuries, and even lead to poor nutrition because they can disrupt the normal digestion and absorption of nutrients.

4.  **Improve brain function.** The brain and entire nervous system control virtually all athletic activity, and a healthier brain produces a better athlete. Improved brain function occurs from eating well, controlling stress, and through sensory stimulation, which includes proper training and optimal breathing.

Those familiar with my other books and essays on fitness and health know that I'm strongly opposed to quick-fix solutions to many of the problems encountered by triathletes, runners, cyclists, and other endurance athletes. Too often, so-called sports medicine experts only consider the symptoms, leaving the basis of a particular problem unattended, only to cause other problems down the road (and sometimes a recurrence of the same problem). Today's practitioners too readily recommend off-the-shelf treatments, including rest, stretching, hot or cold packs, anti-inflammatory drugs, and often surgery. It's a classic case of treating the symptom and ignoring the root cause. This cookbook approach to the human body is indefensible.

Yet there are many exceptional healthcare practitioners in sports, and I devote a whole chapter to how to find one. The better sports practitioners take an alternative view about the best kind of treatment and carefully consider the entire athlete. This is critical because an injury is, with some exceptions, simply the end result of a series of dominoes falling over. For example, one morning, while bending to tie your shoe, you feel a twinge in your hamstring. While that's where the pain is located, it's often not the location of the cause. A comprehensive history and evaluation might discover the cause is in the foot—the result of wearing the wrong kind of running shoe. Some barely noticeable muscular imbalance in the leg might develop, leading to a tilt in the pelvis, with a final stop in the hamstring—the source of the pain.

The remedy? Obviously, ice, anti-inflammatory drugs, or rubbing the hamstring is not going to correct the real problem. Obtaining the right shoe will often quickly allow the body to make its own natural corrections of the fallen dominos.

Generally, the body has a great natural ability to heal itself. When your body gives you a very obvious sign, such as a hamstring twinge, it's time to stop and assess what's going on. If you don't, it may soon be too late. Waiting until you're physically unable to train—the point at which your body forces you to stop—simply results in wasted time, frustration, fitness loss, increased stress, and even depression.

Yes, it's best to view the body in the entire context of physical, chemical, and mental balance. Some call this a holistic approach, or looking at the big picture.

The brain is an influential part of this holistic equation, especially in endurance sports. The brain may be the most forgotten or even neglected aspect of training and competition. I predict that neuroscience will soon emerge as the next frontier in sports research. I'm not referring to sports psychology, which has been around for decades, but the physiology of the brain and how it affects muscles, hormones, energy production, fat burning, and virtually all athletic function.

The brain is the reason we slow down during a race—not too much lactate, or too little glucose or oxygen. As the body's control center, the brain may slow us down to prevent injury or ill health. For example, the body may have some impairment, some "roadblock" that prevents us from going faster, and rather than cause an injury, the brain tells the body to slow down or even stop. With information found in this book, you'll be able to find those impairments before they occur and self-correct them.

*The Big Book of Endurance Training and Racing* also dispels many of the commonly held myths that linger in participatory sports—and that adversely impact performance. These false notions are propagated by common misunderstandings; outdated information about training, competition, and nutrition; and the very worst sins—rampant commercialism and sports marketing. To dispel these myths, I will carefully explain throughout this book the following recommendations:

- Focus on burning more body fat for energy, instead of just on carbohydrates (glucose).
- Train slower, enabling your aerobic system to improve endurance so you can actually race faster.
- Don't use costly, built-up running shoes; instead use the flattest, least protective training and racing shoes to prevent foot and leg injuries.
- Don't stretch; instead, you can obtain significant flexibility through an active warm-up and cool-down, without the risk of injury that can accompany stretching.
- Consume a balance of dietary fats to help build endurance, reduce inflammation, and improve brain function.
- Stay away from refined carbohydrates that can reduce endurance energy, disrupt important hormone balance, and store excess body fat.
- Avoid common dietary supplements that can negatively impact endurance and health.

- Spend time in the sun without sunscreen or protective clothing to obtain more vitamin D to improve athletic performance.
- Recognize and correct overtraining in its earliest stage—long before fatigue, poor performance, or injury occurs.
- Know that age is no barrier to performance. It's possible to go faster in your forties, fifties, and even sixties—with improved fat burning and better slow-twitch muscle function.

## How to Use This Book

*The Big Book of Endurance Training and Racing* will help you individualize your own program. Every athlete has unique needs, and no single program will work for everyone. Most importantly, your primary concern should never be short-term; instead, your focus should always be long-term. By doing so improvements in performance should be consistent for years to come, despite your age or gender.

I've set up this book the same way I personally worked with an athlete—which was one-on-one. Beginning with a general overview, I define common terms in endurance sports, as well as describe some of the key body systems, such as muscle, metabolism, and the brain. I then show you how to put all these ideas into practice with training, racing, and self-testing. Diet, nutrition, and other topics follow, and with each new chapter you'll easily be able to build on a solid understanding. To facilitate this learning process, I have included a number of fitness and health surveys on topics ranging from hormones and stress to diet.

You will also come across brief case histories of some of my former patients and athletes, personal perspectives from those who have followed the tenets of my program, and questions visitors have submitted to my Web site at www.PhilMaffetone.com. I have done my best to answer them in this book. I'd love to hear from you.

In the meantime, enjoy and endure!

—**Dr. Philip Maffetone**

# INTRODUCTION—
## My Personal Journey on the Road to Endurance

Life is a journey of endurance, full of unexpected surprises. Little did I know growing up that one day I would become a holistic practitioner who would spend many wonderful years working closely with endurance athletes, ranging from beginners to seasoned veterans, including some of the world's greatest competitors. These athletes include triathlon champions Mark Allen, Colleen Cannon, and Mike Pigg, world-class distance runner Marianne Dickerson, and the late running guru Dr. George Sheehan.

The irony is that I started out as a high school sprinter competing in the 220-yard event and shorter distances—a far cry from being an endurance athlete myself, or even knowing much about the human body or understanding its potential through proper training, stress management, and diet.

Through years of trial and error, experience, immersion in the literature of exercise physiology, Eastern philosophy, and treating patients and athletes, I continued to refine and expand upon what I consider the big-picture approach to endurance sports. But before offering you a wealth of information on how to become a better endurance athlete, allow me to first recount my own personal story, which reflects the reason why, to this day, I encourage all athletes to never neglect their health for the sake of performance. Both fitness and health are intertwined in a deeply significant way, a fact that became entirely apparent to me soon after I ran the New York City Marathon in 1980.

∽

I started running track in high school in the 1960s, and those twenty-two or twenty-three seconds going all-out on cinders in my spikes represented the full extent of my endurance. Until the end of my sophomore year in high school, I was not physically active; gym class was embarrassing because I was uncoordinated and could not do the things most other kids did. Even my academic world was disastrous, since I was a poor student just barely moving on to the next grade level each year, only thanks to summer school. But puberty and a surge of natural testosterone fortuitously came into my life, and during the last week of tenth grade, our gym class had a fitness test—running 600 yards. Without training or preparation, I beat everyone. The following year I joined the track team and began a streak of nearly undefeated racing that extended all the way into college.

Along the way, I had a few bad races. In my senior year, for example, I was the only runner from my high school to qualify for the biggest meet in New York State. After a cafeteria lunch of the usual junk food, I left with the track coach for the long drive to the meet. Once there, I ran several heats, easily winning each race to keep progressing until I made the finals. But I hadn't eaten anything since lunch. The final race was well into the evening and I was famished. Walking to the starting line, I

felt weak and shaky from lack of food. And, I didn't see my starting blocks, which the rest of the sprinters had already set up. The official told me to hurry across the track and fetch my blocks. As soon as I returned, the race started. I sprinted about 150 yards, and, realizing that I wasn't going to win, I jogged to the finish dead last; the winning time was a slow 23.5 seconds.

After high school graduation, I decided to go to college for one reason—to run track—despite my poor grades. My primary goal was to reach national levels, with thoughts about making the U.S. Olympic team.

Much of my training time at college was spent on my own: an easy warm-up lap or two

*I started out as a sprinter
in high school.*

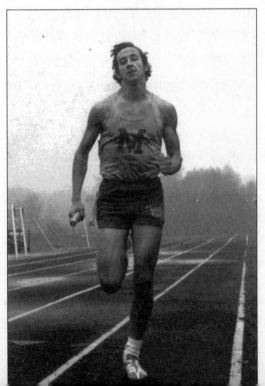

around the quarter-mile track, ten or twelve short sprints, and a cool-down lap. I don't recall many of the smaller track-and-field races with nearby colleges. I would just show up and run fast, winning most of them. With what seemed like too much extra time on my hands, I also wanted to use my leg speed and newfound overall athleticism to play football and base-ball, but was prevented from doing so by my track coach who thought I'd get injured.

I succeeded in qualifying for the nationals during the collegiate indoor track season, having raced on many old wooden tracks to get there. But I had to run even shorter dis-tances like the sixty-yard sprint to accom-plish this goal. At the season-ending race, I was one of three runners in a photo finish—I placed third. But after that race, I lost interest in training and racing. I also dropped out of college. Studying wasn't for me. I was ready to move on with life.

I was now living in the same small upstate New York town where I grew up, ironically near the high school track where I ran so well. I found a good job, with benefits, working for the phone company, which required me to test newly installed equipment inside the tele-phone buildings. I soon got married, started a family, and tried to maintain as much sports activity as possible, joining an amateur foot-ball team as a wide receiver and participating in baseball, playing alternately at most posi-tions. I also swam freestyle, always short dis-tances, and was nearly as good a competitor as in my earlier track days.

During this time I also became interested in exercise physiology and nutrition. Perhaps my childhood contributed to this desire. My mother would often listen to nutrition expert Carlton Fredericks on the radio, and later, my father became fascinated with Rodale's organic gardening ideas and planted a family vegetable garden.

I read Adele Davis's books. In the late six-ties and early seventies, she was recognized as a nutritional sage. I also worked part-time in a health food store and joined a natural foods co-op. I had already been studying Eastern philosophy, and now it seemed even more important, as the only image of health that personally made sense was the holistic one.

One day I had what could only be described as a powerful vision—that I needed to go back to school and become a doctor to help people. It was so strong an epiphany that the next day I gave my two-week notice to the phone company. I planned to complete my undergraduate work at a local college and found an evening job in a restaurant. My grades improved slightly as I learned more about human biology and could relate it to my own health. Eating better was a signifi-cant part of becoming a more attentive stu-dent. Still, my poor grades overall made it difficult to get into any professional school. I met a chiropractor who knew the dean of the National University of Health Sciences in Chicago. There I could study nutrition, sports medicine, and other related topics, and its doctorate of chiropractic would allow me to one day practice as a physician.

Uprooting my family, now with two young children, from New York to Chicago was quite stressful. I found a job as night watchman at a factory, the midnight to 8:00 AM shift, and obtained school loans to pay for tuition and other costs. The school offered the option of a summer semester, enabling students to complete the five-year program in three and a half years, and I opted for the accelerated program. The professional school curriculum was twice as rigorous as that of undergraduate work. The extra study time required overwhelmed me. One could not, for example, learn enough about the body from human dissection class without also spending the entire weekend studying the incredibly intricate details of just where each muscle attached, the delicate structure of the body's joints, and the complex display of nerves running throughout the body.

But it was my disappointment with the philosophy of the chiropractic profession and its narrow range of assessment and therapeutic options that led me to call my old boss at the phone company and ask for my job back. He said my position was there if I wanted it. That evening, while pondering this choice, I went down to the basement of our on-campus apartment complex to do laundry. Accidentally going into the wrong door, I encountered a group of students listening to a lecture on muscles and movement, and how nutrition played a key role. Now I got really excited. Exposure to this kind of information

was the original reason I had sacrificed so much.

Despite the long hours of classes, the graveyard factory shift, and my family responsibilities, it was studying topics outside the regular curriculum that became the priority. Chicago was home to a proliferation of weekend professional seminars regularly offered by medical doctors, osteopaths, chiropractors, acupuncturists, and others who taught about natural hands-on healing, diet and nutrition, and exercise. Exposure to all these topics complemented my studies of anatomy and physiology, biochemistry and pharmacology, and diagnosis. While the National University of Health Sciences was considered overly medical by many chiropractors—because it taught in a very scientific way and included much of what medical students study—it still held to rigid ideological views, an unyielding approach that I was uncomfortable with. For example, the school's curriculum insisted that the spine was the cause of many health problems, and not lifestyle considerations such as nutrition and exercise.

But the learning I picked up at the seminars helped balance my education. The study of anatomy insisted that the bones of the skull were fixed, but now I discovered from osteopathy that the skull's bones could move with the breath and other muscle motions, which offered important therapeutic possibilities. I learned that the brain, if injured, not only could recover but could improve in cognition and function, and with age. And muscles, which commonly get out of balance and can take weeks or months to rehabilitate, can be corrected easily and quickly through various types of hands-on treatment.

Yet even with all that I was learning, both in school and on weekends, I was still missing something: putting all that information into actual practice. I simply could not wait for graduation, so after a short time, I began treating people in my apartment—a sort of underground clinic. My first patients were fellow students, then people from the local community. I would often see this one classmate jog past my apartment to and from his daily workout. He always seemed exhausted upon his return compared to how he looked when he first started. One day I asked him if I could evaluate him, and he agreed. His body was quite beat up after his run—high heart rate, muscle imbalance, poor gait, and knee pain. I began to study how this could happen and became even more interested in exercise physiology.

Unfortunately, in 1976, with less than a year left of school, I physically, chemically, and mentally fell apart. The cumulative stress had caught up with me. One day I found myself in the hospital emergency room, and the physicians were not going to let me leave because I was so sick. My muscles had severely deteriorated, the intestines had shut down, and I was dangerously anemic. Because my immune system wasn't working, my whole body was chronically inflamed. Yet I needed to travel to New York to take the state boards in order to

get my license to practice. After I spent a week in the hospital, the doctors still would not let me leave. So I removed the IVs in both arms, got dressed, and arranged for a ride to the airport. I took the two-day exam, later finding out I passed, but was too sick and weak to return to Chicago and had to be hospitalized in New York.

I now weighed only ninety-seven pounds—a precipitous loss of sixty pounds in less than a year. Despite being bedridden in the hospital, I wanted to watch the Montreal Olympics on television, especially the track events. Yet I was barely able to reach the television switch and was too weak to turn it on. The nurse came in to help me. Jealously watching these Olympic athletes in action, I wondered how my health could so rapidly deteriorate. I wasn't even thirty years old.

Soon after my return to Chicago, I made an appointment with a doctor in Detroit, who had taught a seminar I'd attended. Dr. George Goodheart offered to treat me without charge during my three-day visit, and allowed me to closely observe his treatment of patients, most of whom had flown in from other areas of the country and the world. Dr. Goodheart had developed a form of biofeedback assessment called applied kinesiology, which combined manual muscle testing with a variety of hands-on therapies, such as manipulation, acupuncture, and cranial therapy, with nutrition and other treatment methods. I had already used some of these approaches in my illegal student practice with good results, but never imagined I would see such extreme cases of ill and injured patients getting better in such a short time, including me. My initial blood test showed an alarming blood hemoglobin level of 7.1, low enough to require a transfusion (which never helped). But Dr. Goodheart said my blood test would improve. At the end of the third day, my blood test had reached 11—so unbelievable that, soon after returning to Chicago, I had the blood tested again to see if the result was true. Having studied hematology, I knew that it would take months, not days, to improve the blood cells. But mine was now 11.8! I was even more convinced that the methods of evaluation and treatment I was learning were more powerful than I had imagined. And, it provided me with the enthusiasm and confidence I never got from academic studies. This realization coincided with the beginning of my own physical recovery. In a short time, I further fine-tuned my diet and nutrition, and began to walk for exercise. At first, walking an easy ten minutes was almost impossible. But as I progressed, my muscles started to reappear and I continued improving. I gained most of my weight back.

In 1977, I moved back to New York with my family and entered private practice, once again living near the track where I had excelled as a high school sprinter. I soon began seeing a variety of patients, old and young. Some suffered from joint or back pain or had intestinal problems, not unlike my own for so long. My approach was simple: spend all the time necessary evaluating each patient as an individual, and once it was clear what the causes were, the treatment part was often quick and easy. I had a whole "tool chest" of possible therapies, from traditional physical remedies to diet, nutrition, stress management, even employing exercise as a therapy. It was a matter of matching the most appropriate therapy with the patient's particular needs. Because of my truly holistic approach, and because many of these patients responded quickly, my referral practice built quickly.

The experience of having once been a patient was one of the most important lessons that enabled me to succeed with my own patients. A common complaint of patients is that their doctors don't listen to them, don't take their seemingly irrelevant complaints seriously, and simply treat their symptoms without finding the root cause of their problem. This is exactly what had happened to me when my body shut down. Doctors kept treating my symptoms, the reason I never recovered under their care. In some ways, I felt almost lucky to have experienced being a patient as part of my professional training. Health-care professionals who have never been patients are not often able to relate to certain aspects of what a patient really feels. I vowed to be an exception.

Local athletes began showing up at my office. Typically, an injury had sidelined them and they were looking for help. In fact, many visited me as a last resort after seeing different specialists. My approach was always the same:

spend all the necessary time assessing them, then apply the most effective treatment.

One day, the president of the local Road Runners Club showed up. He was a firefighter who had fallen through the roof of a burning house. He had multiple physical injuries, especially in his back, yet was determined to run in the New York City Marathon, only several weeks away. I was able to fix his injuries and get him running without pain by using many of the therapeutic tools of evaluation and hands-on treatment I'd learned in recent years, especially by balancing his injured muscles. He completed his race with ease.

More and more distance runners from the region began filling up my waiting room as word spread of my successful and unconventional approach to injury treatment. Gradually implementing various biofeedback tools, I began measuring many aspects of human physiology in athletes, from heart-rate changes and breathing to the brain's control over muscle function. I also learned another vital component to my work—that eliminating a simple or serious injury was only half of my job. The other half was knowing how the dysfunction happened and how to prevent its recurrence. This meant understanding how an athlete worked out, taking all the information I learned through my examination and treatment, and using that to make appropriate changes in training and competition.

My exposure to more and more runners led me to take up personal coaching, but I made sure that coaching was nothing like the traditional process of giving athletes training schedules and encouraging them to race harder. Instead, my coaching style was to help them be their own coach while providing objective feedback. They would coach themselves with my input, which helped them become more intuitive and instinctual about their body.

As my own health continued to improve, I entertained the notion of running in the New York City Marathon. By then, I had been walking regularly for more than two years. The marathon was six months away, and that seemed like plenty of time to train for it. So I began slow jogging in the middle of my walks, gradually making more of the one-hour workout an easy run. I monitored my heart rate, wore flat running shoes, and always walked at the start and the end of the session for a proper warm-up and cool-down. Eventually, I got up to two hours for my longest run of the week. While I had a sense of the distances I covered, my training was based on time.

∽

It was a cool, overcast morning on race day for the New York City Marathon. The race started with a cannon blast so loud it shook the Verrazano Bridge. The crowd of 18,000 runners began to move and I was among them. All went well through the first ten miles. The excitement swept me along at a slightly quicker pace than I'd planned, yet I felt great. As expected, by fifteen miles I felt tired but was able to continue. Within the next couple of miles, however, I began to shiver. Despite drinking plenty of water, I felt dehydrated. And I was craving cotton candy. At eighteen miles, I stopped to check my feet. They were numb, and I wanted to be sure they were still there. "My hamstrings are cramping," I said out loud. Suddenly, I realized I wasn't thinking rationally, and all I could remember was my goal to finish the race and prove to myself and others that I was healthy.

Alarmed by how awful I looked, two paramedics tried to remove me from the course. But I wouldn't let them. Somehow, I painfully fought my way onward. I have very little memory of those last few miles, but I'll always remember the finale. It included a minor collision with a television cameraman in Central Park. The crowds got louder, and then I had a clear view of the finish line.

A finisher's medal was hung around my neck. I cried with joy over the ultimate success of passing my four-hour endurance test. But the next moment I discovered myself herded into the first-aid tent. It looked like a war zone. There were casualties all around me. Doctors and nurses were running in and out. Sick-looking runners lying on cots groaned in pain. Ambulances came and went. I thought to myself, "Are these people really healthy? And am I?" I realized then that running the marathon had not proven my health at all. I was fit enough to run 26.2 miles. But clearly fitness was something quite different from good health. This critical concept will be discussed in much greater detail

throughout this book; yes, too many endurance athletes wrongly assume that being super-fit or posting fast times is the same as being healthy.

Soon after the New York City race, I also began lecturing on various topics in holistic fitness and health, first at the local library, an aerobic dance studio, and a health food store, then at running clinics. I also began writing professional papers to present at conferences, where all types of health-care professionals began to adopt my holistic approach and began practicing it with their own patients. Gradually I received more invitations to races, such as the Bermuda Marathon, where I met Dr. George Sheehan, who was also a speaker. A cardiologist and runner, he was a very influential figure in the running community because of his regular columns in *Runner's World* and other publications. He was philosophical and humorous when writing about the curious passions and obsessions of runners. He became intrigued with my implementation of heart-rate monitors. Dr. Sheehan later came to my office to see firsthand my work with athletes.

It wasn't long before I began to be contacted by swimmers and cyclists, and later triathletes. These calls came from all over the United States, including San Diego, California, Boulder, Colorado, and Florida. I eventually set up athlete workshops of varying lengths—a day to a week—in these and other locations, combining one-on-one work, lectures, group runs, and bike rides to evaluate training, and spending time at the pool watching stroke mechanics.

Working with triathletes represented a unique experience compared to single-sport athletes. In this event, an athlete must train in three different activities: swimming, biking, and running. From a physiological standpoint, this type of cross-training has additional built-in benefits over single sports. The three activities are neurologically very different, with the brain responding uniquely to each different sport. Cross-training provided a better-rounded and balanced training response. In addition, each sport could be used to help manipulate the body differently. Clearly, this kind of triathlon training provided more fitness and health potential than the sum of all three sports. Swimming, for example, could also be used to help the body in its physical, metabolic, and other types of recovery following a longer run or bike ride. In particular, a long-distance triathlon was an accumulated increase of physical intensity, maintaining high aerobic activity in the swim and bike, and only becoming anaerobic in the run. These observations became important strategies to help the athletes I worked with succeed.

One endurance athlete who visited my clinic was a young, extroverted, blonde, and supremely talented triathlete by the name of Colleen Cannon. In a short time, she was able to go from a forty-minute 10K to about thirty-five minutes and started performing much better on the triathlon circuit. She also referred other triathletes, including a promising San Diegan: Mark Allen, who had yet to win the Ironman.

Another endurance athlete who came to my office for treatment and coaching was ultramarathoner Stu Mittleman. I had met Stu the day before at the pre-registration for a short-distance triathlon that he planned on entering. But he had a painful foot problem and was going to withdraw from the race. He asked me how long it would take to heal so he could race again. I told him that his problem would be easy to correct, and showed him how, eliminating the pain by manipulating the foot and working on the muscles that caused the problem. The next day, he completed the triathlon without difficulty.

I then began to work closely with Stu. I encouraged him to alter his training, use a heart-monitor, and improve his diet. Like most endurance athletes I've worked with, Stu taught me a lot about human performance. Watching him train made me feel like a scientist studying a human lab animal, especially observing him going round and round the track. Any time I saw a minor deviation in his gait or stride, he would take a pit stop and we'd correct the problem. Together, we prepared for the World Six-Day Race Championships in La Rochelle, France. In this, his biggest ultra event to date, he placed second overall out of a field of the world's top two dozen ultrarunners, reaching almost 100 miles a day for six consecutive days—all while on a 200-meter indoor track. For the entire time he was running, I was stationed just off the track. My job was to keep him balanced as the race progressed—much like the pit-crew in a racecar event. When his energy fell, I would prepare certain food or drink to match his needs. I also monitored his heart rate and breathing, getting feedback about even the most subtle signs and symptoms, and even listening to the sounds of his footsteps as he ran past me on the track. I could associate certain changes in the sounds of his running with specific muscle imbalances.

During this period of working with endurance athletes, I also trained racehorses, using a heart-rate monitor to develop their natural endurance. Despite the obvious differences in structure, horses, if you imagine them standing on their back legs, are remarkably similar to humans. Much of their physiology is similar to human athletes, too. In many ways, horses were easier to treat than their human counterparts.

I was privileged to work with racecar legends Mario and Michael Andretti and numerous other drivers in preparation for such events as the Daytona twenty-four-hour race. I knew that they required significant endurance and fat burning to prevent their heart rates from rising too high during racing. Their brain function was also an important focus, and I helped to improve eye-hand coordination, quick thinking, and focus. I also gave a seminar to the Navy SEALs' basic training instructors, and spent considerable time teaching the endurance pilots who flew the stealth bombers on very long missions. I even got to "fly" the stealth simulator.

Throughout my growing practice, travel with athletes, lectures, and my newly emerging writing career, I continued with my own running, entering many road races from the mile to the marathon, steadily improving year after year to very respectable age-group finishes. I also added swimming to my routine, and biking, competing in some shorter duathlons, triathlons, and swim events.

Yet as my lecturing and work with athletes took me on the road more often, and on longer international trips, such as Europe, Japan, and Australia, it became more difficult to maintain a high level of fitness. By the early 1990s, I stopped competing; even my training was significantly reduced. I finally had to reduce my work on all fronts by reducing my clinic hours and limiting travel to select events like the Ironman in Kona, Hawaii.

The last time I was on the Big Island of Hawaii was in 1995, when Mark won his sixth and final Ironman. I was in the lead media van (which featured the radio broadcast of the Yankees winning the World Series against the Braves).

In 1997, I closed my private practice and continued consulting and lecturing, while I spent a year writing a textbook called *Complementary Sports Medicine*. Soon after this book was published, I had another vision of sorts, not unlike the experience that told me to quit my job at the phone company and become a healer. I woke up one morning with an intense desire to become a songwriter, despite never playing an instrument or singing or knowing anything about songwriting. All I had was music in my head, which had been a lifelong activity. Within a week of this epiphany, I got a surprise call from powerful and influential recording music producer Rick Rubin, who wanted to become a patient. I told him I no longer practiced, but that I had just become a songwriter. We agreed to help each other in our respective endeavors. I was soon spending considerable time with Rick in Los Angeles, one of the great music capitals of the world. I was exposed to many great songwriters and his clients, including Neil Diamond and Diane Warren, and to groups who wrote their own music, such as the Dixie Chicks, System of a Down, and Audioslave. I became Johnny Cash's doctor, trying to save him from declining health and an over-reliance on physician-prescribed drugs. I ultimately recorded my first songs in Nashville. And for a short period, I was the wellness doctor for the Red Hot Chili Peppers, traveling on a world tour with these four great musicians, and treating them like the endurance athletes they were.

During this time I also began measuring brain waves to show music's significant effect on the brain. Not surprisingly, the production of the brain's alpha waves, something humans have strived to do for thousands of years, was not just healthy, but important for athletes—for stress management, increased performance, and injury rehab.

While on the fast track to learning guitar and piano, and busy writing songs, I came to realize that my time living in the Hollywood Hills was much too stressful. I eventually reached a compromise by moving to a small mountain town in southern Arizona within a reasonable drive to Los Angeles so I could continue regular music recording and maintain my holistic work with Rick.

At an elevation of 4,500 feet, the area where I live is beautiful; it's quiet and serene. Planting a large vegetable garden was a wonderful experience, and I continue to work on my music and have so far produced two CDs. Most importantly, I got back in great physical shape by avoiding as much physical, chemical, and mental stress as possible. While I haven't returned to my former level of ability, I feel that I am in the best health of my life. Depending on time of year and desire, I try to do an hour or two of physical activity every day. This might include hiking and biking in the mountains, swimming, or strength exercises.

And, while writing this on a warm winter afternoon, I occasionally look out from the window in my bedroom office at the majestic snow-capped Santa Catalina Mountains. I hear music playing in my head.

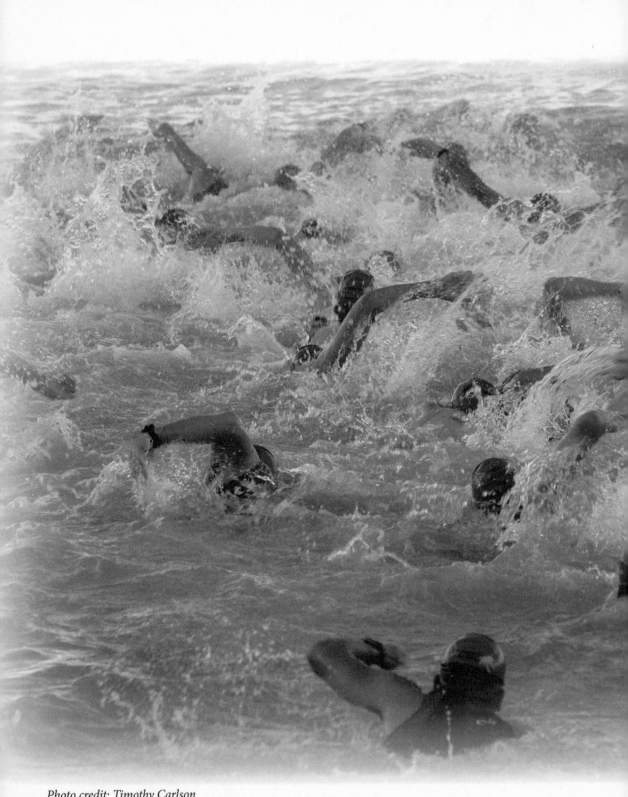

*Photo credit: Timothy Carlson*

# Building Your Endurance Foundation

# CHAPTER 1

# WHAT IS ENDURANCE?

To be human is to possess endurance. It's built into our genes. One of the primary ways we've survived as a species is thanks to the role endurance has played in our own evolution. With bipedal and upright posture, feet designed for walking instead of climbing and hanging from tree branches, and the ability to generously sweat, which prevents the body from overheating, early humans were able to travel long distances without fatigue, heat exhaustion, or injury. The search for food or water could lead to newer life-sustaining environments many miles away.

If, over the course of several million years, natural selection has given us the gift of endurance, it is only recently that sports science has begun to fully examine what it means for an athlete to go far at a consistent intensity. But what accounts for the physical differences among us regarding endurance? Why are some of us faster? Why do some of us excel at shorter distances? Or others race better in longer ones?

While genetics may dictate some of these performance differences, we actually con-trol much of our natural athletic expression through the training and lifestyle habits we choose. Making the right decisions brings out the built-in endurance we already have in our bodies. We increase our endurance by being both fit and healthy.

By looking at the whole body and fine-tuning all of its functions, one can automatically improve endurance. To have great endurance is to be holistic. If you want to achieve optimum endurance—the path to achieving your athletic potential—balancing the whole body is key to bringing out the endurance power within. Many factors contribute to and create our endurance, from muscle function and burning fat, to the various nutrients we consume and the intricate workings of our brain. This book discusses dozens of these factors and shows you how to use them to improve endurance. The optimal working of all these factors is important, and if one is deficient, endurance diminishes. As such, endurance is another individual feature we all uniquely posses. Endurance helps make us more than the sum of our parts.

But what is the meaning of endurance for athletes? Endurance can be defined in many ways. The popular college textbook *Exercise Physiology*, by Ardle, Katch, and Katch, discusses dozens of different aspects of endurance but does not define the term until page 756, and then only in more academic and less practical terms. Other sports researchers and authors define endurance as a form of survival. But you don't want to just survive a triathlon like the Ironman; you want to embrace it, live it, and enjoy it—otherwise, why are you participating? One unique feature of endurance that differentiates it from true sprinting speed is effort: endurance is performed at sub-maximal exertion while sprinters perform at all-out, maximal effort.

Endurance has such a wide range of physical, chemical, and mental functions that I propose several important definitions, specifically for those athletes who engage in training for events lasting more than a few minutes:

- Endurance is our personal human performance; we use it to reach our athletic potential. As individuals, each of us defines our endurance differently—to run a 10K race, swim a mile, or bike a century. Driven by the urge to compete at the highest levels, many endurance athletes express themselves by racing professionally. Riding a bike for three consecutive weeks in the Tour de France, or going strong for eight or sub-nine hours in the lava steam bath known as the Ironman Hawaii, require superb mental and physical conditioning.
- Endurance provides the physical, chemical, and mental tools to enable us to continually power the body over relatively long distances while maintaining higher speeds at sub-maximum effort.
- Endurance is an expression of the body's aerobic system. This key system, discussed below and throughout this book, includes aerobic muscle fibers that burn fat for energy, the nerves and blood vessels associated with the muscles, and all the support mechanisms to put them in action, including the heart and lungs. Properly training the aerobic system can allow a runner to cover five miles in forty-five minutes at a heart rate of 150, then progress to performing the same distance a month later at forty-three minutes. Or, the cyclist who can ride a flat ten-mile course averaging a steady fifteen miles per hour at a heart rate of 140, with proper endurance training can now ride the same course averaging nine miles per hour at the same

heart rate. This feature of endurance is what I call aerobic speed, and is discussed in the coming chapters.

- Endurance is our ability to carry on our athleticism successfully without sacrificing our health. While much of our life, consciously or not, is dedicated to training for more endurance—and for most athletes this includes competition—there's usually much more to do in the course of our long day. Most of us also have other daily chores—career, yard work, family, social activities, and other events that take our time and energy. Endurance sports are not separate from these other activities; balancing everything in our life is vital to building and maintaining the endurance we'll use for training and competition.

∽

We obtain endurance by first developing our slow-moving parts, so to speak. Our aerobic system contains "slow-twitch" muscles that burn fat for energy. Training these relatively slow muscles is the first step to building greater endurance, including aerobic speed, an important component of endurance. Initially, these muscles will move us at relatively slow paces. But as the body can more readily convert fat to energy, aerobic muscle function improves, enabling our endurance to build.

Another important aspect of endurance, and one that differentiates it from all-out speed, is aging. Endurance can persist for many years. Instead, too many athletes lose

endurance with age—not always for lack of training, but for lack of *proper* training, and lack of health. Many endurance athletes can continually improve well into their forties and fifties. Master athletes often outrace younger athletes, despite having a lower maximum oxygen uptake ($VO_2$max). But improvement over time also means that athletes who begin serious training relatively late, such as in their thirties or forties, can perform their best even in their fifties and sixties. And, athletes beyond age sixty and seventy can still achieve remarkable feats, and sometimes still outrace some twenty- and thirty-year-olds.

## Aerobic Speed

One of the best ways athletes can measure their endurance is by regularly testing their aerobic speed. Since endurance is the ability to perform more work with the same or less effort, speed—as minutes per mile, miles per hour, laps per time period, and so on—can be used to keep track of progress. This is done with a heart-rate monitor, testing a sub-maximum effort, such as 75 percent of maximum, during running, cycling, or another activity over a given distance and time.

This is important not only to objectively measure progress in building better endurance, but if this progress is halted, or even reversed, due to some physical, chemical, or mental imbalance, you'll be informed of the problem by a slowing of your pace—often long before you even feel symptoms of any imbalance. This evaluation, the maximum aerobic function test, discussed later, is best performed regularly with the results posted in your training log or calendar.

Traditional tests that supposedly measure endurance include maximum oxygen uptake ($VO_2$max). This test measures oxygen and carbon dioxide, heart rate, respiratory rate, and other factors while an athlete runs on a treadmill or rides on a stationary apparatus. While this test has been the rage for years in the endurance world, it's not a practical application for most athletes, and is not a good measure of endurance performance. Endurance can vary greatly among those with the same $VO_2$max, as many athletes can outperform those with higher $VO_2$max levels. A better evaluation of endurance, similarly performed, is the measurement of respiratory quotient as described below, which evaluates the percentage of fat and sugar burning at specific heart rates.

Endurance athletes include triathletes, runners, cyclists, mountain bikers, swimmers, ultramarathoners, skaters, and cross-country skiers. But others not usually thought of as endurance athletes must possess endurance ability or they will succumb to injury and short athletic life spans. These include basketball, hockey, football, soccer, and baseball players, those involved in racquet sports, and even racecar drivers. I do not necessarily include track-and-field sprinters, downhill skiers, competitive weight lifters, and others in this category of endurance athletes. However, they have many similar needs and can

benefit greatly by following techniques and philosophies described in this book. For example, developing endurance can improve circulation to and from sprint muscle fibers, making them more effective. In addition, sprinters, jumpers, and other track and field athletes often must endure relatively long periods during competition, spending hours or even days waiting to complete their final events. Improved endurance can help prevent a loss of fitness during these periods between events.

Regardless of age, sport, or gender, virtually all aspects of our body and brain contribute to create optimal endurance. This idea can best be understood if we view endurance as an equilateral triangle.

## The Endurance Triangle: The Big Picture

Although the word "holistic" has been overused, abused, and misunderstood for decades, it remains an appropriate term to use when one is referring to endurance. The true holistic approach to developing more endurance is one in which all aspects of the athlete are considered—these are the triad of structural, chemical, and mental fitness and health.

The holistic approach can be represented as an equilateral triangle. Each equal side represents one important aspect of the athlete: the body's structural, its chemical, or mental and emotional state. While this concept is a simple illustration, it does not convey the complex interrelationships that exist throughout the body. For example, the muscles—a dominant part of our body's structure—won't power us through a workout without significant chemical activity to generate energy. And, our hormones, key aspects of our body's chemistry that help guide our training development, are produced in the physical glands stimulated by chemical reactions. The mental and emotional components of sport—in fact, all our thoughts—are produced by chemical reactions within the structure of our brain.

## Structure

This side of the triangle represents all the physical, structural, and mechanical aspects of endurance. The most obvious ones are the muscles, which promote body movement for long periods without fatigue, and support the activities of ligaments, tendons, joints, and bones throughout the body, helping to prevent them from damaging wear and tear. All the muscles are part of a body-wide kinematic chain, with virtually all these structural parts very much dependent upon one another. And, these muscles rely on the bones—in fact, our entire skeleton—for their attachment and to help leverage movement; at the same time, the muscles hold up our skeleton. The bony arches in the foot enable us to run because of the muscles that support these arches. And the physical equilibrium of the bony pelvis, itself dependent upon good muscle balance, has an indirect but significant impact on neck and shoulder movements.

The structure of the brain and all the interconnecting cells (such as neurons) that ultimately tell each muscle fiber when to contract and relax are vital to endurance. Without body chemistry, however, providing fats for use as energy, optimal endurance won't develop. Moreover, if we try to develop endurance only through training our body structure—working the muscles during training—without considering the importance of body chemistry, we won't reach our athletic potential.

## Chemistry

The body is full of complex biochemical reactions taking place from moment to moment even at rest. These are as important as our structure for optimal endurance. These chemical activities have specific effects on other aspects of our body chemistry and on our structural and mental state. For example, the wide-ranging effects of many of the body's

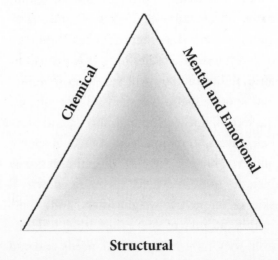

**Structural**

hormones, including testosterone and growth hormone, influence our training. The reverse is also true, as these hormones are also influenced by our physical training. These actions control physical muscle development, the chemical reactions that supply energy, and the body's natural anti-inflammatory chemicals, which promote recovery. These changes also influence our mental state.

Consuming different types of foods can also produce various effects on the body, which influences endurance. This takes place in the brain, muscles, intestines, and other areas. For example, a meal of highly refined carbohydrates, such as pasta, pancakes, or cereal, before training or competition can have an adverse effect on the use of fats for energy and endurance. Or, going on a diet to lose weight can result in structural changes in muscles that can cause an injury or a stress fracture in a bone. Caffeine and other popular drugs, such as NSAIDs (non-sterosidal anti-inflammatory drugs), affect the body in ways that can help or hurt endurance, too. Even the brain's delicate chemistry can influence our muscle function, hormones, and our thought processes through the balance of chemical messengers called neurotransmitters.

## Mental and Emotional

This side of the triangle incorporates our behavior through the activities of the physical and chemical brain. The mental state is also called cognition, and includes our sensations, perceptions, learning, concept formation, and decision-making. These are all important features of great endurance. We must sense our body and its relationship to the environment—such as feeling the ground with our feet as we run instead of blocking that sense with over-supported training shoes. We also sense the water as we swim, and, if we are sensitive enough, how our muscles, joints, and brain respond to training and competition.

The emotional state includes important factors such as pain, moods of anxiety or depression, and motivation to improve our natural endurance. Both our emotional and mental states can produce significant stress, if we allow it, through improper control of our structural and chemical body; this can contribute to poor performance, physical injury, and even overtraining.

The process of educating ourselves about endurance, and how training, diet, and other key features of fitness and health affect endurance is another important example of the mental-emotional side of the triangle. Education is probably the reason you're reading this book. In many cases, reeducation is what takes place, as our society has unhealthy misunderstandings about sport. Many young people think that "playing hurt" is cool because of what they see and hear on television and radio. Many athletes believe that pushing themselves beyond the limit—the myth of giving 110 percent—is necessary for great endurance. Ad campaigns with unreal and unhealthy images are thrown at us and our children on a daily basis, which only perpetuates attitudes and perceptions that contribute to fit but unhealthy athletes. Without an overall balance of fitness and health, our endurance will be less than adequate.

## Fitness and Health

The real lesson from my 1980 New York City Marathon experience was not one of proving health, but rather that I became fit enough to run 26.2 miles. While the terms *fitness* and *health* are often used interchangeably, they are actually two different, but mutually dependent, states.

## Aerobic and Anaerobic

Two of the most important terms used in endurance sports are *aerobic* and *anaerobic*. These will be referred to often throughout this book, not only as they relate to training but also in terms of how they are affected by diet, stress and other factors.

Take a snapshot of the body's metabolism, and the most obvious feature is oxygen. As everyone knows, oxygen is essential for energy production. But not all energy is obtained with the help of oxygen. When oxygen is used to generate energy, it is called *aerobic*, and when the body derives energy without using oxygen it is termed *anaerobic*. But these common academic definitions are not very practical. Instead, a more relevant way to define *aerobic* and *anaerobic* is by the prominent fuels they use to produce energy: fat and sugar, respectively. Let's define each as follows:

- Aerobic: the ability of the body to use more fat and less sugar (glucose) for energy.
- Anaerobic: the ability of the body to use more sugar and less fat for energy.

The chemical generation of energy from fat and sugar occurs in the aerobic and anaerobic muscle fibers, which are important components of virtually all skeletal muscles in humans.

Note: Our body contains three kinds of muscles. Skeletal muscles are used for physical activity, and bulge when contracted; smooth muscle is contained in our intestine and blood vessels, and regulates the size of the passageways; and cardiac muscle is found in the heart, used for its "beating." In this book, most of the time I will simply refer to skeletal muscle fibers as aerobic or anaerobic muscles.

Aerobic and anaerobic muscles perform a variety of activities in addition to generating movement. I will sometimes refer to these collectively as the aerobic system and the anaerobic system.

### The Aerobic System

The conversion of fat to energy—fat burning—takes place in the aerobic muscles (these are sometimes called slow-twitch or red muscle fibers). Humans are well endowed with these muscles and they are the ones depended upon during activity of longer duration—they can function well for many hours and even days in a well-trained athlete.

Aerobic muscles have other important functions too. Three important ones include:

- Physical support for our bones and joints. They help prevent and correct mechanical imbalances that cause injuries.
- Circulation. Literally miles of blood vessels help bring much-needed, nutrient-rich blood to the muscles, bringing oxygen, vitamins, minerals, hormones, and so forth, and removing other products such as lactate and carbon dioxide.
- Immune function. This helps our body's natural defense control excess free radicals to prevent and recover from illness, and help regulate inflammation.

### The Anaerobic System

Sugar (glucose) is converted to energy in the anaerobic muscles. These are sometimes called *fast-twitch* or *white muscle fibers.* They are used for short-term power (such as weight lifting) and sprint speed (such as an all-out 100 meter race). These attributes are used very little in endurance sports. Anaerobic energy is also very limited—relying only on this system won't even allow a 5K race to be completed.

## THE FULL SPECTRUM OF ENDURANCE

Good overall health requires proper balancing of the nervous, muscular, skeletal, circulatory, digestive, lymphatic, hormonal, and all other systems. With this balance comes optimal health and the reduction or loss of common signs and symptoms—complaints that many athletes have, which are often considered normal in the course of training and competition but, in fact, are not. Fatigue, injury, allergies and asthma, frequent colds, and other complaints indicate an imbalance of health, often due to neglecting health and pushing fitness. These aspects of health are also the very systems that provide the activities to build fitness. Athletes who are fit but unhealthy not only have problems on various physical, chemical, and mental levels, but are unable to reach their athletic potential.

Both states of fitness and health should be balanced with each other. Injuries, sickness, fatigue, and so on indicate an imbalance between fitness and health. While these problems are common, especially physical injuries, they are not normal in endurance sports the way they are in contact events such as football or hockey. It is unfortunate that most athletes are willing, consciously or not, to sacrifice health for greater fitness.

**QA** **Question:** In one of your earlier books, you wrote that "aerobic is the ability of the body to use more fats and less sugar (glucose) for energy." And that in events lasting for more than two hours, like the marathon, the aerobic energy used is more than 99 percent of the total energy. If all the above is true, then why do marathon runners become glycogen depleted and hit the wall? If most of their energy comes from fat, then they shouldn't face that problem.

**Answer:** The short answer is that too many marathoners do not fully develop their aerobic systems, and as a result they are unable to burn high amounts of fat for energy during a race. Instead, they must rely on more sugar for energy, often burning too much sugar during the race, including their sugar stores (glycogen), and hence becoming glycogen-depleted.

Even in a properly trained athlete, burning fat is always accompanied by some sugar burning. A runner with a great aerobic system who is capable of burning high amounts of fat can still deplete his or her glycogen stores. This can occur if too much sugar or other refined carbohydrates are consumed before the race (increasing the

We don't normally use only aerobic or anaerobic—or only fat or sugar—during training and competition. For example, the anaerobic system only has about three minutes of energy; and, to maintain fat burning for aerobic activity, sugar burning is also necessary. It's mixture of these two fuels that provides us with optimal performance energy. When an endurance athlete fatigues in a race, it may be associated with the loss of available glucose necessary to sustain the conversion of fat to energy in the aerobic muscle fiber, or due to the inability to burn enough fat because of poor aerobic training.

Depending on your training, diet, stress regulation, and overall state of health, as much as 80 to 90 percent of total energy can

be derived from fat. Unfortunately, too many athletes don't burn sufficient amounts of fat, and because of this may never reach their athletic potential. One of the most important things you'll learn in this book is how to increase energy needs through fat burning to generate optimal endurance. This includes improving aerobic speed—training the aerobic system to get faster.

As the aerobic system improves with proper training, fat burning increases and endurance improves too. This will be reflected in the RQ. For example, if an athlete today can run at a 150 heart rate and burn 50 percent fat and sugar, a month or two later he or she may improve so that, at the same 150 heart rate, now 60 percent of the energy comes from hormone insulin, which can significantly reduce fat burning), by running the first part of the race too fast (which causes more sugar and less fat to be utilized), from excess pre-race stress, especially over several days (which also reduces fat burning), and for other reasons.

Properly training the aerobic system results in a dramatic increase in fat burning not only during training, but during racing and all other times of the day and night. The more you develop your aerobic system, the more endurance you'll have. You still use glucose/glycogen to help burn fat. Think of fat as the logs in the fire (a slow, long-term energy burn), and sugar as the kindling (quick, short term energy that helps fat burn).

For marathon racing, it appears those with the most success run at a pace just faster than their maximum aerobic function. I base this on those who I've trained over thirty years and who are healthy and fit. An unhealthy or unfit athlete will have to compensate for their problem—by running with too high a heart rate, for example—thereby not achieving the best performance and possibly hitting the wall.

fat and 40 percent from sugar. Concurrent to these changes is a faster running, biking, swimming pace, or the same improvements in other activities.

In properly trained athletes I've seen tremendous values for fat burning. The chart to the right was compiled on triathlete Mike Pigg.

## Training

The definition of training may be obvious, but I like to describe it in the form of an equation. Training is the balance of your workouts and your recovery in the form of rest. Simply put:

**Training = Work + Rest**

| Mike Pigg's RQ Values | | | |
|---|---|---|---|
| Heart Rate | RQ | % Fat | % Sugar |
| 127 | .79 | 70 | 30 |
| 133 | .80 | 67 | 33 |
| 135 | .82 | 60 | 40 |
| 137 | .83 | 56 | 44 |
| 141 | .84 | 53 | 47 |
| 146 | .82 | 60 | 40 |
| 153 | .85 | 50 | 50 |
| 155* | .87 | 42 | 58 |
| 164 | .87 | 42 | 58 |
| 169 | .90 | 32 | 68 |

*At 155 heart rate, Mike can run at a sub-5:25 pace.

Regular physical training helps build muscles, improve neuromuscular activity (all those important connections between brain and muscles), increase oxygen uptake, improve fat burning, and other important benefits. Training involves stimulating the body with sufficient stress, but not too much, to provoke these benefits. In physiology this process is called *overload*. In the case of a muscle, for example, you must work it slightly harder than it is normally used to in order to rebuild and improve its function. Training involves programming your body in certain ways, especially through the work of physical activity, to perform better during competition.

Training also requires recovery, which comes in the form of rest. Sleep is the most important way for people to rest. Those who don't rest enough risk overtraining, even if the workouts are ideal.

But work is not limited to just the sum total of your training. It also includes virtually all the physical activities you do in the course of the day, such as yard work and office chores. Throw in taking care of the kids, shopping, cleaning out the garage, and other physical activities, and you have a better idea of all the work you do in the course of a week, month, and year. These activities also require energy and muscle activity, burn fat and sugar, stimulate the nervous system, and other things just like training (although in most cases not as intense). However, these events, while not necessarily helping your training, still require recovery. In fact, they may even take away from

## Measuring Aerobic and Anaerobic Function

With proper equipment from exercise physiology labs or clinics, it's relatively easy to measure the amount of sugar and fat the body is using at various heart rates. A gas analyzer can provide a fairly accurate percentage of these two main energy sources. The respiratory quotient (RQ) or respiratory exchange ratio (RER), measures the amount of carbon dioxide exhaled divided by the oxygen consumed. This is translated to a scale of 0.7 (hypothetically, 100 percent fat burning) to 1.0 (100 percent sugar burning). For example, a ratio of .85 indicates that about 50 percent of your energy is derived from sugar, and the other half from fat.

your training. That's because they increase the need for recovery.

Generally, those who don't rest enough don't recover as well—from training, competition, and all other physical activity. Poor or incomplete recovery can lead to reduced development of the aerobic system, overtraining, and as a result, can prevent people from reaching their athletic potential. Recovery allows the muscles and other working parts to rebuild and prepare for the next bout of training, and it especially prepares the athlete to compete. During recovery, three activities are very important: no training, little physical activity, and sufficient sleep.

For many athletes, the solution to balancing the training equation is to either reduce the daily physical chores, reduce training (and competition), or a combination of all. For professional athletes and others with the benefit of being able to reduce daily chores, more time and energy can be focused on training (although more is not necessarily better). It often means cutting down on training to keep the equation balanced. When this happens, improved performance ultimately follows.

One of my patients, whom I will call Bob, was a good local runner who loved road racing and desperately wanted to improve. But his expanding business and growing family were demanding more time from his busy training schedule. He tried to accommodate everyone and maintain his training. He was waking up earlier in the morning to train, resulting in less sleep. He soon was complaining of fatigue that lasted all day, and eventually developed pain in his knees and lower back. In the middle of a very successful racing season, his performances quickly began to deteriorate. At this point he consulted me. The first thing I recommended for Bob was that he cut his training down by about 40 percent, since he was not able to decrease any of his other commitments. Almost immediately his energy improved and his physical problems disappeared. After about four weeks on his modified schedule, Bob ran a great race and continued racing well for the rest of the season, maintaining his reduced training schedule.

Endurance sports has existed for millions of years in its most natural form, and organized forms only quite recently, with participation in endurance events such as road running, triathlons, and cycling exploding in the past thirty years. Today's endurance athletes, who far outnumber athletes who participate in shorter or sprint events, have been influenced more by the philosophies used to train sprinters than by distance coaches, athletes, and others. This is due, in part, to the presence of many former sprinters, for example, who began coaching in the endurance world. They began training endurance athletes much in the same way they themselves trained. As a result, endurance athletes often hold on to that tradition of sprint workouts. These include track or pool intervals, for example, to increase speed. This relatively new training approach may have contributed to the epidemic of overtraining, chronic injuries, and burnout, and may have prevented many endurance athletes from reaching their potential.

As noted above, endurance is very different from true sprinting: Endurance is performed at sub-maximal exertion while sprinters perform at maximal effort. When endurance athletes train like sprinters, the risk of injury and overtraining rises significantly because this kind of speed is not regularly used in endurance events (and if it is, it can detract from

# MY PERSPECTIVE—BY MIKE PIGG

*Mike Pigg dominated the short-course triathlon scene from the late eighties to the mid nineties, with an astonishing thirty wins in the USA Triathlon Series. Considered one of the hardest-working athletes in the sport, Pigg's multisport racing career lasted for a productive seventeen years. Now retired, he is a real estate broker and lives in Northern California with his wife and twins. Still physically active, Mike is the race director for Tri Kids, a triathlon designed for children ages seven to eighteen.*

✳ ✳ ✳

Train slower to go faster? Is this guy a crazy or what? Phil Maffetone is not crazy, and I feel very fortunate to have met him when I did. I have been a professional triathlete since 1984. When I started my career, I just picked up a triathlon magazine to see what the top pros were doing and then tried to emulate them. The one guy who was a star at the time was Scott Molina. He was doing mega miles in all three sports, plus doing speed workouts for each of the disciplines as if he was just a runner, cyclist, or swimmer only. It looked like a good way to be the best, especially if you had the time to just eat, sleep, swim, bike, and run. Things went well for me during the first three years. In 1988, I was able to work my way up to the top rank. I thought I was invincible. That is when the bumpy road started. I had no control over my progression. I was also starting to lose my love for the sport. It got so bad that I was about to quit and move on. The training became too hard and my results weren't there to justify the pain. That's about the time I ran into Phil.

We sat down and had a long talk. At first it was hard for me to swallow what Phil had to say. What helped me is that I had spent a lot of time training with Mark Allen. What I learned from Mark is that during long bike rides his heart rate was always lower than mine by ten to fifteen beats. During our long rides together, our pace would be even for the first sixty-five miles; then I would start a slow death out on the windy plains of Boulder, Colorado. I was like the hummingbird that needed fuel all the time, and Mark was like a steam engine with an always-ready supply of coals for the fire. He could cruise for hours and hours. Also, I was impressed by how consistent Mark's triathlon career was, with very few flaws year after year. The topper of it all was that Mark had been following Phil's plan for many years.

So I listened to Phil with both ears wide open. After our conversation, Phil gave me one of his books. It was an easy-reading book that had a lot of common sense about how to train and eat properly.

On the nutritional side, I began to reach for whole foods rather than processed ones, especially refined carbohydrates. I increased my protein intake by including more meat and eggs. I seriously took stock of my carbohydrate intake, relying mainly on fruit, fresh or steamed vegetables, and small amounts of whole grains. I also increased my consumption of healthy fats by adding more avocados, butter, nuts, and seeds to my diet. My increased fat and protein intake gave me much more energy.

On the training front, I decided to follow Phil's advice on heart-rate monitoring, using the "180 Formula." It took some time to see the results kick into gear, but once they did, I became a firm believer in his aerobic heart rate training program.

The training seemed slow at first at my designated heart rate of 155. There were times when I had to walk up hills during the run and zigzag on steep bike sections just to stay in my aerobic range. In a little time, however, things started to change and I became stronger at the same heart rate, which became quite exciting. After five months of loyal, consistent training, I saw that the program was working.

Before going on Phil's program, I would sometimes ride to my parents' summer place, which was sixty-five miles away and involved three good climbs. My previous record was set with a good friend of mine. We had this total grudge match all the way to find out who was king of the bike. He would attack on the hills, and I was holding a heart rate between 165 and 182 to establish a record of three hours and fifteen minutes. When we arrived at the cabin, I achieved a total bonk. The best I could do for the rest of the day was eat, sleep, and eat some more, and even that was difficult. Three years later and five months on the aerobic program, I attempted the same course again—this time solo and never going above 155 even on the long climb. The results were interesting—I went 3:09 and felt good enough to go for a ten mile run straight after. Slowly, I was becoming convinced that the theory was working.

My other story comes from the first race of the season while following Phil's plan. It is amazing how I was seeing good aerobic results in my workouts, but I still had doubts about my performance level. You see, I still needed my hammer sessions to build my self-confidence that I was ready to race at a professional level. The season opener was in Australia at the Surfers Paradise International Triathlon. My confidence was so low that I didn't even want to get on the plane. But a swift kick from my wife Marci and I was off. The whole week prior to the race, I was fighting with myself, saying that I wasn't going to do well because of a lack of speed training. Finally, I told myself to shut up and go have a good time. To my surprise I did have a good time, and I won. For some reason the speed and endurance were definitely there. As a bonus, I was able to beat Mark Allen at his own game.

This win marked the start of my total love affair with triathlon—and with staying healthy at the same time. Dr. Maffetone's guidelines are easy. All you need is a heart-rate monitor to listen to your ticker and a little patience. And yes, you can do it just by slowing down and letting your body catch up with your mind.

the race by using up glycogen, over-stressing muscles, and lowering energy).

This doesn't mean that endurance athletes can't train anaerobically, performing faster workouts, such as intervals and fartlek. (*Fartlek* is a Swedish word meaning "speed play." It's similar to a race simulation, where the athlete speeds up and slows down as he or she intuitively feels the body working hard, then needing a brief rest of slower activity. This allows your brain to participate in the workout, so to speak, feeling your body's response to the workout and knowing when to ease up.) But this approach to developing speed is not a priority. Instead, developing aerobic speed, where an athlete can run much faster with the same effort compared to weeks and months earlier, is an important priority.

This not only provides significant speed during training and racing, but it's accomplished with much less stress, so the risk of injury and overtraining is greatly reduced.

Despite this, many endurance athletes expend significant time and energy on intensely hard anaerobic workouts, often neglecting or impairing the aerobic system in the process. This is counterproductive. In a one-hour event, 98 percent of your endurance energy is derived from the aerobic system; in a two-hour event, 99 percent is. Does it make sense to spend so many hours a week on anaerobic work when 99 percent of your race energy comes from the aerobic system? Instead, it's best to first derive your endurance speed from aerobic training, then, as time and energy permits, to add anaerobic training.

# TRAINING YOUR BRAIN, MUSCLES, AND METABOLISM

In one of the most famous photographs of Albert Einstein, taken in Santa Barbara, California, in 1933, the happy-looking genius is having a merry time riding his bike. He was once quoted as saying, "Life is like riding a bicycle. To keep your balance you must keep moving."

Einstein is known for a lot of mind-bending concepts that have altered our understanding of the universe, but he also has a special place in the world of endurance. I bet you didn't know that. It involves the meaning of time. Time is not static. He used the metaphor of a moving clock on a speeding train to help explain the basic principles of time, space, and light. Time can speed up or slow down, depending on how fast you are traveling. For endurance athletes, speed is indeed relative. Furthermore, we have an inner clock mechanism hardwired into our brains.

The same is true for animals. Migrating birds are able to prepare for and successfully complete their airborne endurance events, with some species traveling thousands of miles, by eating properly and storing sufficient fat for long-term energy. Despite not wearing a watch or being given mile splits, birds can pace themselves in a highly accurate manner. Humans also have a highly precise internal clock that runs subconsciously, and during an endurance race it's quite accurate, and even helps us race the final part of the event faster. This clock's

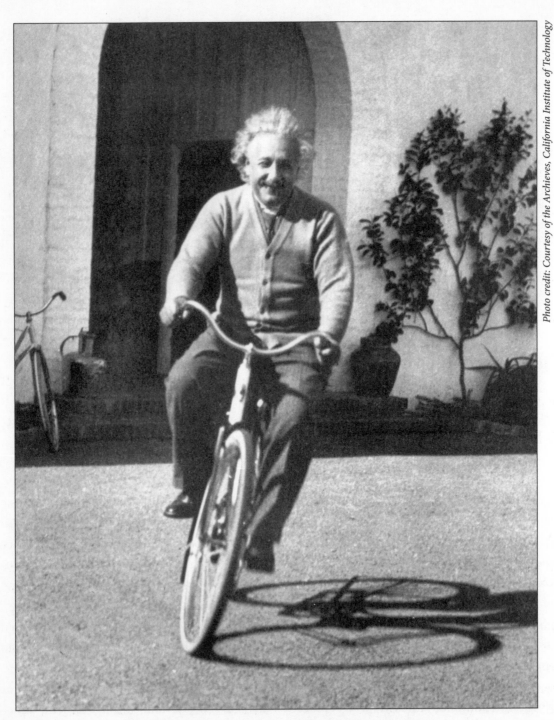

*Einstein once said, "Life is like riding a bicycle.*
*To keep your balance you must keep moving."*

accuracy is based partly on experience of all previous races and training, with seasoned athletes usually being most accurate. Even in a race with mile markers inaccurately posted, for example, the brain's relationship to the passing of time can accurately be maintained in disagreement with the markers. While these relationships are well known scientifically, most experienced athletes are also aware of them, if not consciously, then subconsciously. This is also intricately related to our pacing ability. Most experienced athletes can swim, bike, or run at a given pace just by intuition and feel, and usually maintain good accuracy.

The brain's internal clock is important in a race because it helps us with overall strategy. In particular, endurance athletes should be able to speed up after 90 percent of the race is complete, as the brain has planned for this final kick. This time relationship, called *scalar expectancy theory*, allows the brain to pace the body through this point in the race with sufficient energy to go faster at the end.

Because our diet can significantly influence the brain's chemical messengers—the neurotransmitters—food can have a large impact on our sense of time. A healthy brain that's well nourished without adverse influence from fluctuating blood sugar levels and diet factors (such as vitamin and mineral levels) will function best, and, in the case of racing, will pace the body through the event in the most effective way possible.

While most endurance athletes focus on distance, the time element in training is often neglected. While we consciously train our body, we often forget *to train our relationship with time*, and it can work against us. That's because in most endurance events, time is the primary factor. I'm not just talking about the time for each workout or checking splits, but the big picture of time and how your brain can relate to it in a helpful way.

Whether you're just beginning your endurance career or training for the marathon, Einstein's notion that "time is relative" has special significance. Of course, he was postulating about space and time, not 26.2 miles. A spacecraft leaving earth and traveling near the speed of light for twenty years would return to earth with a different record of time elapsed than that on earth. Comparing two identical clocks, one on the spacecraft and one on earth, the spacecraft clock may show ten years had elapsed, but the clock on earth would show twenty years had passed. Moreover, the passengers on the spacecraft would have aged only ten years while those on earth would have aged twenty years in that same time. This view of two clocks providing us with different times of the same event can be useful in endurance training and competition. We all know the human body can sense and react to time differently in a given situation. A successful race seems to pass more quickly than one in which you are struggling. "Time is not a constant thing by any means," says Olympic marathoner Lorraine Moller of New Zealand. "When you're in a good race, everything comes together. Time flies when you're having fun."

Time can be experienced as a non-flowing, isolated part of any performance; the event does not take place as most see it, but differently. This view of time is most evident when we're falling in love, meditating, or in a trance. As Dr. Larry Dossey observes in *Space, Time, and Medicine,* "These experiences suggest that an alternative to the ordinary means of experiencing time lies within all of us." In our fast-paced society, we always seem to run out of time too easily. That forces us to squeeze training into smaller spaces. This creates unnecessary stress—which is detrimental for all athletes.

"A lot of coping with time," says Lorraine Moller, "is just learning to relax." You might try relaxing in front of a clock with a large second hand that clicks off the seconds. Stare at it. Notice that some seconds seem longer or shorter than others. And if you "play" a little, you may find you can "hold" the second hand in one place for what would seem to be more than one second.

If you're rushing through your workouts, not "taking the time" to enjoy them, this stress may eventually have a negative influence on your overall fitness and health. I once had a patient whom I will call Tim. He had been running regularly for five years, and at age thirty-seven was training for his fourth marathon. He was hoping to break the elusive three-hour barrier, which he had been close to in his three previous marathons. His training schedule included the traditional long Sunday run of two hours, and would soon increase so that his longest run would be two and a half hours.

But how would Tim relate to the time it would take him to run the three-hour marathon? Two hours was a long run, two and a half hours his longest. Was three hours reasonable for him to achieve? I helped Tim modify his training and thinking so that he wouldn't fail to attain his goal. He had to relate both psychologically and physiologically to three hours in a different manner.

Einstein was able to understand and relate to complex issues, but how could I help Tim in such a relatively simple quest as breaking three hours? It required using two "clocks" to control time more effectively.

Tim wanted his marathon clock to read less time than the observed time; in other words, he wanted the race to feel more like an hour. Because he was using his longest run to train for an event that would take more time than the training run itself, Tim had to experience a workout of more than three hours, without overtraining, so the marathon would be relatively shorter. He also had to learn how to manipulate time at will.

Walking was one potential solution to both of these time problems. By adding more time to his long run, by walking the first and the last half hour, Tim could increase the total time of his long training session without risking overtraining. Walking also relaxed him in a way running never did.

After three of these longer workouts, Tim learned how easy it was to manipulate time. His total workout of three and a half hours (a half hour walk, two and a half hour run, and a half hour walk) enabled him to either make the time go faster, or, because he didn't want the now-enjoyable workout to end, go slower. These workouts would reorient Tim, making the marathon shorter, relative to the long workout. On marathon day, he would be able to make the marathon go by quickly.

This is exactly what happened; Tim ran his race in two hours and forty-eight minutes, saying afterward, "It felt like an easy long run."

These identical time tactics helped ultra-runner Stu Mittleman attain his world record in the 1,000-Mile World Championship Run. This event required a modification of the relationship of time to enable Stu to cope with the 1,000 one-mile laps. Averaging approximately eighty-six miles a day, Stu successfully manipulated time so that the eleven and a half days were psychologically and physiologically less demanding. "By the fifth day," said Stu, "if you'd ask me how many days went by, I'd say two."

I used these same time strategies to train Paul Fendler who, in his first-ever ultramarathon distance, became the New York Metropolitan Athletics Congress 50-mile champion in 1987. "All of a sudden, in the beginning of the race, time ceased to be an existing factor," said Paul, "and it was the walk/run workouts that taught me how to control time."

Learning time management is, at its most fundamental level, understanding how

to train your brain. Too many athletes think about only training their muscles. But the three most important facets of performance are the brain, muscles, and metabolism.

# The Brain

Let's start with the brain. It is the most important part of your athletic body, the one most responsive to training and necessary for competition, and the one most neglected. All training and competition begins in the brain. And the brain is not an isolated body part but a key component of the entire nervous system, which includes the spinal cord and all the nerves going to muscles, bones, joints, organs and glands, the intestines, and every square millimeter of the body. All physiological activities are influenced in some way by the brain. The brain also protects us from attempting to exceed our physical limitations; it is the real reason we slow down during a race—or even drop out.

There are many ways we can help our brain function better. In general, this is best accomplished by being a more fit and healthy athlete. For example, the brain is more than 60 percent fat, and the fats we eat influence the types of fats in the brain. Even stimulation of the brain by music, to help produce better brains waves, can help the brain work better.

## Muscle Control

Let's first look at how the brain controls our muscles. There's an important circuit from the brain to the muscle, and another back to the brain. This begins in the area of the brain called the motor cortex, from where nerves run down through the spinal cord to specific muscle fibers; the purpose is to send messages to the muscle, stimulating it to either contract or relax. Virtually all physical activity begins as messages from the brain to some specific muscles to contract, and others to relax (these muscle actions are referred to as "facilitation" and "inhibition," respectively). This same mechanism also controls other features of the muscles, power and strength. The more nerves that stimulate more muscle fibers to contract, the more power the muscle can generate; so it's not the size of the muscle that determines strength, it's how many muscle fibers are told to contract by the brain. Even aerobic muscles can be more powerful than anaerobic ones of the same size because of this phenomenon.

The brain is in constant communication with the muscles, and is also continuously receiving information from each muscle fiber. There's another nerve in the muscle that goes back up to a nearby area of the brain called the sensory cortex. This feature provides important information to the brain about the status of the muscle—everything from its tension and fatigue to energy levels and risk of injury. The brain can then use this information to make appropriate adjustments in the muscle, get help from other muscles, provide more energy or repair, or tell it to slow down or stop working. This "neuromuscular system"—the loop from brain to muscle and

muscle to brain—is very precise, with each muscle's thousands of aerobic muscle fibers having a separate nerve connecting to it from the brain, and one returning to the brain. Thousands of muscle fibers and the same number of nerves participate in each muscle during contraction and relaxation. It's a very large orchestra with the brain conducting.

## Muscle Memory

In addition to the back and forth communication between brain and muscle, and muscle and brain, other areas of the brain can influence our physical activity. For example, observing another person's physical action in your brain's visual center can actually stimulate your own motor cortex to prepare your muscles for the same action—even without you moving. This is called action observation and is associated with stored memories called engrams. This "motor memory" is the basis of the various mental imagery techniques used in sports training. Watching a swimmer who has excellent technique can help you swim more efficiently because your brain has been programmed, through visual input and memory, and your motor area now knows how your muscles need to act. Unfortunately, there are still other areas of the brain that can influence the same memories and actions, including past training where you may have learned incorrect swim technique. So while this can be helpful for many athletes, it's not a perfect training tool for everyone. Watching a marathoner with a great physique and stride may appear like something to imitate, but trying to do that with a body not prepared to run the same way can quickly lead to excess stress on the muscles and joints, and even injury.

Such was the case with Kim, a young distance runner who showed great potential in college. During her summer break she attended a running camp where she was videotaped. The footage, played back in slow motion, accentuated her seemingly imperfect running gait. After being told to lengthen her stride and exaggerate other motions, such as lifting her knees and swinging her arms more like a 400-meter runner, she became very sore after each workout. Within about two weeks, she had leg pain that required days off from training, and eventually knee and hip pain that rendered her unable to train at all. This is when I first saw Kim in my clinic. After hearing her history, and performing an examination, it was clear that the first step was to restore normal communication between the brain and muscles. This was easily accomplished with biofeedback—a technique that corrects dysfunction of injured muscles by encouraging brain-muscle and muscle-brain communication. More importantly, Kim was instructed to stop overstriding and exaggerating her gait, and instead, just run relaxed and allow her brain to dictate the motions. Within a week, the pain was gone and Kim was running again without mechanical problems.

Because the brain remembers everything it experiences, be careful what you put into it. Kim had to unlearn trying to run like a sprinter. In cases of retraining, it sometimes takes a period of adaptation during which you may feel physically inadequate or even experience a falloff in performance until your brain-muscle mechanism gets back in sync.

This was what happened to Sam, a triathlete who I observed swimming laps in the pool. Swimming was his weakest event. One look at Sam in the pool showed why—his technique was poor, and he swam quite irregularly because of a one-sided head-turn and other asymmetrical movements. By improving muscle function, and with the help of a swim coach, Sam was better able to understand correct mechanics, and made great improvements over the following two months. However, this period was in the middle of Sam's racing season, and during this transition to better mechanics, his swim times worsened. Sam could not help going back to his more comfortable improper swim patterns during a race, but in time, as he trained his brain and body to follow better technique, he performed significantly better. Ultimately, his swimming became as strong as his cycling, which was his strongest event.

In summary, proper training includes programming your brain, muscles, metabolism, and all other areas of the body. Training the nerves that attach to the aerobic muscles is key for developing optimal endurance through better fat burning. But you have to stimulate all of these muscles, beginning with the smallest and slowest ones. Over time, as these nerves and muscles are properly trained, they work more efficiently. The result is they'll be able to do more work with the same effort, which translates into more speed.

The brain also plays a role in muscle balance, and adapts the body to muscle imbalance to prevent further injury. Muscle balance is the sum of muscle contraction and relaxation. Muscle imbalance occurs when one muscle group in the front of the thigh—for example, the quadriceps—contracts too much and is tight, and the muscle group on the back of the thigh, the hamstrings, contracts too little and becomes weak. This pattern is a common cause of physical injuries and may be one of the most important factors contributing to fatigue during training and competition. The

brain's role is to sense these potential problems, make corrections, and compensate.

### Race Control

The brain is a very important part of regulating how hard we compete, assuring that we don't consciously push ourselves to injury, or even death. The brain accomplishes this task by constantly monitoring all body activities, from muscle activities to the levels of energy, in particular during the course of a race. It even plans out the course and is aware of our need for a final kick to the finish.

Once the body has undergone a process of training to build fitness and health, you're ready to race. This is sometimes best accomplished by just letting your brain do the work. Instead, too many athletes try new strategies in the middle of their races, surprising their brain, and putting the body under greater stress. Instead, when "all systems are go" as a result of proper training, you can start the race on autopilot. It's proper training of the brain and the rest of your body that best pre-

Photo credit: Timothy Carlson

*The brain is always seeking to perform the best it can in a race but not at the expense of allowing damage to the body.*

pare you to race most effectively, allowing intuition and instincts to participate. An athlete that exemplifies this well is Mark Allen. His intense but relaxed pre-race focus before a triathlon and his knowledge that training provided what he needed helped him to let the brain run the race. Not that strategy is not part of the process. For example, in athletes performing long endurance events, I encourage maintaining high aerobic activity for much of the race, without entering the anaerobic state until later, helping keep the brain functioning well. In Mark's case, the swim and bike leg were aerobic and not until the run did his body become anaerobic, especially for the last 10 percent of the race.

The brain is always seeking to perform the best it can in a race, but not at the expense of allowing damage to the body. Consider a race where you begin at a much faster pace than planned, and one too fast to maintain. The stress on your muscles, ligaments, joints, and bones, and the overtaxing of your various metabolic mechanisms that produce energy, including the reduction in fat burning and rapid loss of sugar for energy, all inform the brain that you're going to be in trouble real soon. The brain offers a subconscious solution: reduce the pace by slowing the various muscles in hopes of recovering for the upcoming miles to the finish. As you notice the pace slow, despite feeling bad, you consciously decide to try to maintain your too-fast effort. Your brain now projects a potential serious problem ahead, since your fitness level won't keep you going without a significant

reduction in speed, but you still won't make the conscious change of pace. In the end your brain wins, and you pull off the road to catch your breath and decide to drop out because you feel so bad. Your brain has saved you from serious damage, except to your ego, maybe.

## Hormones, Memories, and Emotions

The brain also plays an important role in controlling hormones throughout the body, which affects muscle function, energy production, water and electrolyte balance, and other important activities that improve endurance. The pituitary gland, housed in the middle of our brain, produces a variety of hormones that not only affect our muscles and other endurance activities, but respond to how we train. Properly trained athletes maintain an optimal balance of all hormones; overtrained athletes have significant hormone imbalances.

Often referred to as the "master gland" of the body, the pituitary has significant control over our entire hormonal system. In addition, the pituitary is influenced by memories and emotions stored in nearby regions of the brain. Through all these interactions, the pituitary affects adrenal and thyroid hormones, sex hormones, and others discussed below.

The pituitary also secretes growth hormone, which stimulates muscle development. Its production occurs during sleep, making proper sleep patterns an important part of recovery. While growth hormone production is higher in childhood and is reduced as we age, sufficient amounts are still secreted even in older, healthy athletes. Like other hormones naturally produced in our body, poor health may reduce the level of growth hormone. In rare cases, pituitary problems at any age, such as a tumor, might require the necessity of a patient to take a synthesized form of human growth hormone—HGH. Unfortunately, it's become too common for those seeking to restore youth, control weight, or enhance sports performance to also take HGH. However, the use of HGH does not actually guarantee improvements in sports. It's a banned substance in sports, and its use is dangerous. Taking HGH may also reduce the pituitary's ability to produce growth hormone, creating an even more serious problem when HGH injections are stopped. Side effects of HGH include fatigue, muscle weakness, reduced sex hormones and sexual function, blood sugar irregularities, and others.

## The Muscles

Our muscles are composed of a collection of different types of fibers with various functions for speed (fast versus slow), fatigue ability (easily fatigued versus fatigue resistant), physical support, and other features. This neuromuscular variation is one feature that enables humans to perform effectively in so many different sports requiring very different movements at different paces. The ability to swim, bike, and run in one event is an example of this feature.

The different types of muscle fibers are assembled in each of our muscles side by side in a seemingly random order. The different fibers are used when called upon by the brain. For example, during walking almost all the muscle action is from aerobic fibers. If you quicken the pace and even jog, faster moving aerobic fibers are enlisted. As you begin to increase your speed to higher intensity, more anaerobic fibers take over. But with faster activity the slower-moving aerobic fibers reduce their action.

In some animals, like chickens, different whole muscles have more exclusive fiber types. For example, the chicken's leg and thigh contain mostly red ("dark") aerobic muscle fibers; they are used for slow, constant walking. The "breast" muscles, however, are composed of mostly anaerobic fibers—the white meat—used for fast, powerful, short-lived flapping of the wings.

In humans, the percentage of different fibers in a given muscle varies between individuals. Certain muscles of elite endurance athletes contain up to 90 percent aerobic fibers, where sprinters may have as little as 25 percent, with the remainder being anaerobic. Some anaerobic fibers also have the potential for significant aerobic function, as some of the great sprinters can be trained to make even greater endurance athletes. Knowing the percentage of aerobic and anaerobic muscle fibers will do little in ascertaining a person's performance outcome. This is because the muscle itself is not the determining factor in performance, but the sum of the brain, muscle, and metabolic activity and

# THE MYTH OF VO₂MAX TESTING

Traditional sports medicine, as well as most athletes and coaches, dictates that limitations in athletic performance occur because of oxygen, blood flow, lactic acid, or other factors. But these may not be nearly as important as once thought, as it's the brain that monitors and regulates these and virtually all other activities, including muscle function, that limit our performance. For many decades, our maximum oxygen consumption—$VO_2$max—has been the number many worship in endurance sports; but this supposed hallmark of endurance is not as significant as many coaches, scientists, athletes, and the sports press make it. Many athletes have their $VO_2$max tested, and proudly, or frustratingly, display their number like knowing their cholesterol, blood pressure, or other special digit that, by itself, is misleading and insufficient.

Our $VO_2$max is associated with our ability to use the oxygen in the air we breathe—it's the maximum ability of our body to obtain this oxygen. It can be measured as the amount of oxygen (in milliliters) per kilogram of body weight per minute (ml/kg/min). Men have significantly higher $VO_2$max levels compared to women, and both lose $VO_2$max with age. In addition to age and gender, a variety of other factors influence this number, especially training, but in some people training does not significantly increase $VO_2$max. $VO_2$max is also associated with maximum heart rate and with resting heart rate. Other factors, such as breathing efficiency, can significantly affect the outcome of $VO_2$max testing.

There are two problems with making $VO_2$max such an important number. The first has to do with how the test is administered, and a second is its relationship to performance.

A careful look at how the $VO_2$max test is given will help explain why it's not a good measure of human performance or athletic potential. Triathlete Mike Pigg was in my clinic for an off-season checkup, and we decided to visit a facility in New York City where some treadmill tests would measure, among other things, $VO_2$max. The standard protocol was followed, which included telling Mike he was going to run at an increasingly rapid pace until he could not continue. He was not told how far or how long he would have to run. Nor was he given any pre-test meal instructions, and, although he worked out earlier that morning, he would only be given a couple of minutes to warm up. A tube was placed in Mike's mouth, secured with a head strap, which would allow his oxygen and carbon dioxide to be measured; he would not be able to drink water or talk. Then the test began, with the treadmill pace taking Mike on a faster and faster pace, while at the same time the treadmill incline was gradually elevated. In less than ten minutes, the test was over because Mike reached a point of exhaustion and could not continue.

The test revealed how much oxygen and carbon dioxide his body could regulate, his respiratory rate, and other factors. While everyone around was impressed with how fast Mike could run without his heart rate soaring—he ran a sub-5:25 pace with his heart rate at 155—and by the other test results, including $VO_2$max, there was a big problem. Because he did not know how far or how long he was going to run, his brain did not participate, thus making the test an unnatural evaluation. Instead, it was more like a sterile, laboratory measurement providing numbers with little useful information. As a result, his brain could not allow his body to truly mimic a hard workout or race.

While the test was an interesting experience, it contributed nothing to what I recommended for Mike with his training, nor did it give Mike any useful information. In fact, testing Mike on the track, running at his maximum aerobic pace using a heart monitor, provided much more information—giving him confidence that he was getting faster while training only aerobically.

Dr. Timothy Noakes, author of the *Lore of Running* and an exercise physiologist who has been published extensively in scientific journals, has written much about $VO_2$max testing. In an article in the *British Journal of Sports Medicine* (2008) titled, "Testing for Maximum Oxygen Consumption Has Produced a Brainless Model of Human Exercise Performance," Noakes wrote that many people in sport "are apparently wedded to the concept that oxygen delivery alone determines the power output of the exercising limbs, and thus, they appear blind to a converse interpretation." Noakes believes that the development of the $VO_2$max test probably explains why most people in sports seldom consider that the brain's effect on muscle function could be an important regulator of athletic performance. That's because the $VO_2$max test—still a gold standard—evaluates the athlete's body without input from the brain. By not telling the runner being tested, for example, how far or how much time he or she must run, the brain is unable to most effectively monitor and regulate the physical activity. Instead, the test involves running to exhaustion—no endurance event is ever performed in this manner—we always know how far the race will be, and this enables the brain to prepare the body to complete the task in the most effective way possible, and without damaging the body.

The second reason why we should not be over-excited about VO$_2$max is its relationship to endurance performance. Noakes and others are convinced that VO$_2$max is a poor predictor of performance. Older male athletes, whose VO$_2$max diminishes with age, often have lower VO$_2$max levels than younger athletes, yet the older competitors often race better. And, most male endurance athletes have much higher VO$_2$max levels than most women in the same sport, yet a significant number of women outperform these men.

their efficiencies, along with lifestyle factors. For endurance athletes, the lifestyle effect, including training, more than makes up for any individual difference in fiber type and genetics. While your particular fiber makeup is influenced by genetics, your training helps determine the type and efficiency of those fibers. If the goal is reaching your athletic potential, emphasis should obviously be placed on training, diet, and other lifestyle factors.

There are at least seven different muscle fibers, with classifications based on a variety of features, from their microscopic appearance and energy utilization (sugar or fat), to the types of physical actions they produce (relatively fast or slow movement). These categories don't always agree with one another, and as techniques improve even more fibers will be discovered and classified.

To simplify this complex subject, I'll primarily discuss aerobic and anaerobic muscles, with some exceptions to further emphasize how training, diet, therapy, and other factors can significantly affect and change our muscles. For example, there are certain types of muscle fibers that are anaerobic but have the capacity to also function like a fast aerobic fiber. With the increase of aerobic speed, these muscle fibers become very important for gaining even more endurance. In addition, aerobic training, availability of fats for energy, and diets that are lower in refined carbohydrates can help program various muscle fibers to function for better endurance.

Muscle fibers are quite adaptable; in addition to growing in size, some can change from one type to another. A period of low or no training can result in the loss of aerobic fibers due to their conversion to anaerobic ones. Overtraining through emphasis on hard, anaerobic workouts without training the slow aerobic fibers may do the same. This "plasticity" or adaptability in the muscles is, in part, a response to our lifestyle environment—training, competition, diet, stress, and so on. Adaptability also enables older athletes to train and perform surprisingly well in endurance events. With aging comes an increasing loss of anaerobic fibers—one reason we lose speed as we get older. The result is a higher percentage of aerobic fibers in each muscle, making our potential for endurance greater with age. This is one main reason why sprinters reach their peak earlier in life while endurance athletes reach peaks later, often in the third or fourth decade, or beyond, and can still continue to perform at high levels for many years beyond that time.

The adaptability of muscles also enables us to successfully treat common sports injuries, and rehabilitate more serious conditions, often very quickly. This is because most changes in muscles, whether from injury, ill health, or poor training, are not permanent.

### Aerobic Muscles

In the human body, most muscles are made of a combination of aerobic and anaerobic fibers (the exceptions are some of the jaw muscles that are all anaerobic). The aerobic fibers are uniquely different from their anaerobic counterparts. Aerobic fibers are sometimes called "red" because they contain structures called *mitochondria,* which contains the iron-protein, red-pigmented compound myoglobin. It is here, through myoglobin's action in the mitochondria, that oxygen is successfully used in the energy-generating process. The more these muscles are trained, the more mitochondria and myoglobin is produced, and the more oxygen will be utilized to help produce energy. The fuel for the mitochondria's powerful endurance energy is fat.

Also unique to the aerobic muscle fiber is that it is generally fatigue-resistant. This is because the availability of fat for energy is quite vast even in lean athletes. Over time, aerobic muscle fatigue is due to the brain and metabolic aspects. Even after ten hours of racing, there can still be unused glycogen in the anaerobic fibers—unless you used it inadvertently during the event (often the result of too high an effort such as running too fast at the start of a marathon). If this small reserve is still intact, it is quite useful for your final effort, and, even more important is that it helps maintains a relatively high amount of fat burning throughout your training and competitive period.

Another important characteristic of the aerobic fiber is its high concentration of blood vessels, which contributes to its red appearance. Blood coming into the fiber brings oxygen and nutrients, including vitamins, minerals, and fats. On its way out, blood carries away by-products such as carbon dioxide and lactate.

Aerobic muscle fibers are also home to important immune system functions, specifically, that of controlling chemical free radicals through antioxidant activity. (In order for this to happen, antioxidant nutrients must be provided by the diet.) Athletes who are often ill with colds, flu, and other indications of poor immune function typically also have reduced aerobic function.

The aerobic fibers are the most commonly contracted part of a muscle, even in everyday action. Your physical activity at work and home, and doing everyday chores requires aerobic muscle activity. They are also the muscles that support the body's joints, bones, and other areas to help prevent and correct injuries.

### Anaerobic Muscles

The anaerobic fibers come in different types. Some, for example, have a combination of aerobic and anaerobic quality. These fibers are very important in endurance training and competition. When these fibers are highly developed, they are much like a powerful aerobic fiber. Developing their aerobic quality further improves endurance, and most especially what I call "aerobic speed"—the ability to go faster with the same or less effort.

Diet can indirectly influence our body to use more anaerobic muscles. For example, increasing the levels of the hormone insulin, often by consuming products containing refined sugar, can increase anaerobic activity because aerobic function can be significantly reduced (through diminished fat burning). Training obviously can also influence which muscle fibers are used, with harder, anaerobic training promoting more anaerobic muscle function and reduced aerobic function.

### Muscles and Fatigue

Why do we fatigue during endurance training and competition? As we all have experienced, muscles ultimately tire in the course of endurance activity. In some cases, fatigue slows us down, but in other situations it can lead to complete exhaustion. Whether it just slows us down or causes us to drop out of competition, it's a situation that we have control over.

Fatigue itself may be a symptom of other metabolic, neuromuscular, and training problems. And, when we attempt to push ourselves past our limits of fitness, exhaustion may actually be protecting us from more serious damage. Ultimately, as noted above, it's the brain that slows us, not our muscles. But there are various muscle factors that tell the brain to slow us down.

The first reason fatigue impairs our brain and body is the lack of optimal development of the aerobic system. Properly trained, our body is equipped to endure for very long periods because the aerobic system is very resistant to fatigue, as previously discussed. In fact, the aerobic muscles improve function when activated, rather than fatigue. That's why power output of aerobic muscles can be greatest at the very end of competition during the final kick. This requires a properly trained aerobic system, which when highly developed enables us to continue running a marathon at a relatively fast pace with less fatigue.

### Muscle Imbalance As a Cause of Fatigue

Another cause of fatigue is muscle imbalance, which usually occurs from the brain-muscle connections rather than from exercise-related issues of power and strength. To understand this better, let's differentiate between normal and abnormal muscle tensions. In the course of normal activity, muscles become tight as they contract, and more loose when relaxed. When there is an imbalance, muscles become too tight (almost like a spasm) and abnormally loose (often called "weak"). This state of abnormal tightness and weakness is termed muscle imbalance. But it has nothing to do with muscle power, as even a very strong muscle can be out of balance.

Once created, muscle imbalance can persist for weeks, months, or years. The cause may have been an injury from a fall, trauma directly to the muscle, over-stretching, or overuse. But in many cases an athlete may not recall any event that would have caused a problem because it was subtle. And, the severity of the original injury is often not related to level of disability. Therefore, serious chronic pain could be due to a relatively minor muscle imbalance caused by some seemingly minor trauma.

The most common cause of muscle imbalance is for a muscle to become weak, while another muscle, or muscles, becomes tight. This pattern of weak and tight can occur anywhere in the body, on the front and back of the arm, thigh, leg, foot, or other areas. The result is reduced and abnormal body movements reducing overall function, especially in the joints. Despite little or no sensation of muscle imbalance in its early stages, the problem often leads to pain and disability. Muscle imbalance can contribute to significant physical stress such as increased wear and tear on joints, ligaments, and other muscles, and reduces efficiency of physical movement.

Other causes of muscle imbalance include the excess wear and tear of training and competition, inadequate recovery (lack of proper rest), and trauma. Poorly fitting sports shoes can also cause muscle imbalance due to micro-trauma as discussed in detail later. And, muscle imbalance itself can predispose an athlete to further muscle problems and injury.

The brain compensates for muscle imbalance to prevent further damage by increasing the workload of other muscles. So a variety of imbalances can cause many muscles to work much harder than when the muscles are balanced. All of this requires extra energy, which is taken away from performance efforts. The end result is slower physical activity, reduced efficiency of movement (especially important for sports requiring eye-hand coordination), and increased risk for further injury. Because of the added stress on joints, muscles, and other areas, the brain receives more messages regarding body stress, adding to reduced activity and fatigue.

In other words, simple muscle imbalance can cause the body to use more energy to accomplish the same or less work—so without the muscle imbalance more energy would be available for performance. This can be significant in running, cycling, swimming, and activities that require long and sustained movements.

Another way to look at the problems muscle imbalance causes is to consider the cost in terms of oxygen use and heart rate. A hip problem (most are due to muscle imbalance), for example, which can have significant compensation from other large muscles, can dramatically increase oxygen needs—the oxygen cost (the energy required to perform) for activity is directly related to the extent of the athlete's muscle imbalance. In addition, the heart rate can rise substantially with muscle imbalance, with some studies showing almost a twenty-beat increase! The end result is inefficient movement, a higher cost of energy, and reduced performance.

Another example is a knee problem, also commonly associated with muscle imbalance. In most athletes, these problems are usually not associated with an isolated muscle imbalance around the knee. Instead, there are often various other muscle imbalances directly or indirectly related to knee mechanics, often taking place in the foot. The sum total of all muscle imbalances requires an increased effort by the athlete, which can reduce overall performance significantly.

While muscle imbalance is often asymptomatic—the athlete does not always feel the problem—observation of movement (gait) and standing posture will often reveal irregularities caused by muscle imbalance. Throughout my career I traveled to many different sporting events with athletes, with the goal of balancing muscles to help finely tune their neuromuscular system to reduce or eliminate muscle imbalance. This can be accomplished quickly and easily using various methods of manual biofeedback discussed later. Once competition starts, the athlete is biomechanically very balanced and efficient.

In most instances muscle imbalance is self-correcting, just like we heal a cut finger, a bruise, or other common problem. A healthier athlete will correct more of the problems because the body's various systems function better. However, if the body is unable to correct muscle imbalance, due to insufficient rest or less than adequate health, for example, the imbalance can become chronic.

In addition to a poorly developed aerobic system and muscle imbalance, there are other possible causes of fatigue during training and competition, including illness, such as allergy or asthma, anemia, or dietary insufficiencies.

Many endurance athletes focus too much on training the physical muscles and less on the energy they generate or the hormones or foods that influence them. If a muscle's physical attribute was the primary element in endurance, then weight lifting would provide more success than any other training technique, but this is not the case. In a sense, the muscle's physical attributes are just pawns in the endurance game. They are the workhorses, controlled by the brain and dependant on the metabolism that generates energy in the muscle for its action, and other factors, such as hormones that make up our overall metabolism.

## The Metabolism

There are many chemical components to endurance. None are more significant than the metabolic activities that provide energy for muscles, help regulate recovery, control hydration, influence fat burning, and other actions. These are accomplished by a variety of compounds that regulate our metabolism in three ways:

1. hormones produced in our many glands;
2. hormonelike compounds that are created virtually everywhere; and
3. the production of energy by the conversion of food.

These three categories of metabolic activity are influenced by training, by the brain as discussed above, and through lifestyle factors such as diet and stress. In turn, these metabolic activities help build endurance. Let's discuss each category.

### Hormones and Endurance

In the course of training, the normal physical, chemical, and mental stresses have significant influence on athletic performance and overall health. While many factors are associated with this, the hormonal system plays a major role by responding to stress. Some of these hormones are briefly discussed here and elsewhere throughout this book.

A variety of important hormones are produced throughout the body. A number of very important ones are made by the adrenal glands (two small glands atop our kidneys) using cholesterol as a building block to their production. These hormones are important for success in all sports. Cortisol and DHEA (dehydroepiandrosterone) are among the more than fifty hormones produced by the adrenal glands. Three classes of hormones are particularly important for endurance: glucocorticoids, mineralocorticoids, and androgens.

**Glucocorticoids** increase liver glycogen and promote fat and protein metabolism. Cortisol is a key glucocorticoid, and is considered one of the main stress hormones—while a moderate amount is necessary, higher levels can wreck our endurance. Cortisol is elevated more significantly with anaerobic training, competition, and in overtraining (although long-term overtraining can result in cortisol depletion, along with the depletion of many other hormone levels). Too much cortisol can disturb normal blood sugar regulation and cause the body to store fat (especially in the face or abdomen).

Too much training or competitive stress—or too much of any type of stress we encounter in our lives—can produce high cortisol levels. In women, this may cause amenorrhea (the loss of a menstrual cycle) and bone loss. In men, high cortisol can adversely impact reproductive status and muscle mass due to lowered testosterone.

Too much cortisol can also reduce the output of other adrenal hormones, including the *mineralocorticoids*. Aldosterone is an example. This hormone regulates the balance of water and electrolytes (the minerals calcium, magnesium, sodium, and potassium).

The most common *androgen* is DHEA, which makes the sex hormones testosterone and estrogen in both men and women. Testosterone is important for muscles and bones, and overall recovery. In postmenopausal women, adrenal estrogen production occurs to compensate for the ovaries not producing any more estrogen.

The adrenal glands also produce another pair of hormones called epinephrine and norepinephrine. These are important for the "fight or flight" mechanism and glycogen regulation, and they control heart rate, respiration, blood flow, and various aspects of metabolism. In all, these hormones are regulated by the stress we put on our bodies, and by the brain.

Two important hormones produced in the pancreas—insulin and glucagon—are also important for endurance athletes. Any condition that affects these hormones—most notably the quality of the diet—can significantly affect the burning of fat and sugar for energy. For example, a high-carbohydrate diet increases insulin production even in relatively healthy athletes, which can reduce fat burning. High cortisol can also increase insulin levels, as can overtraining, other stresses, or certain drugs such as birth control pills. In turn, high levels of insulin are associated with low DHEA production. With the onset of exercise, glucagon normally increases, and insulin diminishes, a combo that helps regulate glucose and glycogen, and increase fat burning.

### Hormonelike Compounds

Substances produced in the body that are similar to hormones, with equally important functions, also significantly influence our endurance. These include inflammatory and anti-inflammatory chemicals, vitamin D (sometimes called a pro-hormone), and muscle myokines.

During the course of training, competition, and throughout our life, the body repairs and recovers muscles, ligaments, tendons, joints, bones, and virtually all other areas. These actions are regulated by chemicals that trigger inflammation. Acute inflammation is an important part of the healing and recovery process, but only when other chemicals—anti-inflammatory ones—reduce the inflammation to complete the process. When the delicate balance of inflammatory and anti-inflammatory chemicals is disturbed, usually from too much inflammation, we develop chronic problems, including poor recovery, the risk of getting injured, and even the potential for disease later in life.

During all training, especially anaerobic activity, significant levels of inflammatory chemicals are produced throughout the body. This acute inflammatory response, which happens after each workout, no matter how easy or hard, to a great extent, is how we recover. As recovery is completed, anti-inflammatory chemicals are produced to turn off the acute inflammation.

Too many inflammatory chemicals can adversely affect the immune system. Recurrent colds, flu, and other illnesses are common complaints heard from athletes in all sports. During aerobic training, the immune system can actually be enhanced, with immune dysfunction much more common in those who train hard too often, compete too much, and don't recover sufficiently. Even one competitive event, such as a marathon, or a long hard workout, can suppress immune function significantly. That's why many athletes get a cold or flu soon after such efforts. Recurrent infections, especially the upper respiratory type, are often associated with overtraining, even in its very early stages.

### "Vitamin" D

Another hormonelike compound that significantly influences endurance is vitamin D. This compound technically is not a vitamin; it's sometimes called a pro-hormone because it has such powerful hormonelike effects. This substance is so important for athletes than an entire chapter is dedicated to understanding it, and I will just mention its importance here because it's so vital. Vitamin D is produced in our body through the sun's exposure to cholesterol in the skin, with the liver and kidney playing important regulatory roles. In turn, vitamin D helps regulate bone, brain, and immune health, muscle function and many other actions. Without the sun, our body's vitamin D content can often fall far below

acceptable levels, affecting many aspects of our health and endurance performance.

### Muscle Myokines

Hormonelike compounds called cytokines are very important body chemicals that help control inflammation, promote fat burning, regulate glycogen, and affect the immune system. A sub-group of these compounds that are made in our muscles are called myokines. One reason our muscles are considered the largest organ of the body is the immense metabolic activity of these myokines.

Muscle myokines not only influence the muscle itself, but many other areas of the body, including the brain, immune system, fat stores, and other muscles.

During endurance training the contraction of each muscle triggers the release of various myokines. These not only help the local muscles generate energy but assist in recovery; and these chemicals travel through the blood to influence the liver, fat stores, brain, and other areas. Furthermore, myokines may play a role in reducing visceral fat—belly fat (those with higher levels of belly fat may be most in need of building better aerobic function). In addition to helping athletes with their sport, these chemicals help prevent diseases such as cancer, diabetes, and heart disease. Smaller levels of myokines are also produced at rest in aerobic muscles. Moderate myokine production during exercise can be significantly impaired in those taking synthetic vitamin C (contained in virtually all supplements) and high dose vitamin E (the most popular type).

## Testosterone as a Performance Enhancer

Like human growth hormone (HGH), outside sources of testosterone are used to enhance performance. In fact, the use of this androgen may go back thousands of years with the consumption of animal parts containing this hormone, namely the adrenal glands and testicles. This anabolic steroid, as it's called, is the most commonly detected drug in athletes who are tested. A variety of different synthesized testosterone compounds are now produced, many of which attempt to disguise the drug in the testing process. Androgen abuse in men is associated with reduced size of the testicles and very low production of natural testosterone; symptoms include acne and excessive muscularity.

Too much or too little myokine production can be problematic. Higher but still healthy production occurs during lower-intensity training. However, hard training and competition can raise the levels of myokines to dangerously high levels, which can promote inflammation, disturb the insulin mechanism, reduce muscle mass, and reduce the muscles' ability to properly utilize glucose.

Other chemicals called oxygen free radicals are also released during training and competition. While these have great benefits in smaller amounts, anaerobic training and competition can produce much higher amounts contributing to muscle damage and other problems, especially when myokine levels are too low, or too high.

### Where Does Our Energy Come From?

Endurance training and competition require significant amounts of energy over long periods of time. In addition, when we are not training, and even during sleep, moderate amounts of energy are needed to maintain fitness and health. This energy is generated by the body's metabolism with the help of various foods and specific nutrients.

The energy we use for endurance takes a long wondrous journey before we access it. All the energy we use to work out originates as light energy from the sun. Plants absorb this energy, convert it (through photosynthesis), and store it as chemical energy. We eat the plants—and the animals that feed on plants—to obtain this chemical energy through the consumption of carbohydrates, proteins, and fats. Then, we convert it to mechanical energy used for movement. Converting foods into usable energy for muscle action is the job of the body's metabolism. High-quality food and the efficient metabolism potentially produce tremendous amounts of energy for endurance.

Carbohydrates, proteins, and fats are three of our key macronutrients used to obtain energy. When consumed, they are chemically broken down in the intestine and absorbed as glucose, amino acids, and small fat particles, respectively. Eventually, on a molecular level, these substances are converted to ATP (adenosine triphosphate). The energy used for all our body's needs comes from ATP. Different macronutrients can provide varying amounts of energy, with fats contributing more potential energy than carbohydrates and proteins combined.

Traditionally, exercise physiology textbooks discuss three different energy-producing systems in the body. These include:

- The creatine phosphate system for very short-term energy needs
- The anaerobic system for short-term energy needs
- The aerobic system for long-term energy needs

The creatine phosphate (CP) system is the most immediate energy source, but is very limited. For example, at the beginning of a 100-meter sprint, an athlete will use CP for some energy, but it's limited to only about five to ten seconds worth of energy. (This system is only mentioned here because it is emphasized less and its benefits minimized in endurance training relative to the other two systems.)

For energy to be maintained beyond the time limits of CP, the anaerobic system is utilized. Energy from this system is derived from sugar (glucose) in the anaerobic muscles. This energy is used during sprint, power, and is very useful at the end of endurance competition, where a final kick

is needed. It may also be used throughout competition, such as while running a steep hill, a breakaway during cycling, or at the end of a basketball game or tennis match. But the maximum amount of energy the anaerobic system can generate is about three minutes worth of all-out effort, longer if it's used sparingly. If you use up this energy too early in competition, you can adversely and sometimes tragically affect performance at the end, a time when most athletes need a burst of energy.

Since the body has strict limitations on energy gained from the anaerobic system, a third source of energy is available, the main focus for endurance athletes. This long-term energy source comes from the aerobic system, which converts fat in the aerobic muscles to energy. The aerobic system, with its use of fat, may have up to 75,000 kcal of energy available, which is enough abundant energy to maintain training or competition for many hours, or even days.

Triglycerides are the specific type of fat used for energy by aerobic muscles. When chemically broken down in our body's fat stores (they originally enter these stores mostly from carbohydrates and fat from the diet), they enter the bloodstream as free fatty acids, where they are carried to the aerobic muscles and burned in the mitochondria for energy. This process of burning fat is called beta-oxidation. The utilization of some glucose by the aerobic system is vital because it maintains the fat-burning process. During training or competition, if you deplete your sugar and sugar reserves (glycogen stores), you'll also cease burning fat.

Herein lies the endurance game; as the time of your activity increases, more fat and aerobic energy must be generated. But as the intensity increases, less oxygen is delivered for fat burning, so aerobic metabolism is diminished, forcing the body to use more anaerobic energy, which is very limited. If you use up all your sugar, even fat burning stops, along with the rest of your body. Do you refrain from going faster so you can go farther? Can you really go farther and faster?

You can have the best of both; the answer is in proper training. By properly programming your aerobic system to burn more fat for energy, you can develop both endurance and aerobic speed.

The table below indicates how much aerobic and anaerobic energy are used during competition.

### Table Indicating How Much Aerobic and Anaerobic Energy Is Used During Competition of Varying Length

| Time (minutes) | % Anaerobic | % Aerobic |
| --- | --- | --- |
| 1 | 70 | 30 |
| 2 | 50 | 50 |
| 4 | 35 | 65 |
| 10 | 15 | 85 |
| 30 | 5 | 95 |
| 60 | 2 | 98 |
| 120 | 1 | 99 |
| >120 | <1 | >99 |

This is an extremely brief view of the body's metabolism. The chemical activity that takes place in the body every moment during training and competition, and at rest, is very complex. For example, there are at least nine hundred enzymes known to be involved with this metabolism. Just the breakdown of sugar to energy requires nineteen different chemical reactions. And it's not just the metabolism that is complex but all of the body's systems that interrelate with it.

It's also possible to observe the interrelationships between different aspects of the body. As I've watched athletes and measured their improvement during a particular training period, I've seen the brain, muscles, and metabolism respond to progress in slightly different ways. You may experience this too. For example, your perceived exertion at the same intensity may not always feel the same: when you first begin training the aerobic system, the biggest complaint is typically that you don't feel much of a workout because of the relatively slow pace. During that phase, the muscles are more developed than the metabolic components. But in time this situation changes. By developing more aerobic speed, you may now find it's more of an effort to train that fast, even though the heart rate is the same. In this case, the muscular body has not kept pace with the progressing metabolism.

## The Role of Lactic Acid and Lactate

One element that affects each of these three important components of endurance—brain, muscles, and metabolism—is lactic acid. While it's produced in muscles, it ends up in the blood, where it converts to lactate.

We've all heard of lactic acid—that's the so-called waste product that's produced in anaerobic muscles with harder workouts. Lactic acid was thought of as a cause of fatigue and muscle soreness. But a revolution has occurred in this field in the last few years. With a better understanding of physiology, we've come to know these compounds as an important part of our overall fitness and health. In particular, lactate is an important source of energy.

Blood lactate is a normal and important component of our body chemistry. Its metabolism includes production (as lactic acid) in muscles at rest and during all intensities of exercise. Specifically, blood lactate provides us with a variety of benefits; it's an important source of energy, forming glucose, which helps replace muscle glycogen stores when they are diminished; it's an important fuel for aerobic metabolism (to help maintain fat burning); and helps spare blood sugar. Lactate does not necessarily increase fatigue during long endurance activities. And, lactate (or lactic acid) is not directly associated with muscle soreness.

Lactate is also an energy source for many other areas of the body. It provides energy for the heart (cardiac) muscle, the liver and kidney, red and white blood cells, and the brain. Lactate is also important for wound repair and healing. The largest mass of tissue in the body, our muscles, uses considerable amounts of lactate. Let's look at some of these in more detail.

The old view that lactate, beginning with the muscle's production of lactic acid during hard exercise (due to oxygen debt), is a "dead-end" waste product has changed dramatically in recent years. It's not simply an anaerobic metabolite. This is the case when oxygen availability is low, but lactic acid is also formed aerobically in the presence of sufficient oxygen.

Lactic acid is produced in muscles even at rest. The amount can increase significantly with increased exercise intensity. When lactic acid levels elevate, body pH—the acid-alkaline balance—is reduced. This is associated with muscle fatigue, but it may not be the cause, which is still not completely known (although the disruption of calcium and phosphorus metabolism and muscle imbalance are key factors in fatigue). Lactic acid is ultimately diffused into the blood and converted to lactate.

Lactate plays an important role in providing energy to muscles as a source of carbohydrate. During moderate intensity exercise, for example, lactate may become more important than glucose for muscle energy, which may help spare blood glucose. Aerobic muscles utilize lactate for energy as well, helping to burn fat. Lactate accomplishes this by returning to the muscle cells from the blood, and converting to glucose. (Lactate conversion to glucose also occurs in the liver.)

Even without food we can quickly restore depleted glycogen in aerobic and anaerobic muscle fibers with lactate. This is an important part of the "fight or flight" mechanism. (Body fat and even protein can also serve as important sources of energy to help replace depleted glycogen stores.)

Lactate is an immediate (less than thirty minutes) fuel source that helps replenish glycogen following exercise, especially hard efforts. Food sources can also contribute, if consumed immediately (within a thirty-minute window) following a hard workout or competition. Complete repletion of glycogen stores during recovery over the next ninety minutes and beyond is more dependent upon the breakdown of body fat and protein; for example, certain amino acids convert to glucose.

Up to half of the energy needed for complete glycogen repletion comes from lactate, and 50 percent or more from the breakdown of fat and protein. However, new research shows these levels may be conservative and that fat and protein may contribute even more significantly to glycogen replacement.

All workouts and races require recovery. The process of active recovery—the cool-down, discussed later—is especially important for glycogen replacement. This occurs quickly in the anaerobic muscle fibers with the contribution of glycogen from the aerobic fibers. Glycogen, lactate, fat, and protein all provide significant contributions to this process.

### Heart

In the heart, fat is the major fuel for cardiac muscle at rest. During exercise, however, lactate serves as a key source of energy for the heart. Here, lactate use increases proportionally with rising heart rates and increased lactate levels. Lactate may provide 60 percent of the energy for cardiac muscle contraction during training, with other potential energy from sugar (glucose).

Poor lactate metabolism, which may be due to various health problems, including those triggered by poor diet, is associated with various types of heart disease, and occurs in diabetes. Similar reductions in lactate metabolism in the heart are also seen in so-called normal aging.

### Brain

In the brain, lactate is very important in supplying glucose to brain cells (neurons) during exercise, when a significant amount of blood is normally diverted away from the brain to working muscles. In addition, lactate rather than glucose may be the primary and preferred energy source during neuronal activation (brain activity) at all times. Lactate is also produced by certain other brain cells (astrocytes) for use by other nearby neurons.

# MY PERSPECTIVE—BY MAJOR JASON MARSHALL

*Pilots are endurance athletes of the sky. That was clearly evident in the age of Charles Lindbergh and Amelia Earhart. And it continues to be true today for the men and women who guard our skies as part of the U.S. military. B-2 pilots, for example, often fly up to two consecutive days during long-range missions. One of these pilots, and a former decathlete, Major Jason Marshall, recognized that one battle was being lost—the fight against fatigue.*

✳ ✳ ✳

In October 2001, the 509th Bomb Wing at Whiteman Air Force Base in Missouri set a new record for combat-sortie duration in the war on terrorism. Six B-2s led the first few days of Operation Enduring Freedom by destroying some of the most critical targets and clearing the way for other critical combat assets to successfully engage air strikes virtually unchallenged over Afghanistan. One of those B-2 sorties was just over forty-four hours, which made it the longest combat sortie in the history of aviation.

Whiteman's training program and operational innovativeness began reaching out to world-renowned experts in the area of human performance for help. Two B-2 pilots in the tiny cockpit were experiencing micro-naps after twenty-four hours of being awake at the stick. As you can imagine, operating under conditions of extreme exhaustion and going to sleep while flying a $2.2 billion national asset was clearly a problem.

I was the B-2 pilot in charge of flight safety at the time and was determined to figure out how to enable two B-2 pilots to operate effectively for up to fifty hours while airborne. I personally contacted Dr. Phil Maffetone because I had heard of him for years as the "father of sports nutrition" while I competed as a decathlete at the collegiate, amateur, and professional level. When I made Phil aware of the situation B-2 pilots were up against, he cancelled several plans; and although we were ready to fund his expenses to come to Whiteman AFB, he refused and came on his own dime to help. We spent several days immersing him in our environment and constraints.

Phil educated us on the importance of sleep the night prior and helped us to develop a strategy to take turns flying the jet and manage pilot sleep cycles based on our circadian rhythm so we would get the biggest bang for the buck while resting. We scheduled our aerial refueling times around the custom sleep schedules since both aircrews had to be in the seat to get gas while airborne. We were able to get some sleep with this plan, but it was still not enough to reduce fatigue levels below the equivalent of being legally drunk. So more had to be done.

Another problem was that the B-2 didn't have a place to sleep, so we figured out a way to modify a military cot to fit behind the two ejection seats. But altering the cockpit to add a bunk would have cost millions and there just wasn't room. The air vents that control the cockpit and keep all of the equipment cool blow a lot of loud, high pressure, and very dry air, thus leaving the pilots to operate in an environment similar to the top of Pike's Peak—cool and dry with the oxygen equivalent of being at 15,000 feet. Getting the cot and resting position away from the air ducts was another key to giving our pilots the best opportunity to sleep when the opportunity arose.

Phil highlighted the rapid dehydration issues that were occurring as a result of the cockpit's high interior altitude and windy, dry environment. The B-2 was originally designed for a specific Cold War nuclear mission so the toilet was only intended to sustain two pilots for a maximum ten-hour flight. Forty plus hours of drinking the amount of water we needed was another issue we had to work through. Some pilots used "piddle packs."

If the cramped quarters and blowing air weren't enough to make sleep a distant dream, there was the cockpit noise. Phil realized that the noise levels were comparable to, and often greater than, a rock concert. It didn't take him long to convince us that we needed to address this issue. We volunteered our pilots to test the new Bose noise reduction headsets and ear-cup inserts for helmets.

Phil also suggested adding miscellaneous items like full-spectrum light bulbs in the cockpit and posture-perfect seat cushions and lumbar support and more.

Despite all these improvements, we were still not in a position to declare victory. Which brought us to the biggest surprise of all—the effects of nutrition. Phil gave a stunning presentation on the effects of food on performance and how a lifestyle of healthy eating was required to achieve maximum benefit. He pointed out how even just a single meal could have a very significant effect on human and cognitive performance for the next four to six hours. It was frankly embarrassing to most of us when he highlighted that our flight kitchen was restricted to spending less than a few dollars on each aircrew meal to fuel the body of those responsible for flying these billion-dollar machines.

We called our aircrew meals "box nasties" because they came in a thin white card-board box that was probably more nutritious than the food inside. Since everything in the box was mostly simple-sugar-type carbohydrates, pilots were experiencing huge insulin spikes. When a large insulin spike was combined with a lull in the pilot's circadian rhythm, cognitive performance and response times would decrease dramatically. Many of the pilots experienced these so-called afternoon food comas after having a heavy carbohydrate lunch. We tested this in our fifty-hour B-2 simulator missions by feeding one crew whatever they wanted to eat and feeding the other crew meals designed in accordance with the principles Dr. Maffetone taught us. The results were like night and day.

Fortunately, with a little education, the flight kitchen staff worked with us to put together food that would help aircrew to maintain energy levels and not require as much sleep.

The best personal testimony I heard was from our group commander who flew a long mission of over thirty hours. He thought all the nutrition stuff made sense but admitted he didn't expect to experience anywhere near the level of performance increase he later described. He delivered his testimony in a large scheduling meeting with several other commanders. He said he hadn't felt that alert in years and went the entire mission without sleep because he didn't feel like he needed any. He recommended the other commanders get their pilots educated on how to eat like this.

Based on our improved performance at Whiteman AFB due to healthy eating—following meal plans approved by Phil—we soon had people calling us from hundreds of military locations wanting more information on how to engineer these meals.

### The Lactate Shuttles

Among the more interesting features of lactate discovered by recent research is the peroxisomal lactate shuttle, which can provide addition energy for endurance. While about 90 percent of certain fats are burned in the aerobic muscle's mitochondria, 10 percent are burned in other areas called peroxisomes— tiny enzyme-containing components in the muscle. The purpose of this process is thought to be the preparation of fats for burning in the mitochondria. This is a significant amount of potential energy from fat burning that lactate provides. In addition, this energy helps with other important bodily processes such as bile production and cholesterol regulation.

### Lactate and Injury

While I've discussed lactate in relation to its role in the production of energy, lactate can stimulate other activities—especially related to recovery and healing. For example, collagen production, used for physical repair of the body, can double after a workout with rising lactate levels. Physical wounds also produce lactate, accumulating it for healing. Lactate may also promote healing in other ways, by increasing oxygen supply and blood flow to the area. And lactate can even stimulate the production of new blood vessels when necessary. Lactate stimulation following wear and tear, and injury, may also be stimulated by adrenal stress hormones.

The complex physiology of lactic acid and lactate metabolism is still unraveling. In the coming years, new research will reveal even more.

Training your brain, muscles, and metabolism are key aspects to successful endurance racing. Now that we have looked at these three key parts of the body and their interconnected effect on performance, let's continue with our investigation of the "big picture."

# CHAPTER 3

# DEVELOPING MAXIMUM AEROBIC FUNCTION—
## How to Get "Heart Smart" When Building Your Endurance Foundation

The first step in building great endurance is to fully develop the aerobic system, which provides many fitness and health benefits. These include improvements in performance, reductions in body fat, balanced muscles and supported joints, injury correction and prevention, improved immunity, and many others. A fully developed system allows more aerobic speed, which will translate into running, biking, swimming, and going faster in any endurance event.

This occurs even before training the anaerobic system, where additional speed and power may be obtained. A strong aerobic system also improves overall health, and these improvements in maximum aerobic function—MAF—should continue for years.

Over the years, a number of athletes have asked me, "Does MAF also stand for Maffetone, since they are the same first three letters of your last name?" Well, the truth is that this is a matter of pure coincidence. Very early in my career I used another term, "maximum aerobic pace"—MAP—to describe how runners run a faster pace with the same or lower heart rate as aerobic function progresses. But as I began seeing more athletes in the cycling, swimming, and multisport community, the term "pace" was not applicable. In addition, the term MAP is used in exercise physiology—it refers to maximal aerobic power, another name for maximal oxygen uptake ($VO_2$max). The term "function" better describes what is really happening—building more endurance through better aerobic function.

## Aerobic Base

The training period where an endurance athlete focuses on developing the aerobic system is called the aerobic base. I first learned about the concepts of base building in the late 1970s by reading about famed New Zealand coach, Arthur Lydiard, who died in 2004. His idea was that aerobic and anaerobic running should be balanced by specific training. Arthur, originally a distance runner himself, began coaching, and in the 1950s and '60s was a major influence in developing the running boom. He also trained many endurance athletes from around the world to greatness, including Olympic gold medalists Peter Snell (who won both 800 and 1500 meters in the 1964 Olympics) and Lasse Viren (who won both 5K and 10K in the 1972 Olympics), and many of the world's greatest endurance athletes. His extensive travel around the globe left a significant mark on the history of endurance training.

In the early 1980s, while on a lecture tour in the United States, Arthur visited my clinic. While he never complained about any personal aches or pains, we had a lot in common and spent time talking about measuring aerobic conditioning. Learning firsthand from him was much different from trying to read his material. He was frustrated that many in the endurance world did not grasp his concepts. At this time, the "no pain, no gain" myth had already taken hold in endurance sports, consistently popularized by newly created single-sports magazines. The simplistic, unhealthy notion that you must "train fast to race fast" was in full swing, as were the rapid rise in injuries and overtraining. Runners were especially susceptible to this way of thinking; and as the running boon took off, so did the number of leg, knee, hip, and foot injuries.

Arthur and I, along with the very few others who trained athletes "slower" to develop the aerobic system, were considered odd ducks due to our unconventional approach. Acceptance came gradually as endurance athletes learned to recognize the significance of aerobic function. Today, the few remaining coaches and trainers who still might criticize the base-building concept and its application don't understand the basic physiology of the aerobic and anaerobic systems.

By measuring an athlete during all aspects of training, I made the important discovery that anaerobic stimulation, which can come from any anaerobic workout and any physical,

## NO PAIN, NO GAIN . . . NO BRAIN!

The social myth and competitive peer pressure associated with "no pain, no gain"—an attitude that "more is better" regarding more speed, more distance, more weights, and so forth—poses both fitness and health problems. Because when you're fully engaged in this approach, you override your brain's common sense—its instincts and intuition—to slow down during training. Making a conscious effort to go against what the brain wants to do can contribute to overtraining, often with an accompanying injury. And in many cases, the result can be poor performance when this takes place during a race. We can call this "no pain, no gain, no brain" following Dr. Tim Noakes's reference to $VO_2$ max testing as a "brainless model" of exercise performance testing. In both situations, the brain is not able to adequately regulate the most effective body activity, based on what information the brain is given by the body. This is the case when trying to train too hard too often, because the athlete has consciously chosen to override the brain's better judgment. This is an emotional reaction—one that is based on current trends, often started by advertisements and other marketing—and one that can be irrational.

chemical, or mental lifestyle stress, had the potential to interfere with the development of the aerobic system, thereby reducing endurance potential. An important aspect of building the aerobic base, I quickly learned, is that during this process, anaerobic training should be minimized—ideally eliminated—from the training schedule. And, athletes need to become more aware of how stress affects them.

How sensitive is the issue of including anaerobic workouts during aerobic base building? It's quite individual. In many athletes, even an occasional anaerobic run during a base period, for example, may be enough to slow aerobic progress. In others who strictly avoid anaerobic training but have a very stressful lifestyle, the same problem of not fully developing aerobic function can occur. The reason is that the anaerobic stimulation from a workout, and the biochemical changes that follow, can adversely affect the aerobic system and any potential benefits including increased fat burning. The extent of this potential problem varies with the individual. In some athletes, for example, especially those who have been injured or have not performed to their potential, there is a need to spend three to six months building an aerobic base. Others may just need to perform this exclusive aerobic training during a major part of the year. In some cases, an athlete's training is best done aerobically for both performance and optimal health.

While it's clear that anaerobic training can impair aerobic function, a common question is: Just how do anaerobic training, competition, or other physical, chemical, and mental stresses interfere with aerobic development? There may be several mechanisms associated with this problem:

- Stress of any type can interfere with the aerobic system by raising the hormone cortisol. High cortisol can interfere with many physiological processes in the brain, muscles, and metabolism that are necessary to develop aerobic function and endurance.
- High cortisol levels, a common marker of overtraining, also increases insulin levels, inhibiting the fat-burning process necessary for aerobic muscles to work well.
- Anaerobic training can decrease the number of aerobic muscle fibers, sometimes significantly. This can happen in just a few short weeks.
- Anaerobic training raises your respiratory quotient, meaning that fat burning is reduced and sugar burning is increased, encouraging further use of anaerobic function and less aerobic activity.
- Excessive amounts of lactic acid produced during anaerobic training may impair aerobic muscle enzymes, reducing aerobic function.

- Anaerobic training typically causes athletes to consume more refined carbohydrates because of an increased craving for sugar. This can increase insulin levels and further interfere with fat burning, reducing aerobic function.

For many endurance athletes the lack of sufficient aerobic conditioning can cause many problems, including serious physical, chemical, and mental injuries. This problem is not unlike a nutritional deficiency such as anemia. I call the problem "the aerobic deficiency syndrome," or ADS, and it exists in millions of endurance athletes.

## The Aerobic Deficiency Syndrome

As the number of endurance athletes has dramatically increased through the latter part of the twentieth century and into the twenty-first, so has the injury rate. These problems are not just associated with physical injuries, but also those that affect body chemistry and even the brain. Athletes without a good aerobic base typically develop various signs and symptoms. The most common complaints heard from athletes include fatigue, increased body fat, mechanical injuries, hormonal imbalance, inadequate endurance, and poor performance. Carefully compiling these complaints, it becomes evident that these same athletes have one common feature: aerobic deficiency. Moreover, the aerobic deficiency syndrome (ADS) is a primary contributing factor to overtraining. Here are some of the important signs and symptoms associated with ADS:

- **Fatigue.** This is a very common complaint in athletes. This may also be related to numerous problems, but the lack of adequate fat burning due to poor aerobic function is very common. The result is more reliance on sugar for energy—not just during training but at all other times as well.
- **Increased body fat.** This problem is associated with reduced fat burning, causing more fat from dietary carbohydrates and fat to be stored.
- **Chronic inflammation** is one result of higher body fat. Chronic inflammation can also trigger certain injuries and ill health.
- **Physical injuries.** These are often the result of poor aerobic muscle function because these muscles support our joints, bone, ligaments and other structures. Clinical observations reveal the most common areas of injury in athletes with ADS include the low back, knee, ankle, and foot.
- **Hormonal imbalance.** This common problem interferes with many aspects of fitness and health. It is often associated with high levels of cortisol and low amounts of DHEA. High cortisol may trigger insomnia, high body fat, craving for sweets, and blood sugar irregularities, all with the potential to interfere with proper recovery. Low DHEA can result in low testosterone and other hormones. In women, premenstrual syndrome and menopausal symptoms may be complaints, and in men, low testosterone can adversely affect muscles and bones. Loss of normal sexual function can affect both men and women as a result of reduced sex hormones.
- **Reduced endurance.** This is often seen with increasing fatigue, poor performance, loss of aerobic speed, and, in general, overtraining.
- **Nutritional imbalance.** Dietary problems are often associated with ADS, especially in athletes who consume excess refined carbohydrates and have low fat and protein intakes. Other nutritional imbalances may also occur, such as low iron levels which adversely affect the "red" iron-dependent aerobic muscles.

Correction of the ADS is relatively easy. In general, building your fitness and health will accomplish this task. Perhaps the most important correction comes in building a good aerobic base. This is best accomplished by monitoring your heart rate, through the use of biofeedback device called a heart-rate monitor.

Some of this heart-rate monitor information is presented here because it's a foundation of endurance training, with additional information about heart-rate monitoring in the next chapter. The heart rate is an important guide to further help individualize your training, enabling your brain and body to obtain maximum aerobic function, aerobic speed, and other benefits.

## The Heart and Heart-Rate Monitoring

An important training companion to assist you in developing optimal endurance is a heart-rate monitor. This simple device is an important tool that not only guides your training but is part of an important assessment process, and can even be used in some competitive situations. A heart-rate monitor is really a simple biofeedback device. *Dorland's Medical Dictionary* defines biofeedback as "the process of providing visual or auditory evidence to a person of the status of body function so that you may exert control over that function." Unfortunately, most people use their heart-rate monitors only to

see how high their heart rate gets during a workout, or evaluate the morning, resting heart rate.

In the 1970s, I first measured heart rates as a student involved in a biofeedback research project. I observed and jotted down responses in human subjects to various physiological inputs, such as sounds, visual effects, and other physical stimulation, including exercise. The subjects' reactions were evaluated by measuring temperature, perspiration, and heart rate. Through this research, it became evident that using the heart rate to objectively measure body function was simple, accurate, and useful, especially for athletes. I began using the heart rate to evaluate all exercising patients, and by the early 1980s developed a formula that anyone could use with their heart monitor to help build an aerobic base. This "180 Formula" enables athletes to

**Question:** Why does my resting heart rate fluctuate during the day? It's lower in the morning when I wake up, and by late afternoon, it's about ten beats per minute faster. I like running in the late afternoon or early evening after work. Will this have any impact, or should I run in the morning?

**Answer:** It's normal for the heart rate to fluctuate during the day (and even at night during sleep). Heart rate is typically lowest in the morning upon awakening, with higher levels and more fluctuations during the day, due to physical activity and increased function of various body areas including brain and intestines, which rely on high levels of blood flow. The resting rate won't affect your aerobic pace in any significant way, so don't change what's most convenient and enjoyable regarding training schedules.

find the ideal maximum aerobic heart rate in which to base all aerobic training.

For centuries it's been well known that the heart predictably increases and decreases its rate of beating with physical activity and other stimulation sensed by our brain. The Roman physician Galen first described the heart rate almost two thousand years ago. The heart rate—the number of beats per minute—is another example of our physiological uniqueness as we all have different heart rates in response to training, racing, and resting. Observing these changes, through feel (such as sensing the changes in heart rate associated with high levels of exertion), intuition (such as allowing our brain to dictate our response to changes in heart rate), and analysis (by measuring heart rate changes), and the adjustment of our training in response, is a simple form of biofeedback. In fact, humans have a built-in (so-called "hardwired") biofeedback capability that's been in use for millions of years and has been an important aspect of our survival as a species. Today, we continue to use the heart rate to help guide us in training, racing, and recovery. A heart-rate monitor serves as a simple form of biofeedback equipment to help in this endeavor.

The heart rate can provide us with a significant amount of important information—the reason for its extensive use by health-care professionals. The heart rate is directly related to, and a reflection of, the body's oxygen need. The heartbeat, the outcome of the heart's muscular contraction to help pump oxygen-rich blood through the body, is also associated with systolic blood pressure, while diastolic blood pressure reflects relaxation of the heart as measured between beats. The relationship between two heartbeats is associated with heart-rate variability, reflecting our parasympathetic aspect of brain and nervous system function—this being an important factor for professionals to assess heart health and for athletes to evaluate recovery from training and racing.

The heart itself has a built-in mechanism of nerves that controls its own rhythm (to maintain a heart rate of around 70 to 80 beats per minute), but the brain, through the action of the autonomic nervous system and various hormones, controls the wide range of heart rates based on the body's needs. This rate can be as low as 30 to 40 in those with great aerobic function to as high as 220 in young athletes during all-out efforts.

Abnormal heart rates also fall within this range, sometimes making heart rates inaccurate. For example, in the later stages of the overtraining syndrome, the resting heart rate is abnormally low; and those who are too stressed can have abnormally high resting and training heart rates.

Like other neuromuscular tissues in the body, the heart has electrical activity, creating an electrical field throughout the body. This can be measured with an ECG (electrocardiograph), an important tool for healthcare professionals for the evaluation of the heart itself, helping to evaluate abnormal problems in the heart's electrical activity, for example, or damage to the heart's muscle following a heart attack.

Simpler technology allows athletes to obtain the basic information about the heart rate by sensing the beat on the chest and transmitting this information to a wristwatch for easy visual observation. Modern heart-rate monitors have become popular in recent years, with many companies making them, riding the wave of the high-tech revolution. However, without an understanding of how to effectively apply the information obtained from a heart-rate monitor, its use is more like a toy rather than the valuable assessment tool—a true biofeedback device.

### The Pulse

The pulse is felt in the body's blood vessels and reflects the heart's beat. The heart rate and the pulse are the same rate in most instances. The pulse is felt with a slight delay after the heart rate, with those pulses farther from the heart, such as in the foot, taking longer to pulsate. In abnormal situations, the heartbeats are ineffective and don't pump as much blood, such as in some arrhythmias, giving a different heart and pulse rate. In other cases, such as a condition called atrial fibrillation, the heart's electrical system produces a "beat" in the heart without causing a mechanical beat felt in a pulse, also giving different measures.

The pulse can be measured from your fingertip or earlobe with a pulse meter. These devices contain a photoelectric cell sensor.

Because indoor and outdoor light and body movement can interfere with these devices, pulse meters are often not as reliable (as direct assessment of the heart rate from the chest) during physical activity but are useful during rest or on stationary devices. However, quick reductions in heart rate occur when physical activity is stopped, giving inaccurate training rates.

Taking a patient's pulse is one of the first clinical tools taught to all healthcare professionals. Its primary purpose is to assess the heart rate, reflected in various pulses felt on the body, to ascertain whether the rate is too rapid or too slow, the quality of the rhythm, its strength, and, of course, whether the patient is alive. In Chinese medicine, pulse diagnosis is a very important component in evaluating overall body function. As a student, I also learned various other important uses for taking a pulse, including measuring the body's response to certain stimuli. For example, placing your hands in cold ice water, a long-standing evaluation used in Western medicine and research—called the cold pressor test—usually raises the pulse rate, much like when you watch an action or adventure movie, walk a flight of stairs, or are exposed to other forms of stimulation. These typically raise the pulse rate in some predictable fashion, while resting without the same stimulation lowers it.

From my first day in practice, I tested patients' pulses as part of my initial evaluations. This was also important during exercise tests of various types in my office and when

**QA**    **Question:** I have a lot of trouble with my Polar heart-rate monitor. I often get "00" as a reading. It comes and goes during my workouts. As I have really improved my fitness, I want to continue using the monitor. Polar is no help at all. They won't even answer my e-mail.

**Answer:** I can sympathize with you on companies not responding. Sometimes moistening the monitor strap where it contacts your chest is helpful. And sometimes making it a bit tighter can help too. It almost sounds like there's a technical problem in the watch. You might ask the folks at Running Ahead: www.Running-Ahead.com/groups/LOWHRTR/Forum. This is an open online forum of athletes; they are knowledgeable about heart-rate monitors, use all different kinds, and are very responsive.

monitoring the pulse rates of athletes before, during, and after their workouts.

### Manual Pulse Taking

Before using heart monitors, pulse rates are often determined manually and athletes take their own pulses. But I find their accuracy is generally not good when compared to ECG or even finger pulse readings taken at rest using small digital devices. Many athletes who take their pulse manually often find it to be too low. Those who use the thumb to check the pulse have more problems with accuracy as the thumb also contains a pulse—it's best to use the index and middle finger to check the pulse in various locations. When I took an athlete's pulse in some situations, such as after a hard time trial, the same problem occurred. Even a finger pulse unit would be inaccurate in these situations. In many cases, the difficulty in getting an accurate number was not

one of counting or technology, but associated with the athlete's recovering heart rate. Usually, the athlete would have to stop for me to check the pulse, and this would cause the heart rate to diminish quickly, resulting in an inaccurate training heart rate.

One of the most common locations to check the pulse is on the palm side of the wrist (above the thumb) on the radial artery (called the radial pulse). But a pulse can be felt in many other locations throughout the body, including:

- The ulnar pulse on the little finger side of the wrist
- The brachial pulse on the inside of the elbow
- The carotid pulse located in the neck on either side of the midline
- The temporal pulse located on the temple, in front of the ear

- The femoral pulse in the inner thigh
- The popliteal pulse behind the knee
- The dorsalis pedis pulse on top of the foot
- The medial malleolar pulse on the inside back part of the ankle

There is another potential problem with manually taking your pulse. If you place your fingers on the carotid artery on the side of your neck, a location often used by athletes, you can easily find your pulse. However, this area is also sensitive. Applying even moderate pressure here can significantly affect the heart rate, quickly dropping the rate; it can also reduce blood flow to the brain, and therefore oxygen delivery. This is because the carotid area contains nerve endings that normally send messages to the brain indicating blood-pressure changes. Stimulating this area with pressure sends an improper message to the brain, which quickly slows the heart, sometimes quite dramatically. This can be dangerous—the oxygen debt created can cause fainting (or death in an extreme case).

The pulse reflects the contraction and relaxation of one's arteries and in emergency situations is sometimes difficult to feel, even by trained professionals. This is due to the pulse's relationship with blood pressure—if the blood pressure is too low, the artery will not pulsate. For example, if the blood pressure is below 60 mmHg, the carotid pulse, which brings blood to the brain, will not be felt. In this case, the person is usually not alive,

which is the reason this particular pulse is felt in an emergency situation. In a living person, if the blood pressure is below 90 mmHg, the radial pulse on the wrist may not be felt, and if below 80 mmHg, the brachial pulse may not be palpable. Traumatic injury, certain medications, illnesses, or other problems may also cause the pulse to be difficult to detect, even in a conscious person.

### Understanding Training Heart Rates

In my continued attempt to individualize training heart rates, I had several bulky heart monitors in my office, and when athletes worked with me there or on the track, these were used for accurate heart-rate evaluation. Whether the athlete was on a treadmill or stationary bike in the clinic, on the track, or at other locations, I would record a number of pre- and post-workout features. These would include the athlete's gait—their moving posture during the workout—along with standing posture and muscle balance, and I would correlate this mechanical efficiency with heart rate at various points before, during, and after workouts. It was obvious that training at various intensities affected both posture and gait: the more anaerobic, the more distortion of the body's mechanics. These changes are due, in part, to previously existing muscle imbalance and muscle problems that develop during the workout. This is sometimes very subtle and other times more obvious. All this information was correlated, and ultimately, an ideal training heart rate was found that promoted optimal aerobic function without triggering significant anaerobic activity, muscle imbalance, or other problems.

It soon became evident that the athletes needed more consistent training quality, rather than relying on the feel of the workout on the day they used the heart-rate monitor. Soon it became necessary for each athlete to have his or her own heart-rate monitor and train with it every day. The advent of modern heart-rate monitors, which sense the heart rate directly from the chest wall and transmitted the information to a wristwatch, was a great benefit in this regard, with Polar's entry into the marketplace in 1982. One of the most significant observations I made during this period was that athletes who wore heart-rate monitors during each workout felt better and improved in performance at a faster rate than others who trained without a monitor.

It was now possible to find an ideal training heart rate for athletes building their aerobic system; however, it was a relatively lengthy process of one-on-one assessment. My goal now was to find a way that any athlete could determine an optimal training heart rate, using some simple formula.

As I began lecturing and writing more about endurance training, it was difficult to explain the details of all this information on assessment without some simple and specific guidelines. The idea of a formula that would be accurate for an individual and result in a very similar or identical heart rate as my manual assessments seemed ideal. While the 220

Formula was commonly used, the number I found to be ideal in my assessment was often very different from the 220 Formula; it was usually significantly lower. In addition, it was becoming evident that athletes who used the 220 Formula for a daily training heart rate showed poor gait, increased muscle imbalance, and other problems following a workout at that heart rate, and that these athletes were more often overtrained.

## The Old 220 Formula versus the New 180 Formula

Using the traditional 220 Formula, athletes would determine the training heart rate by two steps:

- The first is subtracting their age from 220 to get their maximum heart rate. In reality, most athletes who obtain their maximum heart rate by pushing themselves to exhaustion will find it is probably not 220 minus their age. About a third will find their maximum is above this heart rate, a third will be below, and only a third may be close to what they've calculated. These inaccuracies are often significant.

- The second step uses this so-called maximum heart rate, which is then multiplied by 65, 70, 75, 80, or 85 percent. The percentage most athletes choose is the higher option since most feel the need to train with more intensity to obtain benefits. This results in a relatively high training heart rate. Moreover, the range between 65 and 85 percent is so wide that even athletes who work out without thought of heart rate or intensity will fall into this range.

Since everyone is unique, the 220 Formula never made much sense to me, as it relies on an estimated maximum heart rate which is not very accurate; in addition, this formula is not individualized—it fails to take an athlete's fitness, health, and aging into account.

There are two ways to define age. Chronological age is measured by calendar years, but this may not be a good reflection of fitness and health. We all know athletes who appear much younger—or older—than their chronological age. Some maintain better levels of physical, chemical, and mental function throughout life, reflecting a truer physiological age, while others who are the same chronological age do not. We can evaluate these differences by measuring heart and muscle function, blood sugar, and hormone levels, and by performing other clinical tests. An appropriate questionnaire that asks about fitness and health history is also very useful to assess physiological age, and would better represent "age" in a new and more accurate formula.

Over time, I began piecing together a mathematical formula, taking the optimal heart rates in athletes who had previously been assessed as a guide. Instead of 220 minus the chronological age multiplied by some percentage, I used 180 minus a person's chronological age, which is then adjusted to reflect their physiological age as indicated by fitness and health factors.

By comparing the new 180 Formula with my relatively lengthy process of one-on-one evaluations, it became clear that this new formula matched very well—in other words, my tedious assessment of an athlete and the 180 Formula resulted in a number that was the same or very close in most cases.

Early in this process, I made number of relatively minor changes to the formula. By the early 1980s, I settled on the final, most effective formula and this is the one in use today: 180 minus a person's chronological age, which is then adjusted to reflect their physiological age as indicated by fitness and health factors. The use of the number 180 was and is not significant other than as a means to finding the end number. Plus, 180 minus age itself is not a meaningful number; for example, it is not associated with $VO_2max$, lactate threshold, or other traditional measurements. The end number is an athlete's *maximum aerobic heart rate*. This is the training heart rate that reflects optimal aerobic training, and a number which, when exceeded, indicates a rapid transition to more anaerobic training. Through the use of this 180 Formula, all athletes can obtain their ideal individual aerobic training rates.

## Calculate Your Own Maximum Aerobic Training Heart Rate

To find your maximum aerobic training heart rate, there are two important steps. First, subtract your age from 180. Next, find the best category for your present state of

## MY PERSPECTIVE—BY DR. GEORGE SHEEHAN

*The undisputed philosopher king of running, Dr. George Sheehan wrote eight books and was the medical editor for Runner's World. His most popular slogan was, "Listen to your body." He ran track in college and later became a cardiologist living in Rumson, New Jersey, where he'd run during his lunch hour wearing white long johns. At age fifty, he ran a world-record 4:47 mile. Dr. Sheehan was diagnosed with prostate cancer in 1986 but continued running—and writing about his experiences—until shortly before his death at age seventy-four in 1993.*

✷ ✷ ✷

By teaching "Maximum Aerobic Function," Dr. Philip Maffetone is following the philosophy that has come down to us from the ancient Greeks. Their emphasis was on the cultivation of the self. The maximum function of the body was part of their "art of existence."

We read in Seneca that we should spend our lives learning how to live. Primary to this was the training of the body. Everything a person did was important—exercise, diet, sleep, climate. Even the architecture of the house was thought to have an influence on health.

---

fitness and health, and make the appropriate adjustments:

1. Subtract your age from 180.
2. Modify this number by selecting among the following categories the one that best matches your fitness and health profile:
   a. If you have or are recovering from a major illness (heart disease, any operation or hospital stay, etc.) or are on any regular medication, subtract an additional 10.
   b. If you are injured, have regressed in training or competition, get more than two colds or bouts of flu per year, have allergies or asthma, or if you have been inconsistent or are just getting back into training, subtract an additional 5.
   c. If you have been training consistently (at least four times weekly) for up to two years without any of the problems just mentioned, keep the number (180–age) the same.
   d. If you have been training for more than two years without any of the problems listed above, and have made progress in competition without injury, add 5.

The emphasis on the care of the body is seen again and again in the works of philosophers since the Greeks. We are called upon repeatedly to have a sound mind in a sound body. The great Herbert Spencer, in his treatise of education, writes, "If you wish to be a success in this life you must first be a good animal." And this thought is reiterated by Emerson. "Be first a good animal," writes the sage of Concord.

How best to do that is being constantly amended and refined. A poll of Canadians asking about the rules of health elicited these three items: a balanced diet, a good night's sleep, and regular visits to the doctor. These are obviously not enough. A return to basic principles and personal responsibility is necessary in order to live the athletic life.

Phil not only teaches us how to be athletes but teaches us how to teach ourselves to be athletes. Ultimately, we must become our own individual coaches in this common goal. But first we must be convinced of the importance of everything we do—to or with our bodies. Our bodies are us. Our lives are our bodies in action. So we must live at the top of our powers.

There is no better time to start than now.

For example, if you are thirty years old and fit into category (b), you get the following:

180–30=150. Then 150–5=145 beats per minute (bpm).

In this example, 145 will be the highest heart rate for all training. This is highly aerobic, allowing you to most efficiently build an aerobic base. Training above this heart rate rapidly incorporates anaerobic function, exemplified by a shift to burning more sugar and less fat for fuel.

If it is difficult to decide which of two groups best fits you, choose the group or outcome that results in the lower heart rate. In athletes who are taking medication that may affect their heart rate, those who wear a pacemaker, or those who have special circumstances not discussed here, further individualization with the help of a health-care practitioner or other specialist familiar with your circumstance and knowledgeable in endurance sports may be necessary.

Two situations may be exceptions to the above calculations:

- The 180 Formula may need to be further individualized for people over the age of sixty-five. For some of these athletes, up to 10 beats may have to be added for those in category (d) in the 180 Formula, and depending on individual levels of fitness

**QA**

**Question:** I find that running (or more accurately, jogging) at my MAF (maximum aerobic function) is not fun for me. I feel under-challenged and uninspired to work out at such a low level of intensity. I miss the fun and freedom I feel running at higher heart rates and dislike hearing my heart-rate monitor alarm beep as soon as I start moving at a pace that feels good to me. But biking at my aerobic heart rate is much more fun for me since I can sustain a more stimulating level of perceived effort on the bike. Am I to understand that the aerobic benefits of my bike training will carry over to my running and allow me, eventually, to run faster aerobically?

**Answer:** Look at the big picture. By training "slower" you should be inspired and challenged. Inspired because you've found a major problem (poor aerobic function), which you now have the challenge to correct. You're not only going to be faster (at the same heart rate), but more fit (to race better) and healthier. And yes, the aerobic benefits you build on your bike will eventually carry over to your running. It will be interesting to see how long (or short) it takes for your cycling to become relatively hard to keep at your aerobic pace as you get faster at the same heart rate—just the opposite of what you experienced on your runs. This would indicate that you can start adding some running back into your week. Cross-training is always a great routine—mentally and physically.

and health. This does not mean 10 should automatically be added, but that an honest self-assessment is important.

- For athletes sixteen years of age and under, the formula is not applicable; rather, a heart rate of 165 may be best.

Once a maximum aerobic heart rate is found, a training range from this heart rate to 10 beats below could be used as a training range. For example, if an athlete's maximum aerobic heart rate is determined to be 155, that person's aerobic training zone would be 145 to 155 bpm. However, the more training at 155, the quicker an optimal aerobic base will be developed.

Initially, training at this relatively low rate may be stressful for many athletes. "I just can't train that slowly!" is a common comment. But after a short time, you will feel better and your pace will quicken at that same heart rate. You will not be stuck training at that relatively slow pace for too long. Still, for many athletes it is difficult to change bad habits.

One of my patients by the name of Don was a good runner who usually placed in the top of his thirty to thirty-nine age group. When he came to my clinic with chronic injuries, fatigue, and recurrent colds, one of the first things we did was test him on the track with a heart monitor. At his maximum aerobic heart rate, Don was only able to run at an 8:40 pace—almost two minutes slower than his usual training pace! I recommended that Don train at this slower pace with a monitor for a three-month base period. But two weeks later he called me and said it was impossible to run that slow. I again explained the whole process and how he would get faster. A week later he faxed a letter saying he could not train by my recommendations. But several months later, with worsening fitness and health, and almost unable to race, Don came back to the clinic. Now he was ready to train aerobically. It took several months of dedicated base building, beginning with a slower pace, for Don to increase his aerobic pace until finally he was running his "normal" 6:45 training pace—but this time at a heart rate that was twenty-five beats lower than our previous evaluation.

The accuracy, usefulness, and importance of the formula have been time-tested throughout the years. But by the early 1990s, many of the athletes I'd worked with for a decade or more taught me another important lesson about the 180 Formula. Seeing the changes they made, including some longer than normal plateaus, helped me come to an important conclusion: Those using the 180 Formula successfully for more than five years

needed to adjust their maximum aerobic heart rates down by about two to three beats. They could not keep using the same maximum aerobic heart rate they'd determined years earlier, despite healthier aging. While we age over time chronologically, building fitness and health during the same period results in a slower physiological aging. So in five years of proper (successful) training and improving health, for example, your training heart rate does not need to be lowered by five beats; instead, because you're physiologically not as "old," decrease only by two to three beats. When in doubt, always choose a lower maximum aerobic heart rate. This assumes the factors in the 180 Formula that pertain to medication, illness, and competitive improvements are the same. Otherwise, further reductions in the training heart rate may be necessary.

## The 180 Formula in Different Sports

A frequently asked question is whether different heart rates should be used for different endurance activities. For example, should the maximum aerobic heart rate, as determined by the 180 Formula, while swimming be different when the same athlete is cycling or running? The short answer is no. The 180 Formula holds true for all aerobic training activities. At the same heart rate, different endurance sports require essentially the same levels of metabolic activities. However, other aspects are quite different

## Chemical Benefits of the 180 Formula

Another significant benefit of applying the 180 Formula to heart-rate training is the body's chemical response to training at this lower level of intensity. Normally, the body produces chemicals called oxygen free radicals in response to many stresses, including certain types of training, even at heart rates just above the max aerobic level. While these chemicals can be helpful, too many contribute to inflammatory conditions, over-training, and even diseases such as cancer and heart disease. In addition, increased free radicals speed the aging process. High intensity anaerobic training produces large amounts of free radicals. But even moderate training intensities above the max aerobic heart rate can produce similar levels of free radicals. Using the 180 Formula as your guide, you can minimize free-radical production. Studies show that training at this efficient intensity is ideal when free-radical stress is a concern.

when comparing swimming to running, for example. One significant difference is perceived exertion, which is a subjective feeling the athlete has in relation to the workout. In this case, swimming will "feel" more difficult compared to running at the same heart rate.

An objective factor that makes perceived exertion so different is gravity stress. The difference in this stress between swimming and running is dramatic; there is very little gravity influence in the water, but that same force is maximally affecting the body during running. A great deal of energy may not have to go into countering gravity stress in the pool, but just the opposite is true during a run. And, partly related to gravity stress is the increased volume of muscle activity during running compared to swimming.

The bottom-line clinical reason I don't use different max aerobic heart rates for different sports is that the outcome is better compared to when the heart rates are adjusted for a different activity. Outcomes include aerobic base development, injury rates, performance, and overall health.

Because I've worked with athletes in virtually all sports, my approach to overall conditioning—improving fitness and health and building aerobic function—is very similar. Below are examples of the use of heart monitors in different sports. Once the general idea is clear, applying these methods in any sport will be relatively easy.

### Tennis

As you know there is a significant endurance component in tennis. Consider the length of time—from the start of a warm-up to the conclusion of the final round, especially if it's a long and difficult match. In these events a significant amount of energy (perhaps 50–60 percent or more) comes from the aerobic system. So a tennis player relies heavily on aerobic function to get through an event. And, the more aerobically trained (the more fat burning for energy), the more glycogen will be conserved. In this way, as the player gets to the later games and sets, there will be more anaerobic function for speed and power instead of significant fatigue. We all know that a long tennis match can be won or lost in later sets, and we can recall some of the great matches of Borg, Connors, McEnroe, the Williams sisters, and Billie Jean King that taxed the bodies of these competitors to the very end. It often comes down to who has the most energy left, and not just talent.

By training the aerobic system, tennis players can assure themselves of more than adequate reserves at the end of their matches, and nearly unlimited energy overall, reductions in injuries, and the many other benefits the aerobic system provides.

Using a heart-rate monitor will not only help develop the aerobic system but will provide important feedback regarding aerobic progress. For example, a player starting out may play a one-hour match with an average heart rate of 150, with heart rate peaks hitting 185. After developing a good aerobic system, this same player may now be able to compete in the same match with an average heart rate of 130 and the heart rate never going over 155. This is a dramatic difference, and shows the power of good aerobic function. And, this player will get closer to his or her potential without the undue stress incurred with an average heart rate of 150 with peaks hitting 185. Conserved glycogen, maintained muscle balance (to prevent fatigue and optimize the swing), improved neurological function (eye-hand coordination), improved hydration, and many other benefits follow.

If a tennis player regularly uses a stationary bike or runs to help train the aerobic system, that player will improve in these activities as well (i.e., biking or running faster at the same heart rate).

During the aerobic training period (before the competitive season), a heart-rate monitor should be worn during play and the maximum aerobic heart rate not exceeded. As time goes on, the player will be able to perform much harder without the heart rate going up as much. This reflects increased energy, which allows the rest of the body—especially the brain and muscles—to function at much higher levels.

Of course, the time to start aerobic training for all athletes is long before competition begins—soon after the conclusion of the previous season is ideal. Measuring progress during this period with a heart-rate monitor is important not only for the athlete, but for the coach, trainer, health-care professional, and others involved in the overall conditioning process. Once more sport-specific training begins, the heart-rate monitor can still be used to assure proper warm-up

## MORNING HEART RATE

With proper exercise comes improved aerobic function and increased efficiency in the heart and lungs. This is reflected over time as a decrease in resting heart rate. A simple way to monitor these changes is to check your pulse in the morning. Strapping on your heart-rate monitor will assure you get an accurate reading. Checking your morning heart rate before getting out of bed provides a true resting rate and good baseline, but checking it shortly after getting up after sitting quietly for five minutes can serve the same purpose. Whichever routine you choose, use the same one each time.

The normal heart rate in the morning will vary. It should, however, be within the same range by about three to five beats on consecutive days. A change from one day to another of more than about five or six beats per minute may be an indication that some type of stress is affecting you. It may be an oncoming cold or flu, thoughts about an important business meeting later in the day, or other issues. Perhaps your

and cool-down, interval-type workouts, and overall recovery.

### Basketball

During the off-season, an athlete can develop a great aerobic base through running, biking, swimming, or any endurance workout. During this period, getting on the court can include wearing a heart-rate monitor to perform whatever off-season activity is required, as long as the athlete does not exceed the maximum aerobic heart rate. As the weeks go by, more and more intensity can be gained on the basketball court at the same heart rate, so that as the preseason approaches, a high-level practice game may not bring the heart rate nearly as high as during the start of aerobic training. Here are some examples.

Following a good warm-up, if a twenty-eight-year-old basketball player practices various activities, including dribbling up and down the court, running and shooting, and playing against team members, a heart-rate monitor can guide progress. In this example, a sixty-minute session may bring the heart rate to this player's maximum aerobic level of 152, forcing the player to slow down to prevent exceeding that level. But after a few weeks of developing the aerobic system, the same sixty-minute workout might show an average heart rate of only 131 with peaks not exceeding 152. This player will now have much more energy, better eye-hand coordination, and overall better function, especially in the latter part of game, as a result of these improvements.

diet hasn't been as good in the past couple of days, or you've been allowing your heart rate to get too high on your aerobic workouts. It's a yellow flag and it should make you think about the cause of the elevated heart rate.

There is no "normal" pulse. In a well-trained athlete, the pulse rate may be as low as the mid-30s, but many healthy athletes are in the 50s and 60s. What's more important is how it changes over time. As you progress through your healthy training routine, the pulse will gradually get lower. It may take a few months, but if you check it two or three times a week, you'll see the change over time. The pulse may be stable at an average of 62 for two months. Then it may suddenly drop off to an average of 56 for three weeks. It may stay there for a couple of months and then drop again. Check the pulse often, and keep a record of it.

It's important to note that lower is not necessarily better. In some individuals, as previously discussed, a diminishing heart rate may indicate chronic overtraining.

### Motor Sports

Among the more interesting sports where I've introduced athletes to the use of heart-rate monitors is racecar driving. I've worked with Mario and Michael Andretti, Derek Bell, Al Holbert, and others. Like with many traditional sports, including baseball and football, bringing new ideas into motor sports was not easy. My entry was helped originally after working with a young, unknown driver named Chip Robinson. I trained him like an endurance athlete so his brain and body functioned better behind the wheel going at triple-digit speeds in heavy traffic. He wore a heart-rate monitor during all his preseason endurance training, which included mostly running and walking. He even entered some running races for fun. But behind the wheel during practice sessions,

the stress of driving was evident. So I had him wear a heart-rate monitor during these driving sessions (and even during races). I discovered that his heart rate, which I later confirmed in other drivers, nearly paralleled his driving speed. Chip's, however, was more over-reactive than the other drivers', demonstrating his need to build a bigger aerobic base.

A racecar driver may be running the car at relatively slow warm-up speeds of 90–100 miles per hour, for example, and the heart rate will often be at that level too. Driving poses a certain amount of inherent risk, and a high level of alertness is necessary to perform well and avoid crashes. This all translates into stress, which raises the heart rate—the faster the speed the higher the heart rate. I've seen 180 mph equate to heart-rate peaks of 180.

This was a very interesting finding but not too surprising for me. I had already experimented with wearing my heart-rate monitor while driving on local roads and highways. I found that the faster I drove, the higher my heart rate rose.

For a racecar driver, this information is very important, especially for those who overreact while driving fast, which was one of Chip's problems. If a better aerobic system is developed, the heart rate will not overreact, although it will still rise to "normal" race levels. An appropriate heart rate, considering the stress of driving at very high speeds, improves a driver's ability and makes him or her a better competitor. It also improves overall health, and works especially to improve eye-hand coordination and optimal adrenal function.

After a great aerobic base period, Chip Robinson suddenly won several races with his new team, Jaguar, and his newly developed aerobic system. With this success, the next year he was chosen to be a driver for Al Holbert's Porsche racing team. Al was so interested in Chip's training that he became a patient of mine too. Aerobic base training paid off for the first race of the season, the 24 Hours of Daytona endurance race. The team won, driving almost 2,700 miles in twenty-four hours with a record-setting average of 111 mph. Chip would go on to win many other events, including three championships, before retiring from the sport.

## Aerobic versus Anaerobic Training

Now that the aerobic training state has been defined by heart rate, let's update the definitions of both aerobic and anaerobic presented earlier:

- Aerobic training includes endurance activities performed at or below the maximum aerobic heart rate. The closer an athlete is to this max aerobic rate, the more aerobic stimulation he or she will get from the workout. This includes development of the aerobic system, from increased fat burning and improved circulation to increased aerobic muscle fiber function. Aerobic benefits can still be obtained at lower heart rates. In fact, it's very important to stimulate aerobic muscle fibers that move the body more slowly, corresponding to lower heart rates.

- Anaerobic training includes endurance activities performed above the max aerobic heart rate, whether swimming, biking, running, cross-country skiing, or other forms of exercise.

The only exception to this description of aerobic training and heart rate is when a power workout is performed; this includes lifting free weights, using weight machines, performing push-ups, pull-ups, and sit-ups, and similar activities. These are always considered anaerobic, no matter how slow, easy, or light the workload. One reason, as studies show, is that even easy weight workouts can significantly raise the level of the stress hormone cortisol, and can potentially interfere with aerobic function.

A heart-rate monitor won't provide adequate information regarding the aerobic or anaerobic state during a power workout, such as weight lifting, because of the time factor. In fact, this anaerobic activity often won't raise the heart rate above the max aerobic heart rate. That's because you're not physically active long enough for the heart rate to reach its plateau. For example, as you begin performing a weight workout of, say, fifteen repetitions the heart rate starts to rise. It continues to rise as you reach your limit of fifteen reps and stop. The heart rate will usually remain far below where it would be if you continued lifting the weight—hypothetically, you might not hit the max rate until you got to thirty or forty reps, something you most likely would not be able to accomplish.

In the process of building an aerobic base, it's usually obvious when aerobic function is improving. You'll know this is happening because of several things. First, you'll generally feel healthier. This may be evident because your energy improves, injuries may disappear, and, if your body fat is higher than it should be, you'll get thinner. However, those with a normal, healthy level of body fat won't lose any more because that would be unhealthy—building an aerobic base is not just about getting faster, but healthier. Second, you'll get faster at the same heart rate. For most athletes, this is sufficient proof. But I still prefer to measure, as objectively as possible, this aerobic progress. This can be easily accomplished with the MAF Test, the topic of the next chapter.

# THE MAXIMUM AEROBIC FUNCTION (MAF) TEST—

## Getting the Most from Your Body in Training and Racing

Judging your performance solely by the watch on your wrist is woefully misleading. Those ticking seconds or digital readouts won't tell you how really fit you are. They might indicate how fast you are going on that particular day, but in the long-term, you are much better served by using a heart-rate monitor.

Here's why:

One of the many benefits of using a heart-rate monitor to develop maximum aerobic function is that you will generate more physical function with the same effort. For example, a runner will run faster at the same heart rate as the weeks and months pass. In addition, this same runner, if cross-training by cycling, will also be able to ride faster as well, since improvements to the aerobic system are as much metabolic as physical. In addition to monitoring your workouts to assure you stay aerobic, another advantage of using a heart-rate monitor is the ability to objectively measure these improvements using the Maximum Aerobic Function Test, or MAF Test. I developed this evaluation in the early 1980s so athletes could more precisely monitor their progress, and, even more importantly, be alerted if their training was faltering or leading to an injury or overtraining.

The MAF Test can be performed with any endurance activity. Your goal is to measure how fast you can run, bike, swim, inline skate, and so on, over a given distance at your aerobic maximum heart rate. Alternatively, you can measure how far you can go in a given time frame at the same heart rate. You need not perform the MAF Test in your particular sport. A basketball or tennis player will observe that he or she can excel during play without the heart rate rising as much, but this is difficult to measure. Using other training methods, such as a stationary bike or treadmill, makes for a better MAF Test.

During the MAF Test, use your maximum aerobic heart rate as determined by the 180 Formula. Using this heart rate, determine some parameter such as pace (minutes per mile), speed (miles per hour), or repetitions (laps in a pool) over time. The test can also be done on stationary equipment measuring watts, for example, if the equipment is accurate.

To perform a MAF Test during running, for example, the use of a quarter- mile or a 400-meter running track is ideal. A three- to five-mile distance provides more information. All MAF Tests should be done following a warm-up (discussed later). The following is an actual MAF Test performed by a runner on a track, calculating time in minutes per mile:

## MAF Test of a Runner Performed on an Outdoor 440-yard Track

| Mile 1 | 8:21 |
|--------|------|
| Mile 2 | 8:27 |
| Mile 3 | 8:38 |
| Mile 4 | 8:44 |
| Mile 5 | 8:49 |

As indicated by the above chart, it's normal to obtain slightly slower times with each ensuing mile (which demonstrates a normal fatigue factor). The slower your first mile, the more the time will slow between the first and fifth mile. This is due to reduced aerobic function, which is associated with lower endurance. If your first mile is a 10:17 pace, for example, your fifth mile could be 11:20. On the other hand, if your first mile is faster, the difference between miles one and five is less—if your first mile is 5:50, your fifth mile may be 6:14.

During any one MAF Test, it's normal for your times to get slower; the first mile should always be the fastest, and the last the slowest. If that's not the case, it usually means your warm-up was inadequate. An example of this is if your first mile is 7:46 and your second is 7:39. In addition, as the weeks pass, the MAF Test should show faster times compared to previous tests. The chart below shows typical endurance progress in the same runner from chart above:

The chart below shows typical endurance progress in the same runner from the previous chart:

|        | April | May  | June | July |
|--------|-------|------|------|------|
| Mile 1 | 8:21  | 8:11 | 7:57 | 7:44 |
| Mile 2 | 8:27  | 8:18 | 8:05 | 7:52 |
| Mile 3 | 8:38  | 8:26 | 8:10 | 7:59 |
| Mile 4 | 8:44  | 8:33 | 8:17 | 8:09 |
| Mile 5 | 8:49  | 8:39 | 8:24 | 8:15 |

I refer to these improvements as *aerobic speed*—the development of a faster running pace, cycling speed, or other endurance improvements that occur during the aerobic base training. During periods of anaerobic training, including the competitive season, improvements in speed at the same heart rate usually slow or stop. This means that aerobic development is slowing or stopping, which may be normal and temporary.

Most importantly, and one of the key factors regarding the MAF Test, is that if you don't make progress during this base-building period or, if after some improvements, your MAF Test begins to worsen, it usually indicates there is a problem with your training, diet, stress management, or another factor impairing your aerobic system. This should serve as a significant warning. It may be associated with the onset of a cold or other illness, a dietary problem such as eating poorly during the holiday season, a nutritional problem such as anemia, excess stress from your job, or the early stage of overtraining. Often, an athlete determines an incorrect maximum aerobic training heart rate from the 180 Formula, making the heart rate too high. Even slight elevations—such as three beats—may eventu-

ally cause the aerobic system to not progress. This is a critical aspect of endurance training as the MAF Test is telling you something is wrong. Evaluating your physical, chemical, and mental stresses—from other physical work to diet and mental stress—is essential to not only get your fitness back on track to build endurance, but to prevent your health from faltering.

### The MAF Test in Other Sports

The MAF Test is the most important self-administered assessment tool for endurance athletes. It's something to evaluate about once a month throughout the year. I described how runners can use the MAF Test above. Performing the test on a bike is similar in concept to running, except cyclists have a couple of effective ways to record results. The best and easiest method is to pick a flat bike course that takes about thirty to forty-five minutes to complete. Following a warm-up, ride at your maximum aerobic heart rate, and record exactly how long it takes to ride the test course. As you progress with more speed, your times should get lower. Riding your course today, for example, may take 36:50. A month later it may take you 35:30 and after another month, 34:15. After three months of base work, the same course may only take you thirty-three minutes.

Another option is to ride on a flat course and see how fast a pace you can maintain while holding your heart rate at your maximum aerobic level. This works best in a velodrome

**QA** **Question:** Does a decrease in resting heart rate—it's dropped ten beats to 59 over the five months since I began following the MAF program—mean that I can raise my maximum target heart rate five or even ten beats? I am fifty-one years old and run about four hours every week.

**Answer:** Reduction in resting heart rate is an expected change that accompanies building a good aerobic base. But it does not mean you can raise your max aerobic heart rate (remember, neither resting nor maximum heart rate is factored into the 180 Formula). As your resting rate lowers, along with other aerobic benefits, you'll also see an increased effort such as running pace or faster bike times, which will provide you with a harder effort but at the same heart rate.

or indoors on a training apparatus. As you progress, your speed should increase. If you start at 18 mph, for example, following a three-month period of building aerobic base, you could be riding 24 mph at the same heart rate.

For swimmers, the same idea for the MAF Test is applied. In this case, you can use a pool or open water to evaluate aerobic progress. Because swimming is such a low-gravity-stress activity, you will find that aerobic speed builds quickly and will require more physical ability to keep up with the pace. In other words, you will have to swim much faster to keep your heart rate at the max aerobic rate—in many swimmers with good technique and endurance it may not be possible to maintain the max aerobic heart rate for a forty-minute workout, for example. While this is a sign of good endurance progress, it makes performing the MAF Test dif-

ficult. Until this happens, it's best to maintain faster swimming only if you can maintain good technique.

When you're not able to swim fast enough, or maintain good technique in the water, you have two options regarding MAF Test evaluation:

- First, you can perform your test at a lower heart rate. If your max aerobic heart rate is 150 but you physically can't swim fast enough to reach that rate without your technique suffering, use a heart rate that's more comfortable, 130 for example, if that allows you to swim with good technique.
- A second consideration is to use another activity to monitor aerobic progress. If you also ride a bike or run, use one (or both) of these sports to perform your MAF Test. Progression on a bike, which improves conversion of fat to energy and other

aerobic system aspects, will also allow you to swim at a faster pace.

# Performance: Measuring Progress, Plateau, and Regression

Perform the MAF Test regularly, throughout the year, and chart your results. I recommend doing the test about every three to four weeks. More often than that may result in mental stress; aerobic speed will usually not improve significantly within one week's time. Focusing on the test this often can foster an obsession much like that seen in athletes who are addicted to weighing themselves on the scale daily or even more often. Performing the test irregularly or not often enough defeats one of its purposes—knowing when your training is going off course. If something interferes with your progress—training, diet, or stress—you don't want to wait until you're feeling bad or racing poorly to find that out. Loss of fitness and health will be apparent from your MAF Test sooner than any other method, long before you get symptoms or see poor performances.

As you plot out your MAF Test during endurance training you could encounter three different phases: progression, plateau, and regression. These are quite evident in many athletes, and less so in others.

## Progression

If you successfully develop your aerobic system, you will generate more aerobic speed.

This is the progressive phase of the program; you can perform more work as an endurance athlete in a given time frame. These improvements should continue both short term—for weeks and months—and long term for many years, without regression.

## Plateau

Aerobic training may also have phases of normal plateaus. Initially, your progress will be measured by larger improvements—less minutes per mile, more miles per hour, or whatever parameters you choose to use. As time goes on and development continues, progress occurs at a slower rate, but now you are performing at a much better pace. The graph on the next page represents the general progress of an actual age-group cyclist over a four-year period.

There are actually two different kinds of plateaus, one normal and the other abnormal. A normal plateau will be encountered at some point during progress—almost as if your body needs a rest from the progress it's making. The reason for this is unclear, although it seems like the brain, muscular, and metabolic aspects of the body require a period of adjustment. This may be associated with the need for recovery, much like ascending a long hill during a marathon. These normal plateaus should not last too long—a few weeks to a few months at most. Even slight improvements, as seen in the chart above, should be taken as progress. At the end of that time, progress should again

**Example of Normal Aerobic Progress of Cyclist**

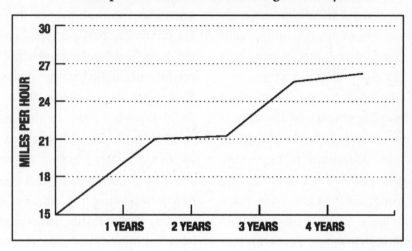

resume as measured by the MAF Test. If you stay on a plateau for too long, it may be abnormal and may mark the beginning of a regression.

An abnormal plateau is due to some physical, chemical, or mental obstacle that prevents progress of the aerobic system. The MAF Test is very useful to help assess an abnormal plateau. Once you find your times have stayed the same for too long, the next step is to find out why. Specifically, some important questions to ask yourself include:

- What is interfering with my progress?
- What changes have occurred in my physical life: new shoes, new bike set up, new training course?
- What changes have occurred in my body chemistry: dietary change, new dietary supplements, over-the-counter or prescription drugs?

- What mental or emotional factors may be causing more stress?
- What adjustments can I make?

There could be many factors, and quite often they are combinations of seemingly minor problems. For example, the combination of a new bike set up that's not quite right for you in conjunction with increased travel for work with the accompanying poor diet can adversely affect aerobic function. In some cases, making an adjustment in your training schedule is the only way to adapt to stresses you can't easily control. An athlete who is also an accountant typically has an exceptionally busy schedule at certain times of the year, often working 50 percent more with longer workdays. In this case, attempting to maintain a normal training schedule can create significant stress; the remedy is to reduce training to avoid excessive stress.

The weather may also be a stress that can halt endurance progression, during extremes of temperature and humidity. The hot, humid months of summer, or very dry extreme heat of the desert, can easily affect performance.

After a marathoner named Karen came and saw me, her progress was rapid—almost from the moment she began building an aerobic base. Her dedication to improving diet and managing stress was quickly paying off. Her first mile MAF Test on the track went from 9:07 pace in September to 7:52 the following June. However, following that improvement, there was a long three-month plateau, but she continued to feel great. Finally, improvement in aerobic speed continued. The next year the same pattern was evident: Her great progress halted abruptly and was followed by three months of no improvements. At first I thought Karen's plateaus were normal. Eventually, I considered the possibility that perhaps her tolerance to the New York summer weather—hazy, hot, and humid conditions—was too stressful, and this was the cause of the plateau. Since Karen could not go to the mountains for cooler weather in the summer to avoid the weather stress, we cut her training schedule down by about 30 percent. Using that strategy beginning in the late spring, Karen continued progressing through the next summer. She also felt even better than normal, and continued racing better than the previous year.

If you think your plateau is abnormal, assess yourself carefully, or get help from a holistic professional who understands the needs of endurance athletes. Find out what may be blocking your natural progress.

**QA**

**Question:** I have just started endurance training using the 180 heart-rate Formula. I am a thirty-six-year-old male and have been consistently running for about five years. I was somewhat saddened to find out that I can only maintain a 12–12:30 pace at an average 140 beats per minute, and find that my pace per mile has to slow down even more when running beyond 14–15 miles in order to maintain the 140 rate. I am currently logging approximately 40–50 miles per week. My goal is to maintain this training for a minimum of eight to ten more weeks. Should I expect to realize a minimum level of improvement over the course of this training period?

**Answer:** Your pace of 12–12:30 indicates that the level of your aerobic function is poor. Everyone, in all sports, slows down during the course of a training workout. You should expect an obvious improvement in speed over your ten weeks of base building, and if not, something is wrong with your health and/or fitness. It could be a problem with your diet, nutrition, stress, or another issue.

If you are a triathlete, you may plateau for one event but not the others. In this case, if you are measuring progress in swimming, biking, and running, you may see your swim and run times improving while your bike improvement has reached a plateau. After a month or two, this may change with swimming and cycling showing progress while your running maintains an even level. The reason for this is unclear, but I feel it is a normal part of progression in healthy athletes.

### Regression

An abnormal plateau resulting from some type of stress or other factors mentioned above will eventually cause your MAF Test to get worse each time you check it. If this happens, your body is in a "red alert" and you should be very cautious. This is the time when you become most vulnerable to injury and ill health. In this case, one recommended strategy is to cut your training, even by up to 50 percent. This will ensure more rest and recovery, and give your body a chance to recover from whatever stress is affecting it. At the same time, however, it's important to reevaluate all your training, diet and nutrition, and other lifestyle factors. If you are performing anaerobic training, this would be the first change to make—stop all anaerobic workouts, including racing. The most common cause of reduced aerobic function is anaerobic training, and/or too much racing.

During the early stages of regression, you may not necessarily feel bad or notice an injury or other health problem. Those obvious signs and symptoms occur in the later stages of deteriorating endurance. There may not be any early symptoms. Blood, urine, and other standard tests may also appear normal. The two most common signs that may (but don't always) appear with a worsening MAF Test are an elevated resting (morning) heart rate and slight elevations in the stress hormone cortisol. But in most cases, the only sign that something is wrong may come from your MAF Test.

If you do not respect the advice of your body, which during a worsening MAF Test indicates you are regressing, you may ultimately be seeking symptomatic relief from complaints such as fatigue or exhaustion, physical injury, sickness, or some other breakdown, possibly including one on a mental level such as depression. Regressing endurance parallels poor health.

The most important aspect of performing your MAF Test regularly is to record the results. Make a graph, chart, or just write your results in a diary. One of the first things I did when athletes visited my clinic was to look at all the MAF Test results they'd recorded since the previous visit. In many athletes, this was one of my most important assessments.

## Factors That Affect the MAF Test

The MAF Test can be applied to any endurance activity. However, there are a number of factors that may affect your test results. When running, for example, the type of track surface may have a slight influence on your pace. The modern high-tech track surfaces result in the fastest pace, whereas

## THE MYTH OF THE PEAK

Periods of significant changes in fitness in endurance athletes—the highs and lows that frequently occur during the training year, are so common that some athletes and coaches think they're normal—but they're not! This notion has falsely given birth to the myth of "the peak," a belief that asserts you build up your endurance, progress to a high level where performance is optimal, and then you fall off. When you decline from this peak, you perform poorly.

The concept of "peaking," as it's been used through the years, isn't healthy for endurance athletes. As I've seen it in practical application, it usually involves a gradual overtraining. In this first stage of overtraining, performance can actually improve just before more common signs or symptoms of overtraining begin. However, this increased performance window is short, and athletes quickly enter the second, more serious stage of overtraining where injury, ill health, and performance loss occurs.

The problem with the concept of the "peak" is twofold. First, pushing yourself to hit a peak in performance is obviously unhealthy if it's part of the overtraining

the old cinder tracks will slow your pace at the same heart rate. Most athletes who run with heart-rate monitors are aware of this, especially when running on very soft surfaces such as sand. One study showed that just walking on sand required 1.8 times the energy of walking on a hard surface at the same speed. This is reflected in a higher heart rate and, if you're maintaining a specific max aerobic rate, it slows your pace.

Uneven tracks also result in slower MAF Test times compared to perfectly flat surfaces. The ideal situation is to have an indoor track. But beware, shorter tracks, such as 200 meters, will generally cause a slightly slower pace due to the increased turning compared to longer ones (400 meters).

On your bike, a velodrome is ideal but not accessible to most athletes. The roughness or smoothness of the road surface, its varying grades, and traffic will all affect your test results. The net result of hills usually is a worsening of pace, unless there are significantly more downhills. A good option is to use a wind trainer or rollers indoors.

Usually, these factors, and the others described below, can make a difference of five to eight seconds per mile on a track, or two to three miles per hour on your bike, possibly more. While this may not seem significant, it's best to be consistent. Use the same course or method each time you perform the test. In the event that you change your test course, be sure to note it in your diary or chart.

syndrome—and it typically is. Overtraining in any form is not an approach I recommend or that any health-care professional should endorse because it's harmful. Second, with proper training an athlete can attain just as high a level of optimal performance, and for a much longer period. A well-trained healthy athlete will always perform better for a longer period than any other approach.

Rather than a performance peak, I promote one of continued improvement throughout the competitive season, with each event producing better results than the previous one. An athlete will typically perform best as the season progresses, with the best performances at the end. I then recommend taking time off after the racing season. During this period, where training is reduced, sometimes significantly, fitness will also reduce, but not in an unhealthy way; this is different than having your fitness reduce due to overtraining. I would not call this a peak, just part of a training strategy that makes fitness and health a priority. Mike Pigg would take three weeks off after his last triathlon of the season, and during this period he would train very little. As a result, his MAF Test declined slightly. But with the onset of aerobic base training, his fitness would quickly increase, as indicated by a faster MAF Test.

Other factors that can potentially interfere with your MAF Test include the weather, altitude, hydration, and your equipment, including shoes and bike. Most of these factors can work against you by increasing your physical effort, which increases the heart rate. Since you are working at a specific heart rate, the result is a slower pace. Again, the minimal amount of influence should not pose a real problem. Rather, you should just be aware of these factors.

Many of these factors are controllable, including hydration, shoes, and overall health. For example, the weather affects some people more than others—the difference is the body's thermoregulation, which is under control of the brain and metabolism, and, more specifi-cally, water and electrolyte regulation under adrenal gland control.

## Climate: How It Affects Your Physiology

The weather can influence your body in various ways that will often leave you feeling perplexed. You might be wondering why your times are slower, you feel sluggish, or have an elevated heart rate. So let's look at some of the key meteorological factors:

- A sufficient enough headwind will physi-cally counter your forward motion, raising your heart rate. A good tailwind will have the opposite effect—you'll go faster at the same heart rate.

- Temperature may also be a factor during your test. High heat and low cold will raise your heart rate, forcing you to slow down.
- High humidity can act much like a headwind. It is a physical barrier of water that you must work through. The increased effort raises your heart rate and results in a slower test.
- Rain and snow are similar to humidity and headwinds. Going through rain (and to a lesser extent snow) requires more effort. In addition, if the surface you are on is wet with water or, especially, covered with snow, additional physical effort is required (much of this is the brain being overcautious as you bike, for example, with increased tension in your muscles while riding in case of a fall).
- Barometric pressure can also have a slowing effect on your MAF Test. Low barometric pressure results in a slightly lower oxygen uptake. The result is less oxygen getting to your muscles and your body compensates by raising the heart rate.

Often, weather stress is not the result of a single factor. A combination of cold and wind, for example, can elevate the heart rate significantly. Summer heat, humidity, and low pressure, sometimes referred to as the "dog days of August," can also stress your body and raise the heart rate. The dew point is also an important factor. Relative humidity is a measure of how humid it is; the dew point temperature measures how much water vapor is in the air. High dew points that approach 75°F are most noticeable when training or competing outdoors—the air feels thick with moisture because the water vapor is very high. For these reasons, if you arrive at your MAF Test day and the weather is extreme, wait a day or more until the weather stress has lessened.

Altitude can have a significant effect on the body and MAF Test, especially if you have not had a chance to adapt to a new altitude. If you're headed for the mountains to train for a period of time, wait at least a week or more until you adjust to the altitude before performing your MAF Test. Even then, your times generally slow when you ascend to higher altitudes. When descending to lower altitudes after adapting to high altitudes, your MAF Test usually improves.

These weather factors not only affect your MAF Test, but all training, racing, and, in fact, virtually all human performance, including chemical function, such as hormone balance, and mental activity, such as scholastic test-taking. The end result of much of this weather stress is human error; there are more accidents associated with certain weather changes, for example, including low barometric weather systems affecting the body.

## Other Factors Affecting Performance

Hydration also affects your aerobic pace. Even slight dehydration can slow you down. Once you dehydrate, it may take twenty-four hours or longer to rehydrate, no matter how much water you consume. It's important to drink smaller amounts of water all day rather than large amounts a couple of times a day.

Your equipment can also affect the outcome of your MAF Test. The two most significant items are your bike and running shoes. Your bike set-up and positioning, the pressure and wear on your tires, and any other factors that change drag, such as clothing, can slow your MAF Test results. Make a note in your diary if your test is done with a different bike set-up, more clothing, or other factors that may change the test.

Running shoes will also affect the results of your MAF Test. In general, shoes with more cushioning and support and heavier shoes slow you down. Lighter shoes, including racing styles, generally allow you to run faster at the same heart rate.

While most of the above factors will raise your heart rate and slow your pace or speed, performing the MAF Test for longer rather than shorter times will help compensate for these natural variables. For running, this means five miles, for a bike test, a total of about thirty to forty-five minutes or more.

One other factor that will affect your MAF Test is worth mentioning here: ill health. When you are sick, or starting to get sick, your body's immune system is working very hard to recover, and it needs all the energy it can get. The last thing your body wants to do is work out, especially when you have an elevated temperature. In this situation, don't

train or compete. If you've ever attempted this, and worn a heart-rate monitor, you know what happens: your heart rate elevates, sometimes drastically. The same happens if you are anemic: less oxygen is delivered to the muscles, with the resulting MAF Test results being slower.

Since these and other factors can affect the results of your MAF Test, they can also influence your performance during competition. The best defense is, of course, being as fit and healthy as possible so all compensatory mechanisms in the body are functioning optimally.

## MAF Test and Measuring Performance

I began working with Linda just after her successful fall racing season. Her first MAF Test in early December was about an 8:25 pace for the first mile. I explained that this aerobic pace was related to her average pace for a flat 5K race, which a week previous averaged around 6:50 per mile (and a finishing time of 21:10). As Linda's MAF Test began improving through the winter months, she was feeling better overall with more energy, better sleep, and fewer allergy symptoms. Her MAF Test improved to 7:45 for the first mile just prior to her spring racing season. Her first race in early April, after only training aerobically through the winter, was a 5K, and she ran a personal best of 18:57. The important point is that as Linda's aerobic function improved, as demonstrated by her MAF Test, so did her race pace.

The MAF Test is directly related to your competitive performance, including race results. As your aerobic system and MAF Test results improve, so will your competitive ability.

Beginning in the early 1980s, I collected a lot of MAF data on runners. After hundreds of tests and several racing seasons, it was evident that the pace a runner could perform at his or her max aerobic heart rate—the MAF Test—was positively correlated with race pace. I collected more data for 5K and 10K distances and charted this information (see right). Through the years it also became obvious that performance in all endurance events—triathlons, marathons, cycling events, swimming—could be improved by developing a faster aerobic pace. Even athletes involved in basketball, soccer, tennis, and other events that required significant amounts of aerobic efforts could improve.

| MAF Test vs. Running Race Pace | | |
|---|---|---|
| MAF Pace | 5K Race Pace | 5K Time |
| 10:00 | 7:30 | 23:18 |
| 9:00 | 7:00 | 21:45 |
| 8:30 | 6:45 | 20:58 |
| 8:00 | 6:30 | 20:12 |
| 7:30 | 6:00 | 18:38 |
| 7:00 | 5:30 | 17:05 |
| 6:30 | 5:15 | 16:19 |
| 6:00 | 5:00 | 15:32 |
| 5:45 | 4:45 | 14:45 |
| 5:30 | 4:30 | 13:59 |
| 5:15 | 4:20 | 13:28 |
| 5:00 | 4:15 | 13:12 |

**QA**

**Question:** I have been playing with heart-rate monitor training for a little while. I am intrigued with your ideas. One thing that I am concerned with is the 180 Formula that relies on age. I am forty-three years old, in good condition from years of martial arts training. My max heart rate while running is 193 (tested doing intervals on hills). The standard formulas for predicting max heart rate predict significantly lower than my actual max heart rate. According to your formula, 180–43=137. I am on a low dose of HCTZ for a slightly elevated blood pressure, so subtract 10. That makes the number 127. I have had a cold this year and a stomach bug (might have been food poisoning, not sure), so I guess I miss out on the +5. This seems pretty low.

**Answer:** Remember, max heart rate is not factored into the 180 Formula. Be conservative. The 180 Formula is incredibly accurate, albeit sometimes difficult because it slows you down, but only initially.

## MY PERSPECTIVE—BY MARIANNE DICKERSON

*In 2009,* Running Times *magazine wrote, "Marianne Dickerson is a good candidate for the title of the Marathon Medalist That History Forgot." The only American woman ever to win a World Championship marathon medal, she took the silver in 1983 in 2:31:09. It was only her third marathon. Now retired from road racing, Dickerson prefers competing in Ironman triathlons as a sub-twelve-hour enthusiast.*

✳ ✳ ✳

In 1974, as a fourteen-year-old freshman, I began running as a member of my high school track and cross-country teams. I quickly excelled as a middle-distance runner competing in the half-mile and mile events. The improvement I made during my four years of high school competition was dramatic, primarily driven by high-intensity interval training during the competitive season. I continued my track and cross-country career as a college scholarship athlete training year-round. During the course of my college career, I migrated toward longer distances, competing in races up to ten kilometers. As a result, both my weekly mileage and intensity continued to increase. My training paid off as I achieved collegiate all-American honors in both track and cross-country.

Following graduation in 1983, I decided to train for the marathon with ambitions of making the U.S. Olympic team in 1984. My training intensity and mileage continued to increase, with my typical training week consisting of over 100 miles with two days per week dedicated to intense interval training on the track. My improvement over a six-month period from January 1983 to August 1983 was nothing short of miraculous. I competed in the 1983 Avon Woman's Marathon Championship in May of 1983, placed third, and qualified for the USA Track & Field team to compete in the first ever World Championships of Track & Field. Ten weeks later, I competed in the World Championships in Helsinki, Finland, and placed second (quite an accomplishment for a twenty-two-year-old newcomer to the sport of marathoning!). I was literally "on top of the world" after signing a contract with one of the leading running shoe companies, thinking this was just the beginning of a promising career as a world-class distance athlete. After all, the 1984 Los Angeles Olympics were right around the corner.

Little did I know that my Cinderella story was about to end. A mere six weeks after the World Championships, I sustained an injury to my lower back. I was out for a long run and noticed sharp pain in my sacroiliac joint. I saw numerous orthopedic doctors over the course of the next twelve months to no avail. After months of getting cortisone injections into my sacroiliac joints, taking anti-inflammatory pills, and getting chiropractic adjustments, I was still unable to run without pain. I did however continue to maintain a high-fitness level through cycling and swimming.

I met Dr. Phil Maffetone in August of 1984 at an event we both appeared at, and the experience was life-changing. Dr. Maffetone told me my problem was due to adrenal stress caused by too much "anaerobic" training. At first I was skeptical, but Dr. Maffetone had me go to the nearest track and run a mile with a heart-rate monitor set to my aerobic threshold. I was shocked to see that I could not run a mile under eleven minutes aerobically: this was unbelievable given the fact that twelve months prior I had run over twenty-six miles consecutively at an average pace per mile of 5:48!

Naturally, I was a bit suspect of Dr. Maffetone's diagnosis, but at that point I was willing to try anything. Over the next eight weeks, I followed a structured dietary and training plan that he had laid out. The dietary plan basically consisted of incorporating good fats into my diet, eating lots of good protein such as eggs, and avoiding sugar and hydrogenated fats. My training plan consisted of "building an aerobic base" with all workouts (forty-five- to ninety-minute runs) conducted wearing a heart monitor with a focus on keeping my pace to a level where my heart rate would not exceed my aerobic threshold range. Each week, I noticed my pace became quicker as I was able to run faster within my aerobic limits. After eight weeks of base building, he had me enter a 10K race. I was shocked at how easy the race felt. And my finish time was a personal record of 33:02. *Miraculous*, I thought, given that a mere eight weeks ago, I could barely run a mile under eleven minutes aerobically and now I was running 6.2 miles at an average pace of 5:18 per mile!

I had a few more successful years of running but then decided to return to college and focus on my career. I retired from serious running in 1988, though I've continued to be a participant in endurance. Despite working a demanding full-time job as a business consultant that involves extensive travel and long hours, I've completed three Ironman triathlons in the last five years. I still follow Dr. Maffetone's training philosophies religiously in preparation for these events, conducting all my workouts under my aerobic threshold level and have finished all of these Ironmans under twelve hours—and feeling great!

Comparing the first mile of your MAF Test, for example, and running race times as noted above reflects normal aerobic and anaerobic functions. If these relationships are not balanced, it could indicate an imbalance between the aerobic and anaerobic states. Consider the runner whose mile one MAF Test is seven minutes per mile and who races a 10K with an average mile pace of 5:45 per mile; this may actually reflect an imbalance between an overactive anaerobic system and aerobic deficiency. In other words, this runner may be in the early stage of overtraining, where "over-performance" appears at the expense of an unhealthy aerobic system. While these situations may not seem so bad since the athlete is performing relatively well, they most often reflect a significant imbalance associated with early stages of overtraining. When this type of athlete retrains and builds a good aerobic base, he or she very quickly returns to this same level of competition—but with much lower heart rates—and quickly improves beyond it.

The MAF Test is a very important assessment tool for all athletes to monitor the progress of the aerobic base. It also helps indicate potential training and competitive imbalances such as the earliest stage of overtraining, aerobic deficiency, and other common problems that can lead to injury, ill health, and poor performances. Additionally, the MAF Test can provide a prediction of your race performances—the better your MAF Test, the better your racing will be.

# CHAPTER 5

# WARMING UP AND COOLING DOWN—
## The Two Key Critical Elements of Every Workout

**I** learned about warming up and cooling down in a most peculiar way, and without even realizing it. During my first summer off from college, I worked at a small, local moving company. The owner, a big muscular former marine, would bring his small crew of three or four to a house to pack up the truck and order us to begin with the smallest items.

I found this rather odd—here we were bringing out the smallest and lightest boxes and other items. Gradually he had us bring out larger and heavier items. Toward the end, we began bringing smaller and lighter objects out to the truck again, so by the very end we were hardly carrying much at all, just like in the beginning. I believe this was what he had learned worked best, though perhaps didn't know why

nor analyzed it. I thought it was quite odd until later in my studies when I learned more about circulation, muscles, and the process of warming and cooling the body.

While in practice, whenever I would go to the track with athletes, we would see others come and go to do their workouts. We would slowly jog to warm up to our training pace, watching others do the traditional stretches

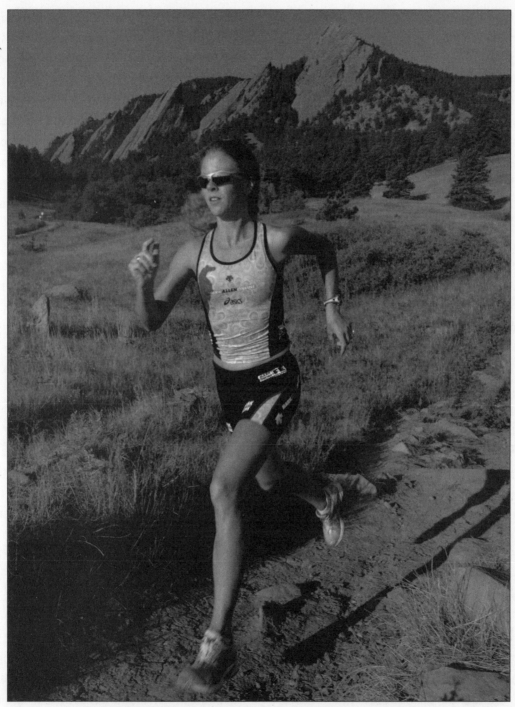

*Make sure you properly warm up before working out;*
*it will lessen the risk of injury.*

on the ground, bouncing around for a bit, then get up and start running fast. Others would be stretching in the parking lot, using their cars as if trying to push them, to help stretch their tight calves and other muscle groups. When most of these athletes were done, they would stop their fast pace and hop back into their car. We were just starting our cool-down. What's wrong with this picture? Plenty!

The aerobic system can provide you with two vital components for all training. By preparing your brain and body for a workout, and by initiating the important first stage of recovery afterward, you can improve the quality of your workout, get more benefits, and reduce the risk of injury.

When the topic of warming up is mentioned, most people think of stretching. While stretching may be important for those who participate in certain sports like track and field, gymnastics, and ballet, it does not produce a true warm-up and cool-down. Stretching is much less significant a need for endurance athletes, and it can even be harmful. A physically active warm-up and cool-down is ideal for endurance athletes—they don't require extremes in ranges of motion but significant improvements in flexibility.

## Warming Up

An active warm-up refers to easy physical movement that prepares the body for activity, and should be an integral part of every training session and competition. A proper warm-up can decrease the risk of injury and is an important "therapeutic" aspect of physical exercise; it can also reduce the muscle soreness associated with the early stages of a new part of your training program. The lack of a warm-up can cause bodily stress and result in abnormal heart function (as indicated by an electrocardiogram), reduced oxygen to the heart muscle (myocardial ischemia), and poor blood pressure response following exercise, even in healthy, fit individuals.

Warming up prepares the body for training or competition. The "warming" occurs partly from an increase in blood circulation. Normally, as you begin a workout, the muscles quickly require much more oxygen and other nutrients, and quickly develop byproducts that must be removed. This need by the muscles is accomplished by an increase in blood flow. The aerobic muscles are well endowed with blood vessels, and most of the circulation is directed there.

If the muscles are receiving more blood, where does it come from? The answer to this question is a very important aspect of warming up. At rest, your body devotes much of its circulation to the brain and nervous system, organs and glands, intestines, and other systems. From a standpoint of blood circulation, this resting state is just the opposite of working out.

When you begin your workout, the muscles require greater blood circulation. More than half of the blood flow going to the rest of the body gets detoured into the working muscles. During an anaerobic workout, for example, up to 80 percent of the blood is shifted to the muscles. While this satisfies the muscles' demands, the organs and glands suddenly have much less circulation for their optimal function. In many ways, it is a major stress to the organs and glands when the shift occurs too quickly.

The way to satisfy the whole body has to do with timing. If the systems slowly relinquish their circulation at the same time the blood flow to the muscles is gradually increased, there is no stress. It allows brain, organs, glands, intestines, and other areas to adapt to reduced circulation while providing the muscles with proper nutrients. This can take at least twelve to fifteen minutes and is accomplished by much slower activity than the workout ahead. This period is called a warm-up.

After the first stage of the warm-up, which is a slight elevation of body temperature, a number of significant benefits occur, including:

- Increased blood flow to working muscles
- Increased oxygen availability
- Greater mechanical efficiency of joints, muscles, tendons, and ligaments
- Increased range of motion in joints
- Release of stored fat to be used for energy in aerobic muscles
- Increased breathing (lung) capacity
- Improved neuromuscular activity

In order to accomplish this, the muscle activity—the level of workout intensity—should begin very easy and gradually build up. Often, athletes start off a workout with too much intensity, which shifts the blood flow away from the nervous and metabolic systems too quickly, potentially causing stress.

A heart-rate monitor is a very helpful tool for warming up because it allows you to properly gauge the warm-up process. Let's use the example of an athlete starting an hour aerobic workout with a maximum aerobic heart rate of 140 (with a range of 130–140). Initially, the starting heart rate is 60. For this athlete, a proper warm-up means going from a heart rate of 60 to 140 over a period of fifteen minutes, the heart rate is slowly raised from the 60s to the 70s, 80s, and so forth until the 130–140 range is reached after fifteen minutes. For training lasting more than about ninety minutes, the warm-up should be extended—perhaps to about twenty minutes or more. And for a three-hour or longer workout, more warm-up time is usually needed.

Ideally, your warm-up should be tailored to your body's needs. Once you get used to warming up properly, you may notice your body requiring more warm-up time, even for a short workout. If this is the case, heed your body's signal and extend your warm-up time. Never assume, however, that you need less than a twelve- to fifteen-minute warm-up. This seems to be the physiological minimum.

## Cooling Down

An active cool-down refers to easy physical activity at the end of your workout—just

**QA** **Question:** I understand the advantages of warming up by walking to elevate the heart rate steadily. I've seen that starting to run too soon without my body being properly warmed causes a spike in my heart rate of maybe thirty to forty beats. Typically, when this occurs I resume walking and start running when a little warmer. Anyway, a few weeks ago, when the outside air temperature was about 65°F, twelve minutes was sufficient warm-up time before breaking into a jog. A week later the temperature dropped to 50°F, and this time I had to walk twenty minutes before I could start running without my heart rate spiking. This weekend the temperature dropped again to 40°F. This time, it took thirty minutes to warm up before I could start running. The difficulty is that when air temperatures are low, it's hard to warm up when suitably clothed for running. As you know, running attire is typically lightweight and designed for easy movements. If I were to keep warm by wearing additional clothing, this would make running very uncomfortable. Interestingly, I'm finding it's much easier to control my heart rate in the second hour of a run when my body is very warm. Do you have any tips for dealing with this issue? Is there a way to warm the body quickly? I've toyed with the idea of riding an exercise bike indoors before setting off on a run but the problem here is that the warm-up and run would be separated by fifteen minutes in a car.

in the opposite order of the warm-up. This is in contrast to passive recovery, which means you suddenly stop your workout and sit or lie down to rest, like my friend George who, when asked how he cooled down, said he would sit down on his front lawn with a beer.

Worse is the idea that you should sprint the last several hundred yards of your run. This is a recipe for disaster because, even though your muscles are warmed up, you now put them back in high gear with more stress, requiring even more of a cool-down.

The most important reason for a cool-down is that it begins a key process of recovery

from the workout. The cool-down slowly allows the heart rate to descend. While you will not reach your starting or resting heart rate, you may come within ten or twenty beats of it. Let's use the same example of the athlete above who began the workout with a heart rate of 60 beats per minute and ascended to 140. Fifteen minutes before the end of the workout, the heart rate is gradually reduced by slowing down, until it approaches 60 beats per minute (although a proper cool-down may bring you back to 70–80).

This slow descent in intensity, monitored by the heart rate, prevents physical and

**Answer:** Your idea of riding an indoor bike is perfect, and one I often recommend. Once you warm up indoors, the warm-up effect will last much more than the fifteen minutes it takes you to start running. Any indoor warm-up would work, such as a small trampoline, stationary bike, or other way to perform an active, aerobic warm-up. Also, warming up indoors on a cold day will keep you from needing too many layers of clothing during your workout. This is normally okay as you want to avoid getting too cold or chilled, but as you warm up further, it's important to remove the excess clothing to avoid overheating—a potential stress. Overheating can impair the physiological function of certain fat stores, reducing fat burning. In addition, overheating during longer workouts can increase the risk of dehydration and raise your body temperature too much. So if you wear layers, remove each one as you get warmer.

For most situations, cooling down even in cold weather is more practical. In some situations where it's difficult to perform a good, active cool-down, you can do the same as your warm-up, just in reverse. But in this case, consider a shorter cool-down outside, then get home to complete your cool-down indoors.

chemical stress, especially within the cardio-vascular system and the muscles. It helps oxygenation and circulation in the muscles and helps remove blood lactate (even during an aerobic workout). These are all vital parts of the process of recovery.

For most workouts, spend about fifteen minutes cooling down, and, for longer workouts, such as those of two, three, or more hours, increase this time to at least twenty to thirty minutes.

The warm-up and cool-down are really whole-body workouts. As such, you need not be restricted: you can warm up using a different activity from your main workout. For example, you can ride a stationary bike for fifteen minutes to warm up, then go for your one-hour run. You can even cool down by doing something different, like say, swimming. This is helpful during certain periods of bad-weather stress. On a cold winter morning, training can start with an indoor warm-up before going out to run in the cold. If your indoor tennis session begins and ends with an easy jog, you'll accomplish a proper warm-up and cool-down.

The time spent warming up and cooling down should be included as part of your total workout—it is a very important portion. So, if you plan on doing a "one-hour aerobic run," spend fifteen minutes warming up, fifteen cooling down, and a half hour in your aerobic training zone.

Don't be fooled into thinking that because you don't feel like you're getting much of a workout that the warm-up and cool-down don't count as part of it. Tremendous health benefits are obtained through these aspects of your training. A lack of warming up and cooling down can even contribute to over-training. Nagging injuries sometimes disappear when a long enough warm-up precedes the workout. And, competition can improve when the body is properly warmed.

## Stay Away from Stretching

Many athletes associate stretching with warming up. But stretching does not accomplish what a real warm-up does. Many also think stretching will prevent injury and improve performance. Not only is this untrue, but often just the opposite can occur.

It's very important, however, that athletes increase their flexibility. This can be done just as effectively, and without risk of harm, with a proper warm-up. Even patients with arthritis can improve flexibility with an aerobic warm-up, as much as by stretching.

There are two basic types of stretching, referred to as "static" and "ballistic." Static stretching is a very slow, deliberate movement, where you lightly stretch a muscle and hold it statically for ten to thirty seconds. When properly done, this activity promotes relaxation of the muscle being stretched. Optimal static stretching requires that each muscle group be sequentially repeated three to four times. It also demands that the activity be done slowly and not rushed.

Static stretching can be done actively or passively. Of these, active is much safer than passive.

**Graph of 1-hour workout including 15-minute warm-up and cool-down**

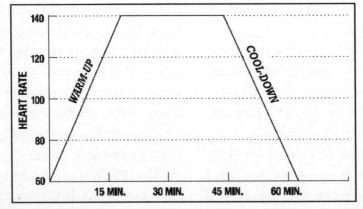

**QA**

**Question:** I am a 17:19 5K racer and want to break 17:00. I'm using your MAF method but I am slow: 9:30–10:30 miles with some walking. I have been overtrained for the last year so this is all new to me. I have been used to 80-mile weeks. My question is: How much volume should I be doing in order to race again at a high level? Should I train twice a day with three long runs per week, or should I cut it back since I have been overtrained?

**Answer:** Overtraining is a serious condition that must be fully corrected before resuming competition. The relation between your aerobic pace of 9:30–10:30—over thirty minutes for 5K—and your 5K race time of 17:19 demonstrates how much of an imbalance you have. This is a typical pattern seen in overtraining. Fully correcting overtraining is done best by building a great aerobic base and making the appropriate dietary and lifestyle changes for your particular needs. I suggest focusing on time and heart rate, instead of miles and pace. This provides the brain and body with a more realistic approach and helps bring out intuition—our natural response to training is associated with the time we're doing it and the intensity, not miles and pace. With full recovery and a great aerobic base, it sounds like your goal of breaking 17:00 is not only realistic, but improvement far beyond that may also be possible.

- Active stretching is accomplished by contracting the antagonist muscle (the one opposite the muscle you're stretching). For example, to actively stretch the hamstring muscles, the quadriceps muscles are contracted.

- Passive stretching uses gravity or force from another body part or person to move a body segment to the end of its range of motion or beyond—the reason this form of stretching can so easily cause injury.

The second basic type of stretching is called ballistic. This is a "bouncing" method and is the most common type of stretching done by athletes. It makes use of the body's momentum to repeatedly stretch a joint position to or beyond the extreme ranges of motion. Because this method is more rapid than static stretching, it activates the stretch reflex, which increases tension in the muscle, rather than relaxation. This can result in micro-tearing of muscle fibers with resultant injury.

Ballistic stretching is the type most athletes say they don't do but most realistically employ. That's because most athletes are in a hurry when stretching before or after

## WALKING: THE OTHER ENDURANCE WORKOUT

Most endurance athletes think of walking as something that's done during a bad race. But walking is a powerful tool that can further help in the process of warming up and cooling down and help build even more aerobic function. Walking can trigger the use of many small aerobic muscle fibers that are not used during training—turning these muscles on increases fat burning and additional circulation. Walking is also very useful during rehabilitation from injury, an important way to extend long workouts, a vital part of training for ultramarathons, and a tool for cyclists, swimmers, skaters, and other non-runners to implement a cross-training effect. Through cross-training, athletes can expand the fitness and health benefits of training.

Walking can be useful for all endurance athletes before and after competition. Even more important is that during the pre-race period, walking can help an athlete relax—an important habit to develop for more successful racing as this can help prevent too much stress which will trigger too much sugar burning and reduce fat burning.

As part of a cool-down, walking can help complete the process and begin recovery. Walking is especially helpful following competition as many athletes don't feel like running or biking, for example, but walking is usually not only comfortable, but once they've tried it, most athletes realize how important it is for better recovery.

training. Pre-race tension tends to make one stretch in a more stressful and quick, and hence more ballistic, mode.

### Flexibility Is Different from Stretching

Flexibility refers to the relative range of motion allowed by the muscles around a joint. This is related to the tension in the muscles that move or restrict the joint. Muscle balance may be the most important aspect of flexibility, with muscle imbalance producing reduced flexibility in a given joint. Overall, a healthy body is more flexible.

Aerobic function improves flexibility because of its effect on muscle function. Those with a greater aerobic base generally have more flexibility—not too much or too little. Those with too much flexibility also risk injury as the muscles allow joints to move too far from their normal ranges of motion.

Too much or too little flexibility is associated with injury. The risk of injury is also increased if an imbalance in joint flexibility exists between left and right, front and back, or sides of the body.

### Dangers of Stretching

A study of U.S. Army recruits found that the least flexible and the most flexible were

There are also three types of endurance athletes who use walking as a primary component of their competition:

- Olympic race walkers compete in both 20K and 50K distances, walking at speeds of less than seven minutes per mile.
- The modern road-racing trend has given birth to a very large group of recreational walkers who perform at much slower paces. These athletes compete in distances as short as 5K and as long as marathons and beyond.
- Ultramarathoners run distances beyond the 26.2-mile marathon, with the most common ones ranging from 50K (31 miles) to 100 miles. Some are based on time rather than distance, with events such as the twenty-four- and forty-eight-hour races and six-day races, where the athlete who accumulates the most miles wins. While most ultra athletes train by running, without adding a significant amount of walking to the training schedule, the time spent walking in a long event may not be as effective, or as fast. When training Stu Mittleman in preparation for his six-day races, I encouraged him to focus on walking, which he did, attaining speeds of eight minutes per mile with a normal walking gait (not Olympic-style race walk).

more than twice as likely to get injured compared to those whose joints had moderate flexibility. Endurance athletes who stretch generally are injured more frequently than those who don't stretch. That has not only been my observation over the past thirty years, but the opinion and observation of many other professionals, and is supported by scientific studies.

One common example used to show the increased injury rate in stretchers versus non-stretchers is the hamstring muscles. It is both the most frequently injured muscle group and the most stretched. Studies show that stretching exercises do not make tight hamstrings less stiff.

A recent study published in *Research in Sports Medicine* reviewed the previously published research on static stretching and injury prevention. They concluded that there is "strong evidence that routine application of static stretching does not reduce overall injury rates."

In the October 2009 issue of *Journal of Strength and Conditioning Research*, two different studies were published on the potential harmful effects of stretching. The first showed that muscular force was diminished

## MY PERSPECTIVE—BY BILL KATOVSKY

*Bill Katovsky is a two-time finisher of the Ironman Hawaii triathlon (1982 and 1993) and founder of* Tri-Athlete *magazine, which he later sold and the title became* Triathlete. *He is also the founding editor of* Inside Triathlon. *In addition, he's written several books on fitness, media, and politics. His most recent book is* Return to Fitness: Getting Back in Shape After Injury, Illness, or Prolonged Inactivity.

✳ ✳ ✳

I am like so many others whose flawed, wayward path eventually led them to Phil's doorstep. I should have listened to his counsel ages ago. I should have memorized the holistic message contained in his writings. I should have improved my diet. I should have used a heart-rate monitor. I should have done a lot of things. But I didn't. And boy, did I ever pay the price for being such a stubborn numbskull.

I have known Phil since 1993. I was the editor-in-chief of *Inside Triathlon* when a colleague sent me a copy of Phil's first book, *In Fitness and In Health.* I admit to just skimming it, but there was plenty of useful stuff about training and racing, so I asked Phil to write for the magazine.

I later left *Inside Triathlon* and headed over to *Triathlete* as editor. Phil followed me there as a columnist. We got along fine—but I felt like a heretic in Phil's company. I was a recreational multisport athlete who sporadically trained about seven hours per week and regularly binged on junk food. Many long bike rides began with a quick stop at the local 7-Eleven, where I loaded up on a custard-filled chocolate donut, Odwalla protein smoothie, and a small bag of potato chips. I didn't seem to suffer all that much from this haphazard regimen and lifestyle. When you are in your thirties, you can get away with cutting corners and gorging on sweets and carbs; the body is more forgiving.

But once I reached my forties—by then, I had left *Triathlete* and begun writing books—matters started falling apart, both physically and mentally. My body began to crumble, like a house with an unsound foundation. I got edema and dermatitis in each leg. I was bedridden for months. I had chronic insomnia. I became addicted to over-the-counter sleep and pain aids. I became depressed. I stopped working out. Muscles disappeared. I lost all motivation to exercise. I didn't bike or run for almost a decade. I felt hopeless and adrift with my declining health. Forget about fitness. I didn't break a sweat during that entire ten-year period.

In total desperation and panic, I reached out to Phil, with whom I had stayed in touch. I wanted to reclaim my health, fitness, and sanity. But I didn't know how or where to begin. We talked. We reviewed my options. He put me on a better diet—one with more vegetables and protein. I threw away every single bottle of Tylenol, Advil, and Aleve. The dermatitis eventually went away. But when it came to working out, I kept smashing into the same unyielding wall of adrenal fatigue. The cycle repeated itself. I would gradually build up the running mileage and then overdo it by charging up hills at an anaerobic pace for several consecutive workouts. Then the inevitable would happen. Legs went soft, unresponsive, buttery. The body would say, *"No más."* My breathing would become labored, even on short ten-minute runs. I was a classic case of adrenal burnout—a somatic system meltdown from within. Instead of being able to run for an hour, I could barely jog a mile. I would then have to wait three or four months before I could start working out again. Frustration is an understatement to describe my darkening mood during each forced hiatus. Why was my body rebelling?

Phil fixed this problem as well. He suggested that I start training with a heart-rate monitor. As someone who is hyper-phobic of technology, I resisted his recommendation for the longest time. But after my third episode with overtraining and adrenal burnout, I finally bought a monitor, and using Phil's 180 Formula, I rebooted my training from the beginning. The results went exactly as he has wisely outlined in his books and writings. I went slowly at first, making sure to keep my target heart rate below 128 whenever I went running. On hilly sections, my "running" seemed more like a fast walk. But I was a respectful and obedient slave to my Timex Fitness HRM master, always maintaining an aerobic pace. Within several months, I was comfortably running up to ninety minutes—including hills. Best of all, I hadn't experienced any adrenal burnout. I was injury-free. (I run in thin, flat-soled Nike Frees with the insoles removed—Phil told me to do this.) I felt reborn. I also started mountain biking again. Six months went by. My aerobic base was solidifying. To test my fitness one rainy day, I went trail running for five hours, with a 2,000-feet elevation gain. I was surprised by how easy it felt. My recovery also went smoothly. Four days later, my legs felt fresh and ready for a forty-five-minute run.

By listening to Phil, I learned to listen to my body. I now expect to have many years of fitness ahead.

in those who performed static stretching just before activity. This was performed on female athletes in their sixties. Another study performed with younger male athletes showed that sprint ability may be compromised following static stretching.

Dr. Richard Dominguez, author of *The Complete Book of Sports Medicine* and orthopedic surgeon at Loyola University Medical Center, says that among the specific stretches that are most damaging to the body are the yoga plow, hurdler's stretch, toe touching, and the stiff leg raise.

The types of injury created by stretching may be in the muscle itself, the tendon, and ligament associated with that muscle, or even the joint controlled by that muscle.

Exercise repetition from swimming, biking, running, and other endurance sports results in an already slight over-stretched state. In addition, the chemical reaction to stretching, whether from a normal workout or the act of stretching, increases the production of inflammatory chemicals. Adding more stretching only increases the potential for increased inflammation.

Many athletes stretch because they think it will help performance. But as noted, studies show this is not the case. Static stretching not only does not improve athletic performance, but may actually hinder it.

For those who require a very large range of motion for performance, however, proper stretching may be necessary. But these athletes include dancers, sprinters, and gymnasts, and not endurance athletes.

I had one patient named Randy who came to me with lower back pain and chronic asthma. He was a serious amateur cyclist. He'd begin his morning with ten minutes of stretching, especially what he perceived as his "tight" hamstrings. Then he'd head outside for his ride. He lived in a hilly area, so the first fifteen minutes of his workout were spent climbing hills. When he first used a heart-rate monitor, his heart rate surged to 170 within five minutes. But he could not imagine how any of that was contributing to his lower back pain. By performing manual muscle testing, however, I discovered that Randy's hamstring muscles were over-stretched and weak, not helping to support his lower back. Therefore, my first recommendation was to stop stretching his already over-stretched hamstrings. Within a couple of weeks, his lower back had significantly improved. This was followed by the difficult task of adjusting his morning ride to avoid the hills. The only solution was for Randy to ride indoors on his rollers for about fifteen minutes before going outside, then riding very slowly until getting past the hills. When he was able to accomplish this, his chronic asthma also disappeared.

### What About Yoga or Pilates?

Yoga and other "whole-body" flexibility activities are very different from stretching as I've described it above. When properly performed using a very slow, deliberate, and easy motion, whole-body flexibility activities are healthy, safe, and very effective. However, most athletes I've observed doing yoga, Pilates, or other activities to improve flexibility, do them improperly—too fast and too hard. In addition, since these activities don't provide a sufficient warm-up, an active warm-up should precede them to allow the athlete to gain the most out of the workout.

# CHAPTER 6

# OTHER AEROBIC AND ANAEROBIC TRAINING METHODS

**I** had a patient I will call John. He was a thirty-two-year-old triathlete and in his fourth year of building a winter off-season aerobic base. I first tested his maximum aerobic function while he ran on a track; he went 9:45 per mile at a heart rate of 152. Of course, his first comment was a complaint: "I can't train that slow." Yes, it was a change from his regular effort of around eight minutes a mile.

But that slow pace of 9:45 quickened as the months went by and the aerobic system improved. Four years later it was 7:10 per mile. Along the way, John had gone from complaining about his "too slow" aerobic training runs to saying his aerobic bike rides were getting to be a tough workout, to almost complaining that his now faster running pace of 7:10 (for his first MAF Test mile) was a bit too fast for everyday running.

In the process of building an aerobic base, several important training features will become evident. Although your aerobic training may feel too easy initially, and you'll wonder if you're even benefiting, your effort will quicken in time, and it will ultimately become more of an effort to achieve your maximum aerobic heart rate. This may happen in a matter of months depending on many factors, including training consistency and discipline, keeping to your maximum aerobic heart rate at all times, diet, and especially stress. For many, this stress comes in the form of working a regular job or dietary imbalance. *If you do not see improvements in your aerobic base after a short period—certainly after the first month or two—something is probably interfering with your aerobic system.* It's your job, sometimes with the help of a coach or healthcare professional, to find out what the problem or problems may be.

When all the training ingredients are in place, and your diet and stress are under control, the aerobic base will develop and your pace will increase as shown by your MAF Test. As your workout pace increases, you develop more aerobic speed. This means you'll be able to swim, bike, run, skate, or ski at a faster pace with the same effort or heart rate. And, you're successfully developing your metabolism so you convert more fat to energy. In addition, as your aerobic system functions better, you'll be healthier.

With more aerobic speed, two training techniques can be added to your aerobic base routine. These can even be performed during the anaerobic phase of training if it fits your schedule. These include downhill workouts and aerobic intervals.

## Downhill Workouts

While building your aerobic base, you can help develop more leg speed without the need to train anaerobically by doing downhill workouts. I refer to them as such because I first

employed them with athletes running downhill, but this workout can be used for many activities—running, biking, cross-country skiing, or skating. This workout allows you to go at a faster pace without the heart rate rising. The increased pace is accompanied by a quicker leg turnover, in the case of running.

For example, at a heart rate of 145, if you can run at a 7:45 pace on flat ground, then running down a hill at the same heart rate will force you to run much faster, perhaps at a 6:55 pace depending on the hill's slope and distance. A cyclist may be cruising at 17 mph, and on a nice long, but moderate, downhill can average 28 mph at the same heart rate.

Using a long downhill that's not too steep, you can train your brain to turn the legs over much more quickly than would ordinarily occur during a run on a flat course—all while staying aerobic. If you have a long steady downhill that takes you ten minutes or longer to complete, you can derive great neuromuscular benefits. It's important to be sure the downhill is not too steep a grade, which may force a runner to overstride, putting too much mechanical stress on the feet, knees, hips, and spine. Even on the right grade, your stride length should be about the same as if you were on level ground.

If the downhill run is short, such as five minutes, you can do downhill repeats, walking or slowly running up the hill while staying aerobic to start your downhill interval again. Some treadmills can be adjusted to slant downhill, which is a nice alternative for runners.

I often suggest one or two downhill workouts per week, not on consecutive days, during the base period. Even though you're aerobic, this workout does add more good stress to your body, and it's best to assure recovery by not using the technique on consecutive days. When properly done, most athletes don't feel much different from any other workout, but some may feel a slight or mild soreness in some muscles indicating the new activity. This workout need not be very long—runners can go forty-five minutes while cyclists up to an hour and a half, including warm-up and cool-down. These workouts will also help you further develop more aerobic speed.

### Aerobic Intervals

Once you have achieved a higher level of aerobic speed by building a more effective aerobic system, it may be difficult or impossible for you to reach your aerobic maximum heart rate, depending on the type of workout and the course. This is due to an improved aerobic system enabling you to perform faster at the same heart rate—the increased fat burning provides you with more energy for running, biking, and so forth. This is most true in swimming, cycling, skating, or cross-country skiing. Some runners will also feel the difficulty in maintaining a six- or seven-minute-per-mile pace everyday. At this stage of your development, you may be ready to add what I call *aerobic intervals* to your program.

Aerobic intervals enable you to train at your maximum aerobic heart rate for short periods despite the difficulty in maintaining that level of activity. You'll know when you're ready for aerobic intervals; riding or swimming, for example, at your maximum aerobic heart rate will be physically challenging—your heart rate won't exceed the maximum aerobic level but you'll physically have a difficult time maintaining it, or even reaching it because you'll have to ride or swim faster

**Q&A**

**Question:** I "suffer" from above-average maximum and exercise heart rates. I have been exercising one hour, two to three times per week, for the last fourteen months. I had a stress test a year ago with a "no risk, reduced exercise tolerance" result. At fifty-four years old, my maximum aerobic function test at the maximum aerobic heart rate of 126 only allows a steady walk at 3.3 mph, no running possible. When I slow-run at 4.0 mph, my heart rate rises quickly to my age-predicted maximum (166), and when I run at 6.2 mph, my heart rate levels out at 186, and I feel a bit queasy the rest of the day. I can run for ten minutes at 4.5 mph if I ignore my heart rate then recover for three minutes and run three minutes/walk three minutes forever. Any suggestions how I can be a "runner"?

than your comfort level. This is exactly the opposite of what you felt when first starting out with the MAF program and thought that the pace was too slow.

Since you won't easily be able to maintain your maximum aerobic heart rate for the whole workout, or if it's just too challenging for an everyday activity, you can perform a short interval at or near your maximum aerobic heart rate, then slow down for a period of time, then go back to the maximum aerobic level. This is much like traditional interval workouts, except it's all aerobic.

For example, if your maximum aerobic heart rate is 152, and you want to do an aerobic interval session on the bike for ninety minutes, here's a sample workout:

- A twenty-minute warm-up
- Ten-minute segments consisting of five minutes at a heart rate of 152 and five minutes at 120, repeated five times for a total of fifty minutes
- A twenty-minute cool-down

## Your Brain on Aerobic Intervals

In some instances, aerobic intervals can be performed fartlek style. In this case, following your warm-up, bike at your maximum aerobic heart rate until your brain tells you to slows you down; then ease up for a break from the higher intensity, speeding up again when you feel ready. For many, the fartlek workout is a relief from the burden of the track and clock, or some predetermined workout that seemed interesting at the time but that may not match your body's specific needs during the workout on that particular day. Fartlek is a great way to individualize a given workout on a particular day.

Combining both the downhill workouts and aerobic intervals can also be done when running or biking, for example, on a hilly course. On the downhill part of the course, try to maintain your maximum aerobic heart rate, using the flat parts (or even uphill) as an easy section.

**Answer:** This is a more extreme example of an aerobic-anaerobic imbalance. Your aerobic system appears to obviously be in very poor condition since you can't run at the slowest of paces without exceeding your maximum aerobic heart rate. While you can physically run at faster paces, it puts significant stress on your whole body as indicated with the extreme rise in heart rate (and the all-day queasy symptoms you get following the workout). You could be well into the second or even third stage of the overtraining syndrome. Building the aerobic system is the first step, and, just as important, consider all dietary and stress factors. Most importantly, if you don't see improvement in your MAF Test, there are still dietary, metabolic, stress, or other factors that need improvement.

## Anaerobic Training

An anaerobic workout is training above the aerobic maximum heart rate and includes *all* types of weight training, in addition to push-ups, pull-ups, sit-ups, and crunches. Ideally, you should not train anaerobically until you've developed a very good aerobic base, typically after three or four months, or even longer. Even after a good aerobic base has been developed, some athletes are unable to tolerate the stress of regular anaerobic workouts. This may be the case even while performing anaerobic workouts without any physical problem only to find out a week or month later that an injury has been brewing. Many endurance athletes find that training only aerobically is the best formula for success since most of their competitive energy (usually more than 95 percent) comes from the aerobic system. In this situation, they rely on racing to successfully provide anaerobic stimulation. Others find anaerobic training helpful for training and competition. Once anaerobic training begins, however, one might see the aerobic system plateau. In some athletes, this occurs after a brief period of improvement. The plateau typically continues through the race season and aerobic function usually won't improve (per the MAF Test) until the next aerobic base period. Any regression in aerobic function during an anaerobic or race period should serve as a warning sign that an imbalance—in the form of the overtraining syndrome—is developing.

With careful planning, the potential benefits of anaerobic training include physical changes such as building anaerobic muscle fibers and increasing your muscle power. While power can be helpful in some events, it's not a primary factor in endurance sports (otherwise, the strongest athletes would always be the top finishers instead of those with the best endurance). Anaerobic training can also produce metabolic changes that help a variety of chemical factors including the hormonal system. Mentally, many endurance athletes are convinced that anaerobic training is important. But be careful and prudent, since most injuries, ill health, and other aspects of overtraining occur during the anaerobic phase.

Most of your anaerobic benefits may occur within three to four weeks of the onset of anaerobic training. This is associated with the *overreaching* state—one that may precede the first stage of overtraining. Carefully monitoring your signs and symptoms, and MAF Test, is very important—a normal plateau is acceptable but a regression in your MAF Test is not and may be your first indication you've crossed the line to overtraining.

Studies also show an increased risk of overtraining after about three weeks of anaerobic training. If the MAF Test shows a decline in aerobic function, anaerobic exercise should be stopped. This may indicate that you have obtained adequate anaerobic stimulation, perhaps as much as your body can tolerate, and further anaerobic training is unnecessary.

# IS AEROBIC TRAINING BENEFICIAL FOR STRENGTH ATHLETES?

Many strength athletes—weight lifters, body builders, football players—avoid aerobic training because they fear it will adversely affect their power development. This idea comes from older studies that demonstrated this potential problem. However, newer, more objective studies addressing this issue have shown that strength develops regardless of the combination of aerobic and anaerobic training. In fact, anaerobic benefits can increase when the aerobic system is developed. Consider the important benefits of improved aerobic function: more circulation, better lymphatic drainage, improved recovery, increased mechanical support of joint, tendons, ligaments, and bones, and other improvements in health. All of these will help you if you're a power athlete.

Power athletes should make every effort to maintain a balanced training program that includes anaerobic and aerobic components and, most especially, a proper warm-up and cool-down.

I had one patient named Ed who was an Olympic weight lifter. Much to his disappointment, he had not improved in competition for more than two years. This seemed like an eternity for him since he was only twenty-six years old. He consulted me because of continuing health problems with asthma and allergies, chronic muscle and joint pain, and fatigue. With great reluctance in the wake of my first recommendation, Ed ceased all weight training to build an aerobic base. He chose walking, jogging, and riding a stationary bike. His aerobic function and overall health improved significantly during the nearly five months of base building. Then, he began weight lifting again, adding a proper warm-up and cool-down. He also performed aerobic work four to five days a week in between his weight workouts. In his first three competitions, Ed lifted more weight than he had in the past two years and achieved several personal records. He began scheduling a four-month aerobic base period each year and continued to improve in competition.

It may also indicate that there is some imbalance preventing the body from progressing further. In either case, it is important to cease all anaerobic workouts.

During anaerobic training periods, significant aerobic activity must be maintained. This can occur during anaerobic workouts as part of the warm-up and cool-down, and

## FINDING YOUR MAXIMUM HEART RATE

Another example of individuality is each person's maximum heart rate. Even within a group of athletes of the same age, gender, and ability, the maximum heart rate can vary considerably. There are two ways to find your maximum heart rate. One is by trial, and the other by formula.

The best approach is by trial. Your maximum heart rate for specific activities can be determined following about three to four minutes of maximum (all-out) training, with running being the most effective way to bring the HR to the highest level.

The best formula for determining your maximum heart rate—for healthy adult male and female athletes not on medication—is as follows: 208 minus 0.7 multiplied by age (subtract the result of 0.7 times your age from 208). It's different than the traditional formula of 220 minus age, which is not as accurate. But even using this or other formulas, athletes usually won't find the same maximum heart rate as performing a trial. In most cases, actual maximum heart rates are higher.

It should be noted again that your maximum heart rate is not factored into the 180 Formula in obtaining the maximum aerobic heart rate; 180 minus your age is *not* your maximum heart rate but just a means to obtain your max aerobic rate.

through participation in aerobic training on days without anaerobic sessions. If you're cross-training, you can also maintain swimming, for example, as a regular aerobic workout.

### Performing Anaerobic Workouts—Keep Them Simple and Short

By keeping the workouts simple and short, I am referring to the specific types of workouts in each sport. Some anaerobic-interval track workouts, for example, have become so complicated that you almost need a computer to follow them (and, in fact, computer pro-

grams are now available to provide you with such schedules).

After decades of assigning hundreds of different types of anaerobic intervals in many sports, I have concluded without a doubt that all of these different methods result in the same or very similar benefits when it comes to endurance athletes. Whether a runner does 400-meter repeats, uphill repeats, step-ups, or fartlek, the anaerobic stimulation will provide very similar, if not identical, results for most racing needs. If the swimmer does varying distance intervals with any number of specific patterns offered by the many successful

Maximum heart rates vary between different types of activities. Running would produce the highest maximum heart rate compared to cycling or swimming in the same person, due to the increased amount of muscle mass associated with more gravitational stress that accompanies running compared to other activities.

Maximum heart rate may also vary slightly due to a person's training and stress levels (well rested or tired), nutritional status (such as hydration), weather (high or low humidity), and other factors. This produces a wide variety of maximum heart rates. In a group of forty-year-old athletes, for example, a normal range of maximum heart rates can be 160 to 200 beats per minute. In addition, maximum heart rate diminishes with age in athletes, by about five to ten beats per decade; this, too, can vary considerably with one's fitness and health.

Despite the inexact science, maximum heart rate has been shown to change with training. In particular, maximum heart rate can decrease with successful aerobic training. This is due to increased efficiency of the heart, improved changes in blood volume, and other factors. It's also been shown that maximum heart rate can increase during periods of no training, such as during a period of injury when training is reduced.

coaches in the sport, he or she will obtain very much the same benefits for endurance races. The most useful anaerobic benefits come when you perform them similarly or identically to what you do in competition. This includes runners training just faster than the pace they seek to race with, cyclists riding just faster than their race speed, and so on.

Regarding anaerobic workouts for activity other than weight lifting, your heart rate should not exceed 90 percent of your maximum heart rate. If you're doing intervals on a track, use the heart rate as your primary guide, along with total workout time. Betsy, another endurance athlete patient, was a track runner in high school and always enjoyed training on the 400-meter oval. Her choice was to perform one-mile repeats for anaerobic sessions following her four-month base period. With a PR of 41:10 in the 10K, her goal was to eventually break forty minutes. I suggested that she run her mile repeats around a 6:30 pace with an easy quarter- to half-mile recovery at the low end of her aerobic range of 140 to 150. This pace also corresponded with a heart rate in the low 180s at the end of her mile intervals. (Betsy's maximum heart rate of 197 was determined in a one-mile race six months earlier.)

The main question is this: How is maximum heart rate useful for athletes? While many athletes focus on their maximum heart rate believing that higher is better (which is not necessarily true), there are at least two uses of maximum heart rate. First, I recommend using a percent of maximum heart rate to obtain a general guideline for anaerobic training. This may be the best training intensity that produces maximum training benefits, with training above this heart rate producing little or no additional benefits while adding potentially harmful stress. This figure is 90 percent of maximum heart rate, and can be employed during interval training, hill repeats, and other anaerobic workouts (except weight training, of course).

A second use of maximum heart rate is to compare your actual rate as determined in training to the formula above that predicts maximum heart rate (which generally underestimates the actual maximum heart rate). Athletes who don't come close to their estimated maximum heart rate could have a problem with their autonomic nervous system, the brain's control of the heart, blood vessels, or another area. In extreme circumstances, significant differences in the actual versus formula maximum heart rate can even indicate a heart problem and an increased risk of sudden death—these cases are sometimes associated with very low maximum heart rates.

The same type of workout can be performed in other events too. Cyclists, for example, can ride three-, four-, or five-mile distances at their anaerobic effort and slightly faster than the speed of a race. Regardless of the sport, allow your heart rate to come down well into the aerobic zone during the interval recovery. The most significant concern with anaerobic workouts is this: while they must cause a certain amount of stress to be beneficial, they should avoid creating excessive stress. Unfortunately, athletes are often impatient and want to improve too quickly. This only leads to the excess stress associated with overtraining.

After reading an article I wrote on the importance of the aerobic system, Dan, a runner, contacted me. He had just completed a successful winter aerobic base period and was ready for spring track work. Like Betsy, his favorite race distance was 10K, and this year his goal was to break forty minutes. He decided to work out with a friend, and he began his track sessions with quarter-mile repeats at seventy-five seconds each, with a quarter-mile jog in between. When race time came, his times were only a few seconds faster than the previous year. What's worse, his race times got slower as the season wore on, and he never came close to breaking forty minutes.

Why was Dan doing his intervals so fast? He had not yet broken forty minutes for 10K, so his interval pace of seventy-five-second quarters was far beyond his racing ability—the speed of a runner going at a five minute per mile pace! He would produce much less stress and potentially obtain more benefits if his quarter-mile repeats were ninety seconds instead. This was my recommendation when seeing Dan in my office for the first time.

In addition, running a quarter-mile in seventy-five seconds brought Dan's heart rate well into the 180s, which was almost his previously determined maximum heart rate. Running the same quarter mile at ninety seconds would bring his heart rate to about 170, closer to 90 percent of his maximum heart rate, and a much more effective level of intensity for anaerobic training: it's lower in stress, offers significant anaerobic stimulation, and still allowed Dan a slightly faster pace than his racing goal.

I've not seen the need for long anaerobic training sessions in endurance athletes. It's relatively easy to stimulate the anaerobic system to obtain benefits and, unlike aerobic training, shorter bouts of anaerobic workouts are very effective. So, the second principle of anaerobic training is to keep it short. This relates to both the total time of each workout and the number of weeks these workouts are maintained. Both longer anaerobic intervals in a training session and anaerobic training that continues for too many weeks (or months) are common causes of overtraining and injury, and together

they can be quite problematic for an athlete's health.

Your brain, muscles, and metabolism have a limit on what they can gain from a given individual anaerobic workout. And I do mean *limit*: forty-five minutes for high-stress activity such as running, sixty to ninety minutes for other activities like cycling, skating, and swimming. This is, however, more than sufficient time to get substantial benefits. And remember, these times include your warm-up and cool-down. So after this workout, don't expect to come home ready to collapse; it's not necessary.

How long should you continue doing the anaerobic part of your schedule? That depends on a number of factors. The biggest is stress—specifically, how much stress do you have in other areas of your life? Since stress and anaerobic workouts are basically the same because of the hormone cortisol, the more stress in your life, the less anaerobic training you can perform without overtraining.

Another important factor is time. How much time do you have in the course of the day and week, especially considering the increased need for recovery from anaerobic workout (plus all your other aerobic training)? Remember the training equation: **Training = Work + Rest.**

It takes longer to recover from anaerobic sessions, and if your days and evenings are generally busy with other commitments, you may not have the luxury of doing much anaerobic work.

## MY PERSPECTIVE—BY RICK RUBIN

*Rick Rubin, forty-seven, is one of the most influential record producers in America and the co-head of Columbia Records. In 2008, Rubin won the Grammy for Producer of the Year based on his work with the Dixie Chicks, Michael Kranz, Red Hot Chili Peppers, U2, Green Day, and the late Johnny Cash.* Time *magazine has called him "Hit Man" and the* Washington Post *nicknamed Rubin the "Song Doctor."*

✳ ✳ ✳

I met Phil in 2003, and since that time everything in my life has changed. I used to live a late-night, sedentary, carb-dense vegan life. Through Phil's suggestions, and combined with controlling my calories, I have lost 135 pounds. I can't remember ever feeling this good. My days are now filled with physical activity: I swim, bike, jog, and stand-up paddle. I eat lots of protein all through the day and spend a great deal of time in the sun. It feels like I'm starting an entirely new life and one I never dreamed possible. It's been interesting to watch the "far out" ideas that Phil's been teaching

The best way to answer the question of how long you should continue anaerobic work is by performing the MAF Test. If you see a slowing of your pace at any time during your anaerobic training phase, it's time to stop all anaerobic work and return to aerobic base training. A worsening of your MAF Test would indicate you've done too much anaerobic work. As many athletes find, only a few short weeks of anaerobic training is all that's required. (Of course, any abnormal indication that the anaerobic sessions are not healthy should also bring the same conclusion—these include disturbances in your sleep, pain, extreme fatigue, and others.)

For most endurance athletes, the maximum time for anaerobic work is about six to eight weeks. But this is the maximum, and more of an exception. For the average endurance athlete who works a forty-hour workweek, especially if he or she has a family, five weeks may be quite sufficient and effective. Want to play it safe? Most athletes can obtain maximum anaerobic benefits after three to four weeks. But for many, *no* anaerobic training is best. Finding the right scenario for your particular needs is very important, and requires an honest self-evaluation, and not just following other athletes or the latest article in popular sports magazines.

By now, you're asking yourself the customary question: "How will I get fast if I don't train fast?" Let me emphasize as I did earlier, and assure you that most endurance events for all these years finally becoming mainstream science as well as finding their way into the culture.

Barefoot walking and jogging on the beach was considered taboo—you needed support, orthotics, and cushioning, said the "experts." Now Harvard has just published a scientific paper extolling the virtues of exercising barefoot, exactly how Phil has been preaching it. There have been many, many examples of this just in the few short years I have followed Phil's advice. Another one is getting in the sun daily. Dermatologists would have had you believe the sun was poisonous even in small doses. Now a prominent dermatologist has come out saying it's worth the risk of being in the sun to get vitamin D to prevent osteoporosis and bone loss.

The tide again is turning toward Phil's teachings. Using the heart-rate monitor, I have gone from not being able to swim one lap to swimming a mile. From barely being able to walk for five minutes, I can now comfortably walk for hours daily. When I decided to start jogging, the time I could go without stopping multiplied almost daily. Phil's methods work!

rely on the aerobic system—not the anaerobic—for 95 to 99 percent of the body's energy needs. You will increase your speed by getting more efficient through aerobic training.

Going through a yearly schedule without anaerobic work is a dramatic break from tradition for many who have been in endurance sports for a long time. But once you've done it, and seen the positive results, you'll have no trouble creating a new habit. Actually, a better question will then be: "How will I get my anaerobic stimulation?" The answer is by racing; you are performing anaerobic work when competing. For many athletes, that's just enough hard input to keep the body balanced and working well. Consider Mike Pigg's

1994 triathlon season—one of his best and certainly one of the greatest single seasons of any multisport athlete. He won most of his races and finished high up in most of the rest. He did not perform any anaerobic work until mid-September, when most of his races were completed.   When anaerobic training is included in your schedule, there are a few basic rules to follow:

- Including competitive events, do not exceed two to three anaerobic workouts per week; for most athletes, one to two is sufficient.
- Most athletes will reach maximum anaerobic benefits after three or four weeks of anaerobic work.

- Workouts the day before and after an anaerobic workout should be easy aerobic ones, or off days.
- Never perform anaerobic workouts on two consecutive days.
- Try to mimic your race environment during anaerobic workouts. This includes running on the road, cycling with a group, or swimming open water.
- Focus on relaxation and breathing to increase your mechanical efficiency. If you're uptight and stressed (or fatigued), do an easy workout or take a day off, and try again the next day.
- Try to do your anaerobic workout in the morning or about the same time as the start of your regular competitions.
- Be sure to warm-up and cool-down sufficiently.
- Treat your anaerobic workout mentally and physically as if it were a race.
- Be sure to eat and drink enough fluid before and after your workout, and during as needed.

### Weight Lifting and Other Anaerobic Workouts

Working out with weights is anaerobic, whether you're lifting low weights and using high repetition or the reverse. Included with these types of anaerobic activities are push-ups, pull-ups, sit-ups, and similar workouts. Everything I discussed about anaerobic workouts also applies to weight training, especially keep it short and simple, and warm up and

cool down using whatever easy aerobic activities you want.

As noted, don't expect to see your heart rate increase beyond your maximum aerobic level during a weight session. In most people, the muscles you are working fatigue before the heart rate reaches its peak level. Since you stop lifting at that point, your heart rate never reaches its highest level so using it as a guide is not accurate.

Weight lifting and similar workouts can help endurance athletes if the schedule permits it. For example, improvement in gait can follow proper weight workouts assuming adequate recovery.

But weight lifting obviously adds some amount of muscle bulk. This added mass induces weight gain, sometimes significantly, which can be a negative factor during competition in most endurance events. Some feel the added muscle gained during lifting will protect them from injury. But it's the aerobic muscle fibers that perform this task much more than the anaerobic fibers. Others feel weight training improves power, which is does. But this power is not used nearly as significant as aerobic function in endurance events.

Most importantly, the average endurance athlete already has a tough schedule: training, working, family or home responsibilities, and perhaps other obligations. Finding time for another workout—especially two or three times a week—adds further stress to an often busy week. If your schedule permits two or three added workouts per week, and you have built as good an aerobic base as possible, consider weights as an added anaerobic workout. If necessary, make room in your schedule by reducing other training. In addition, if you have lost muscle mass, due to reduced training or injury, then weight lifting can serve a valuable purpose. Or, if you're in your thirties or older, and you're just starting to work out, adding weight training after establishing your aerobic base may benefit you.

Think of *all* anaerobic training, including weights, as an investment. It's a high risk—one with a small return. Fortunately, most endurance athletes can obtain all the anaerobic stimulation necessary from competition. A competitive season following a good aerobic base should result in great performances.

# CHAPTER 7

# TRAINING STRESS—
## The Good, the Bad,
## and the Ugly

Stress affects many endurance athletes but not always in an identical fashion. I once had a patient named Bruce. After watching his girlfriend compete in a local bike race, Bruce got excited about the idea of training for duathlons and triathlons. A former college swimmer who was working out at the gym for fitness using weights and a stationary bike, Bruce started jogging outdoors and soon bought a road bike.

After several months, improvements were notable; Bruce was running about fifteen miles a week and riding twice that amount while maintaining his three-times-a-week weight sessions at the gym. The excitement maintained his enthusiasm. But an acute back problem brought him to my clinic.

Bruce's personal history turned out to be the most important part of my evaluation. He was a single parent with two children. His busy job required a forty-five-minute commute each day that left less time for training than he wanted. So he got up an hour earlier each morning and went to bed an hour later than usual. Having virtually no leisure time was rapidly catching up to Bruce's body and brain. His stress hormones were waking him at two in the morning each night. He drank more coffee in an attempt to overcome fatigue. Basically, Bruce was sacrificing his health for more fitness.

One of the secondary symptoms from all this stress was his worsening back pain. But before his back could improve, he first needed to reduce the rising level of stress in his life. Since little could be done with his work schedule and family life, attention was directed at his training schedule, along with his diet. By significantly reducing his training schedule, including eliminating weight training, and using a heart-rate monitor to train more effectively, Bruce quickly felt his energy return. In addition, within two weeks he felt no back pain. While he complained about the slower training pace, changing to time rather than distance provided a different perspective on working out. A month later, Bruce said his running and biking were noticeably faster at the same heart rate.

Improvements from training are, to a great degree, the result of stress. We apply sufficient physical, chemical, and mental stress to the body, and it develops endurance as a result, leading to better performance. This is an example of good stress. But apply a little more of those same stresses or combine them with other stress, and benefits can quickly disappear—an example of bad stress. In sports, bad or excess stress often leads to overtraining.

Excess stress is not only the most common problem I've seen in athletes, it's also the problem most neglected and underestimated by them. If you want to reach your athletic potential and optimal health, a better understanding of stress is the first step.

Stress is such an incredibly powerful influence that even if you are doing everything right in terms of training, diet, and nutrition, it can still crush your fitness and health efforts. Enough excess stress can contribute significantly and directly to injury, reduced aerobic function, and poor performance. And it contributes to many health conditions, ranging from reduced quality of life to deadly diseases such as cancer, heart disease, Alzheimer's, and others. It can also contribute to fatigue, bacterial and viral infections, inflammatory-related problems, blood-sugar problems, weight gain, intestinal distress, headaches, and most other disorders. Stress-related problems account for more than 75 percent of all visits to primary-care physicians and are responsible each day for millions of people needing to take time off work and school. So stress comes with a monetary price tag as well as a toll on your fitness and health.

Charles Darwin wrote not that it's the fittest who survive, nor the most intelligent, but those who can best adapt to their environment. Proper adaptation to your training schedule is just one example of how stress can help you perform better.

It's important to remember that stress is a normal part of fitness and health, and excess stress is not without a remedy. It's a question of adapting to, or coping with, stress. The body has a great coping mechanism for stress—the brain and adrenal glands. However, when the adrenal glands are overworked, body-wide problems can result. And when the brain is overly stressed, you won't achieve your endurance goals.

There are effective ways to help protect yourself from bad stress. So let's begin by addressing the three main types of stress: physical, chemical, and mental-emotional. These types of stress generate many different effects throughout the brain and body. Moreover, each athlete responds differently to various combinations of these stresses.

## Physical Stress

Physical stresses are strains or exertions on the body, something athletes take for granted. Overworking your muscles is an example of physical stress. Slight physical stress is what makes training beneficial and is an example of good stress. However, too much physical stress, or that same good stress without adequate recovery, can potentially result in a variety of problems. A common example of physical stress is riding a particular hilly course on your bike that you're not used to, resulting in sore quadriceps muscles; this stress can then affect your lower back, causing pain. Likewise, something unrelated to athletics, such as dental stress, can affect more than your mouth, often causing stomach dysfunction, shoulder, neck, or head pain. Other physical stresses include irregular gait, poor posture, eyestrain, and many other situations that adversely impact the mechanical body.

## Chemical Stress

Many chemicals from our environment can adversely affect the body's natural chemistry and cause stress. This can adversely affect your immune system, intestines, breathing, heart rate, and other areas. Dietary and nutritional imbalances such as too much sugar or too little vitamin D, for example, could be chemical stresses. In addition, drugs obviously influence body chemistry; examples of bad stress include excess caffeine or the side effects of prescription or over-the-counter drugs. Other sources of chemical stress include chemicals in the air—second-hand smoke, indoor and outdoor air pollution, and many others. Reducing harmful chemicals from air, water, and food, and improving diet quality are key ways to reducing stress. Chemical stresses can also affect physical and mental-emotional problems.

## Mental and Emotional Stress

The stresses most people are familiar with are of the mental and emotional types, which include tension, anxiety, and depression. Mental stress may contribute to pain, moods of anxiety or depression, and loss of enthusiasm or motivation, and can lead to physical and chemical problems as well. Mental stress affects cognition, including sensation, perception, learning, concept formation, and decision-making. These are all very important factors in sports. For example, mental imagery and the ability to form an effective racing strategy are hallmarks of great athletes.

All three forms of stress are often associated with training and competition. But stress can also come from your job, family, other people, your emotions, infections, allergic reactions, and even the weather. Most people are affected by more than one form of stress, and frequently by all three types. And, stress is cumulative; the response to a physical stress from the weekend's long training may be amplified by Monday's chemical stress of too much coffee and poor eating, further compounded with a family-related mental stress on Tuesday and another with the boss on Wednesday. All of this will affect your performance at a competitive event on Saturday.

The weather is a potential stressor, as previously shown in its relationship to the MAF Test. Weather stress can affect us physically, chemically, or mentally. Seasonal Affective Disorder (SAD) is a good example of how the weather at certain times of year, typically in the fall and winter in the northern hemisphere, can have a dramatic adverse effect on people.

Some people accumulate so much stress that they lose track of it. When I ask a patient to list their stresses, for example, they may recall three or four—but if I ask, "What about this or that?" they say, "Oh yes, that too." When you're ready to deal with stress, the first thing to do is make yourself aware of it. The best way to do this is write it all down as a stress list.

## Stress List

Athletes are certainly not immune to stress, and reducing even some of it can have a significant impact on overall training and racing. Reducing or eliminating individual stresses is easier if you write them down on paper. Here's an example:

- On a page, make three columns, one each for physical, chemical, and mental stresses.
- In each category, write down what you think are your stresses. This may take several days to complete since you probably won't think of all your different stresses right away.
- When you're done, prioritize by placing the biggest stress of each category on top.
- Then, work on reducing or eliminating one stress at a time. Or, if you can handle it, work on one stress at a time from each category.

Reducing or eliminating unnecessary stress from your life will give your body a better chance to cope with other stresses you may not be able to change right now.

As you make your list, put a star by the stresses over which you have some control. This may include unhealthy eating habits like rushing or skipping your meals, drinking too much coffee, or not taking time to warm-up or cool-down properly during training.

Simply draw a line through those stresses that you can't control. If there's nothing you can do about them anyway, don't worry about them for now. Many people expend lots of energy on stresses they can't—or in most cases *won't*—do anything about. This may include job stress or the weather, though in reality almost any stress can be modified or eliminated—it's just a question of how far you're willing to go for optimal fitness and health. As time goes on, you may want to reconsider some of the items you've crossed off. You'll realize, for example, that changing jobs is a must, or moving to a more compatible climate will significantly improve both fitness and health.

Once you can "see" your stress listed on paper, it will be easier to manage. Start with your starred stresses first, because you have more control over them—not that it's always easy. Circle the three biggest stresses from the starred list and begin to work on them. You may be able to improve on some and totally eliminate others. Some will require habit changes. It's a big task, but one that will return great benefits. When you've succeeded in eliminating or modifying each one, remove it from your list and circle the three next most stressful ones, so you always have three to work on.

In addition to self-managing your stress list, here's some other strategies for dealing with stress:

- Learn to say "no" when asked to do something you really don't want to do.
- Decide not to waste your time worrying about the past or the future. That's not to say you should ignore the past or not plan for the future, but live in the present.
- Learn some relaxation techniques, and perform them regularly. The most powerful one is respiratory biofeedback, described in chapter 28. This is especially valuable around the time of competition.
- When you're concerned about something, talk it over with someone you trust.
- Simplify your life. Start by eliminating trivia. Ask yourself: "Is this really important?"
- Prioritize your busy schedule: do the most important things first, but don't neglect the enjoyable things. Before getting out of bed in the morning, ask yourself: "What fun things do I have planned for today?"
- Know your passion and pursue it.

What's most important about stress is that too much of it interferes with rest. Or more accurately, recovering from excess stress requires more rest. If you don't get enough rest, usually in the form of sleep, the effects of stress will continue accumulating. One of the questions to ask yourself is whether you're getting enough sleep, considering the amount of stress you have. As you will see, one of the symptoms of excess stress is insomnia. In fact, too much of the stress hormone cortisol can interfere with sleep, waking you in the middle of the night and causing difficulty returning to sleep. A disturbed night's sleep not only is a stress, but reduces recovery.

By learning to take control of the various types of stress in your life, you can improve the quality of your training, perform better, and be healthier. This will also help your adrenal glands regulate other stresses better.

## Stress and the Adrenal Glands

No matter what type of stress you encounter—whether it's physical, chemical, or mental and emotional—your body has an efficient mechanism for coping. This is the important job of the adrenal glands. On the top of each kidney, these small glands work with the brain and nervous system to regulate important coping mechanisms, including the "fight or flight" reaction. The adrenal glands accomplish their work through the production of certain hormones, making them not only essential for stress coping and optimal human performance, but also for life itself. These hormones help with stress regulation, sex and reproduction, growth, aging, cellular repair, electrolyte balance, and blood sugar control.

As noted earlier, cortisol is the key adrenal stress hormone and commonly measured by simple blood and saliva tests. Saliva is a better way to measure cortisol in most instances because having a needle thrust into a vein in your arm evokes stress—and cortisol production—sometimes making the blood test quite inaccurate. A saliva test only requires a small sample of your saliva in a small test tube during the normal course of your day. And, since cortisol fluctuates throughout the day and night, a saliva test can easily be taken four different times throughout the day for a more accurate evaluation.

When your body is under high stress, cortisol level can increase dramatically, and when the stress passes, the level returns to normal. In chronic stress states—the continuation of stress without relief—high cortisol levels can become dangerous. This can adversely affect the brain, including the pituitary gland, and especially reduce memory, impair aerobic function, create blood sugar problems, reduce fat burning, suppress immune function, lower the body's defense against not just cold and flu but any infection, and cause intestinal distress. Long-standing stress can result in a "burning out" of adrenal function, with a serious loss of normal hormone production. In this state, cortisol levels become dangerously low, along with other hormones made by the adrenals.

Sex hormones, including estrogens and testosterone, are also important adrenal hormones that help both males and females to maintain proper sexual function and reproductive health. In addition to gonadal sources, these sex hormones come from another important adrenal hormone, DHEA. When stress raises cortisol, DHEA is often reduced.

Excess stress is also the cause of the overtraining syndrome discussed more fully in the next chapter. Whether we call it burnout or overtraining, it's the same problem. While our understanding of overtraining is relatively new, adrenal stress patterns were discovered nearly a century ago, along with the

## THE ATHLETIC OR "RUNNER'S" HIGH

Most athletes would say that working out is the best way to reduce stress. The so-called "runner's high"—a feeling of euphoria during exercise—is often discussed as a way for an athlete to escape. This occurs not only during running, but biking, swimming, and virtually any other sport. What really is this "high"?

We don't really know exactly what runner's high is or why it occurs. In past decades, research has associated this state with natural opiates in the brain, or a cognitive state of dissociation. This usually centered on a discussion of endorphins—different types of hormonelike chemicals produced in the brain; some may even be produced in the skin, associated with sun exposure and vitamin D. More recently the so-called runner's high has been associated with the same brain receptors for substances like marijuana. While these receptors in the brain are still being studied in the lab, and undoubtedly other chemicals will be discovered that might better explain that elusive feeling gained from working out, the brain is far too complex to pinpoint just one cause for an "elevated state."

I believe the runner's high phenomenon is an important state of consciousness. Normally, when we're sleeping, in a business meeting, or in the middle of a great workout, our brain produces certain brain waves. When we're mentally relaxed, unstressed, and doing something that takes us to our own private world, such as that workout, our brain produces alpha waves. This state also can be promoted by listening to music, mediating, prayer, and other activities. Unfortunately, not all athletes experience the high because, for some people, stress can overpower the enjoyment of the workout, impairing the ability to make alpha waves. A further discussion and practical application of brain waves is found in chapter 28.

well-documented three stages of stress, which correlate to the three stages of overtraining.

### The Physiology of Stress

Our knowledge about stress and adrenal function began in the 1920s, when famous stress-research pioneer Hans Selye began to piece together the common problems resulting from excess adrenal stress. They include poor immunity and intestinal dysfunction, which in turn can trigger hundreds of other problems—like a domino effect. Selye eventually showed how the adrenals react when confronted with excess stress. This General Adaptation Syndrome has three distinct stages:

- *Stage 1*: The first stage begins with the alarm reaction, when we're initially hit with a stress. This increases adrenal hormone production to help the body cope with the stress. This is what commonly occurs during anaerobic training and the competitive season, but much less during aerobic training. The purpose of this first stage by the adrenal glands is an attempt to battle and adapt to the increased stress. If it is successful, and the stress is reduced, we recover; adrenal function returns to normal, especially with sufficient rest. If this stage is of sufficient length, a variety of mild symptoms may occur: noticeable tiredness during the day, mild allergies, or even some nagging back, knee, or foot pain. If, over time—a few weeks or months—the adrenals fail to meet the needs of the body to combat the stress, they enter the second stage.
- *Stage 2*: During this period, also called the resistance stage, the adrenal glands themselves get larger through a process called hypertrophy. Since the increased hormone production of the first stage couldn't counter the stress, the glands enlarge in an attempt make even more cortisol to do the same. During this stage, more advanced symptoms may occur, including fatigue, insomnia, and more serious back, knee, or foot pain, or poor recovery. Most athletes with stress problems are stuck in this stage, often for months or years. They usually no longer see their best performances, and injuries or ill health are common. If athletes in this stage continue to push themselves, thereby maintaining high levels of stress, the adrenals eventually can enter the third stage, called exhaustion.
- *Stage 3*: An athlete who enters this stage is exhausted, often with chronic injuries and most likely is not able to compete near the same level of effectiveness. The adrenal glands are unable to adapt to stress and are unable to produce adequate levels of hormones, including cortisol. The person is usually more seriously ill—physically, chemically, or mentally.

But this discussion is not just about adrenal disease; rather, it concerns the gray area between normal adrenal function and disease. Addison's disease occurs when the adrenal glands are unable to produce sufficient cortisol to sustain life. It can occur in men and women of all age-groups; symptoms include severe weight loss, muscle weakness, fatigue, low blood pressure, and sometimes darkening of the skin. The disease is also called adrenal insufficiency or hypocortisolism.

## Diet and Adrenal Function

Adrenal stress can be caused or aggravated by the consumption of refined carbohydrates and sugar. This includes hidden sugars in many foods. How much is too much? Less is best.

Caffeine is a common source of adrenal stimulation—one of the main reasons people consume it. Coffee, tea, and cola are the main sources. If you have an adrenal problem, assess your caffeine intake. For many, no caffeine is best; for others, a single cup or two of coffee or tea may be tolerable. You must determine this, as objectively as possible, by listening to your body to see how much caffeine you can tolerate. Feeling jittery and high-strung, a rapidly rising heart rate, or queasiness in your stomach may indicate you've consumed too much caffeine.

Breakfast is always the most important meal of the day, but most especially for those with adrenal dysfunction. A healthy breakfast includes protein but is void of refined carbohydrates. An egg-based meal can be the cornerstone of an ideal breakfast.

People with adrenal stress often need to snack between the three main meals, as much as every two hours, in the early stages of recovery. Healthy snacking means eating healthy food in small portions.

### Nutrients and Adrenal Function

Your nutritional needs may vary with adrenal stress. These include factors to help the immune system, intestines, and the adrenal glands themselves. Most, if not all, nutrients should come from an optimal diet. Below are some possible supplemental nutrient needs:

- For many types of adrenal stress, especially those that cause insomnia, zinc may be useful. Studies show this important mineral can help lower high cortisol levels that accompany adrenal stress. Taken right before bed, for example, zinc may improve sleep patterns associated with high cortisol.

- Choline is a nutrient commonly needed by some people with adrenal stress, in part due to the relationship of choline with the brain. Individuals who are always on the go, overworked, and trying to do too much are examples of those who may benefit from choline. A smaller dose several times a day, rather than one or two higher doses, may be most helpful. Those with exercise-induced asthma may need higher doses. The best source of choline in the diet is egg yolks.

## Training and Adrenal Function

Building a great aerobic base can be a significant strategy for improving adrenal function. Anaerobic training can worsen existing adrenal problems. Once adrenal function is improved, anaerobic exercise can be resumed, though the balance of aerobic and anaerobic exercise must be maintained.

## Natural Hormones

All hormones play a major role in one's physical, chemical, and mental well-being, and are important for all athletes. Three important hormones, produced by both men and women, include a group of estrogens, testosterone, and progesterone. As we age, and with increased stress, the production of

## ADRENAL STRESS CHECKLIST

Ten common symptoms of adrenal dysfunction are listed below. Note those that pertain to you. While any of these can be caused by other imbalances in the body, together they make up the most common complaints heard by those with adrenal dysfunction.

- *Low energy.* This is common especially in the afternoon, but could happen anytime, or all the time. The fatigue can be physical, mental, or both. When the adrenals are too stressed, the body uses more sugar for energy but can't access fat very well for energy use. This can significantly limit your energy for daily chores, training, or competition.
- *Dizziness upon standing.* Standing up from a seated or lying position, or just bending over to pick up something from the floor, can make you dizzy because not enough blood is getting to the head quickly enough. Check your blood pressure while lying down and then immediately after you stand. If you suffer from adrenal dysfunction, you will often notice the systolic blood pressure (the first number) doesn't rise normally—it should be higher when you're standing by about six to eight millimeters.
- *Eyes sensitive to bright light.* Adrenal stress often causes light sensitivity in your eyes. You may feel the need to wear sunglasses even on cloudy days or have difficulty with night driving because of the oncoming headlights (often misinterpreted as bad night vision). Some people find their nearsightedness (ability to see distances) worsens with adrenal stress.
- *Asthma and allergies.* Whether you call it exercise-induced asthma, food allergies, or seasonal allergies, they are all similar symptoms of adrenal dysfunction.
- *Physical imbalance.* Problems in the low back, knee, foot, and ankle are particularly associated with adrenal problems. They can produce symptoms such as low-back pain, sciatica, and excess pronation in the foot, leading to foot and ankle problems.
- *Stress-related syndromes.* What we call burnout, being stressed out, overtraining, and nervous breakdown are virtually the same and are usually the result of adrenal exhaustion. While occasionally these problems become serious enough to warrant medication or hospitalization, adrenal dysfunction occurs long before this point.

- *Blood-sugar stress.* With adrenal dysfunction, the body is unable to properly regulate blood sugar. Symptoms include constantly feeling hungry, being irritable before meals, especially if meals are delayed, and having strong cravings for sweets or caffeine.
- *Insomnia.* Many athletes with adrenal dysfunction fall asleep easily (from fatigue) but wake in the middle of the night with difficulty getting back to sleep. This may be due to high levels of cortisol occurring at the wrong time (levels should be low during sleeping hours). Many people say they wake up in the night to urinate, but it's usually the adrenal problem that awakens them, and then they get the urge to urinate. Rest is a key factor in recovering from adrenal dysfunction. Are you getting at least seven to eight hours each night? If not, you may need more sleep. Adrenal stress increases the need for recovery.
- *Diminished sex drive.* This is a common symptom of adrenal dysfunction due to low levels of the hormone DHEA, which makes estrogen and testosterone. Medications such as Viagra just dilates the blood vessels and does not affect the hormones.
- *Seasonal Affective Disorder (SAD).* This is a common problem, occurring in the colder months. As the hours of daylight lessen and the temperature drops, many people go into a mild state of hibernation. The metabolism slows and the body and mind become sluggish, sometimes resulting in a mild or moderate depression. (This corresponds with a combination of stresses: the weather, lack of sunlight and vitamin D, and even the start of the holiday season—people don't eat well, are less active, and weight gain is common.)

Recognizing these ten common symptoms of adrenal dysfunction can be useful in your self-assessment. You may also want to test some of your adrenal-hormone levels with the help of a health-care professional. The best initial test for adrenal function measures cortisol and DHEA in saliva, and is performed over the course of a typical day and evening, rather than just once.

these hormones is diminished. This occurs especially when cortisol rises, diminishing the production of DHEA, and subsequently diminishing the estrogens and testosterone.

Since the hormonal system is very complex, it's recommended that you seek the input of a health-care professional to assess and treat any hormonal imbalance. The use of natural hormones is on the rise. Most health-conscious individuals rely on natural hormones instead of synthetic versions, which often have dangerous side effects. However, many healthy people can restore normal hormone balance by improving adrenal gland function. When this is not sufficient, natural hormone supplements may be the next best option.

## Estrogen

This most well-known of hormones is actually a group of about twenty compounds. The most important estrogens are estrone, estradiol, and estriol. The different estrogens have unique roles in the body. For example, estradiol is the most stimulating to the breast, potentially increasing the risk of breast cancer. Estriol protects against breast cancer. Normal production of both by the body is the right balance. A variety of benefits are attributed to the effects of natural estrogens, including prevention of hot flashes, better memory and concentration, slowing of the aging process, and reduced depression and anxiety.

Hormone replacement theraphy (HRT) with estradiol places you at high risk for breast cancer. This is due to the fact that it's not broken down in the liver as quickly as your own natural estrogens (affecting the cells for a longer time). Premarin, made from the urine of pregnant horses, simply doesn't function exactly like the estrogens made in the human body. In addition to natural estradiol, other natural estrogens have synthetic companions and are marketed under various brand names.

One of the common risks of HRT is the higher dosage of estrogen compared to what your body would normally produce. The most common symptom of too much estrogen in your system is water retention. This can lead to breast tenderness and swelling, weight gain, and headaches. Excess estrogen can also lower blood sugar and increase your cravings for sweets. Too much estrogen also increases your risk of uterine cancer and gall bladder disease.

While the idea of HRT is often "sold" to patients by touting the benefits of building strong bones, estrogen doesn't actually do this. Rather, it decreases the rate of bone loss that occurs naturally throughout life. The hormones that have the greatest impact on new bone growth—something your body is always doing—are progesterone and testosterone.

## Progesterone and Testosterone

Unlike estrogen, which is a group of hormones, progesterone is the only hormone in its class. It improves sleep, builds bone mass, protects against breast and uterine cancer, improves carbohydrate tolerance, helps burn fat, prevents water retention, increases sex drive, and in many people has a calming effect on the nervous system.

Provera is a commonly used synthetic version of progesterone. However, it doesn't have the same functions as the natural hormone. While natural progesterone acts like a diuretic, Provera can increase salt and water retention and body fat. Too much of this syn-

## MY PERSPECTIVE—BY DR. STEPHEN GANGEMI

*Dr. Stephen Gangemi, a chiropractor who lives in Chapel Hill, North Carolina, with his family, has pursued advanced training in applied kinesiology, nutritional biochemistry, functional neurology, acupressure and meridian therapies, and other holistic body therapies. Dr. Gangemi is a six-time qualifier and finisher of the Ironman Hawaii World Championship Triathlon. He has completed fifteen Ironman races as well as countless other triathlons. He has been an all-American triathlete twice, in 1997 and 2004.*

**✳ ✳ ✳**

I first heard of Phil in the early 1990s after visiting a local chiropractor who insisted that I read *In Fitness and In Health.* Phil's book inspired me, as I was becoming interested in health care, not disease care, while still in high school, and I was an avid athlete, starting to race in triathlons. Like many others, I figured my heart-rate monitor was either broken or just didn't work for me, because my heart rate was much higher than I could have expected. I wore it but didn't train according to Phil's principles; it was more of a reference device to see how hard I could push myself.

My diet consisted of what most athletes ate in the late 1990s—the high-carb, low-fat, pasta and bagel diet. I raced well, but I was constantly injured. I eventually had them all—low back pain, neck pain, plantar fasciitis, heel spurs, iliotibial band syndrome, shin splints, muscle aches. There was always something wrong going on, one injury after another. I was a hard-core highly conditioned triathlete, so I pushed through the injuries either by seeing various doctors who knew nothing more than to look at my symptoms or by treating the ailments myself. Anti-inflammatory drugs were a staple, and healthy fats were to be avoided. After all, I was taught they'd make me fat and slow me down.

Then about five years later I began longer distance racing—half-Ironman and Ironman distance races. At this time I was also in chiropractic school and became fascinated with applied kinesiology and the link between biochemistry and neurology. I ran into Phil at the popular St. Anthony's Triathlon in Florida. He took my

thetic hormone can cause bloating, depression, fatigue, increased hair on the body, or increased weight gain. Provera can also cause your body to diminish its own production of natural progesterone, forcing you to rely more on outside sources. Other synthetics can cause birth defects, epilepsy, asthma, and heart problems.

then-vegetarian wife and me out to dinner that night to a sushi restaurant! She was pissed, to say the least. I knew Phil was a good coach by the time we left. My wife had gone from being on a 100 percent "nothing-that-was-once-alive" diet for over ten years to leaving that restaurant having eaten raw fish.

Fast-forward fifteen years to 2010. I have had the unique perspective of putting Phil's principles to work not only as an athlete, but as a health-care professional. I've completed fifteen Ironman races as well as countless other endurance events throughout the United States, all without any major injury or illness. Proper training principles and dietary guidelines have been the reason for such success. Rarely do I train without a heart-rate monitor.

I think the main message behind Phil's teachings is this: Do whatever you can to reduce stress and optimize your health and fitness potential. It's not just about training. It's not just about your diet. It's not about fitness or race performance. It's about achieving your maximum physical and mental health, and it can't be done by just practicing one principle. You can exercise aerobically your entire life and still be aerobically deficient if your diet is riddled with refined carbohydrates. You can have major hormonal imbalances, particularly high cortisol and low sex hormones, if you're under significant mental stress, even if you eat a diet that is high in good fats and high-quality protein. It's all got to come together. I see this time and time again in my practice dealing with patients who are under a significant amount of stress.

You've got to change what you can in your life to reach the maximum potential available to you at the time. In other words, if your job is extremely stressful and you've adjusted to it to the best of your ability, then diet and exercise become even more critical to balance out the work stress. Though your body will crave caffeine and refined carbohydrates, which are most likely readily available in your workplace, adjusting your diet as Phil describes will have a huge impact on your overall health and make the work stress much more manageable. So whether you are looking to cut some body fat, cut some minutes off your 10K, or cut your chances of developing any of the many diseases lurking out there, following an aerobic lifestyle is the foundation for it all.

It's important to note that both estrogen and progesterone work together. In a real sense, they balance each other when in their natural state. Taking one form without the balance of the other often creates stress.

Testosterone is also a naturally occurring hormone made by both men and women. It's important for healing, helps build and maintain muscles and bones, increases sex drive and overall energy, and is a very important hormone for other areas of the metabolism. The synthetic version is methyltestosterone, with side effects including hormonal imbalance, intestinal distress, increased cholesterol, hair loss, depression, anxiety, and others.

All these hormones, and others made by the body, are important for optimal endurance and health. The ideal scenario is to have your body make the types and amounts of hormones necessary for you. That amount varies from day to day and year to year (even from minute to minute). If reduced health interferes with this delicate mechanism, imbalances can occur.

If you have signs and symptoms related to hormone imbalance, measuring your hormone levels by testing your saliva is very important. A reevaluation of the same tests will help you know whether improved lifestyle habits or any replacement therapy is successful.

It's important to ask your health-care professional about these alternatives as many are by prescription. And, it's important to understand the legal ramifications of using natural hormones in sport. For more information, contact the Women's International Pharmacy (800-279-5708, www.WomensInternational.com), Hopewell Pharmacy (800-792-6670, www.HopewellRX.com), or another reliable source.

Some non-prescription hormone products are also available. Pro-Gest, for example, is a natural progesterone cream that can be absorbed through the skin rather than taken by mouth (your liver breaks down much of the natural hormone taken orally). For those who require both natural estrogen and progesterone, a cream product called OstaDerm is also a non-prescription preparation of both natural hormones.

For menopause, premenstrual syndrome, or other hormone-related imbalances, the use of natural hormones can improve your quality of life. What's most important is to understand that no one has to live with the pain, displeasure, and discomfort that too many doctors have told patients are normal with aging.

I can't emphasize enough that preventing and correcting hormone imbalance by improving adrenal function and overall fitness and health is the most effective and best first option. And, athletes with hormone imbalances often have an undiagnosed overtraining syndrome.

# CHAPTER 8

# THE OVERTRAINING SYNDROME

Overtraining is the most common problem that prevents endurance athletes from reaching their potential. It's also the most common cause of injury and ill-health for millions of athletes. And overtraining is a problem that many athletes, coaches, and health-care professionals don't recognize until it becomes a more serious condition.

As a result, overtraining is not recognized soon enough to prevent loss of training time, injury, ill-health, or poor performance. In other words, overtraining is too often remedied in a reactive way, after it's happened, rather than preventatively. Overtraining is the accumulation of various physical, chemical, and mental stresses.

Overtraining has been traditionally described as diminished performance that results from an increase in either training volume or intensity. Let me emphasize this point again: Overtraining is an imbalance in our simple endurance equation:

## Training = Work + Rest

Overtraining has multiple causes and effects—and all are associated with brain, muscle, metabolic, and other problems. Because of this complex overlapping, it makes better sense to use a broader term known as "overtraining syndrome." This condition can vary considerably from one athlete to another, including its signs, symptoms, and onset.

Prevention and correction of the overtraining syndrome begin with careful, ongoing assessments. Observing subtle symptoms in their earliest stages are crucial to the prevention of further regression. You might be experiencing increased stress. The MAF Test is also a powerful tool for assessing overtraining as it begins to develop and may provide the first objective sign—a red flag telling you to pause, listen to your body, and make appropriate changes. Otherwise, the next indication, one more obvious, will be a physical injury that impairs training, illness that interferes with racing, or worsening performances.

## The Big Picture

Let's look at the big picture of overtraining, not just its more obvious components. This is a holistic approach. And to do so, we first need to take a look at how our nervous system works since this will have a profound impact on how the body responds to training.

Understanding the details of the brain and the rest of the nervous system, and all its components, including the autonomic system, can get quite complicated. So here's an analogy. Consider a house with all the many wires going throughout, some wires being different types for specific purposes. All these wires represent different parts of the nervous system. Some go to switches and lights, some to large users of electricity like air conditioners and refrigerators, still others to phones and modems, while others to low voltage devices like doorbells. The brain would be like the main electric box, and the autonomic system comprised of a cable of two wires, like those used for phone lines: one wire for sympathetic and another for parasympathetic.

The sympathetic part of the autonomic system raises your heart rate and blood pressure, increases muscle power and speed, and other actions used in a race, for example. We feel this as pre-race tension, an important way to prepare for competition. The parasympathetic part is important for recovery, relaxation of muscles, slowing the heart rate, and lowering blood pressure. And it activates the intestines for better digestion.

The sympathetic has been compared to the accelerator in your car, making things go faster, while the parasympathetic component is likened to the brakes, slowing it down.

While the autonomic system functions automatically, we can influence it through lifestyle. The sympathetic part tends to be ready to go into action much of the time, so we often control autonomic function through the addition of more parasympathetic activities to balance both. We can do this by choosing to relax, by meditating, and by avoiding too much caffeine (a sympathetic stimulator).

When autonomic imbalance occurs, it's usually associated with too much sympathetic and too little parasympathetic activity; with chronic imbalance, as seen in the third stage of stress, just the opposite occurs: the sympathetics "burn out" and can't function well, and the parasympathetics take over. Overtraining follows this pattern and, the same as Selye's General Adaptation Syndrome, has three stages of stress.

The negative consequences of overtraining are often gradual. The body is quite good at masking the earliest symptoms. But overtraining is a canny adversary. The problems it engenders will triumph in the end, unless changes are made to training, diet, and stress level.

- *Stage 1 or functional overtraining.* The onset and earliest stage, very subtle indicators can clue you in that you're heading for more serious problems.
- *Stage 2 or sympathetic overtraining.* Brain and nervous system and hormonal imbalances cause a variety of signs and symptoms.
- *Stage 3 or parasympathetic overtraining.* A serious condition, it results in exhaustion, severely affecting the nervous system, muscles, and hormonal levels.

The overtraining syndrome typically results in poor athletic performance, structural injury, such as in the foot, knee, or lower back, secondary to muscle imbalance, and metabolic problems, such as fatigue, infection, bone loss, sexual dysfunction, altered mood states, and brain and nervous system dysfunction. The signs and symptoms go beyond training and competition problems; they can even affect a person's quality of life, sometimes for many years. More importantly, in the earliest stage many of the problems of overtraining are somewhat vague and indistinct unless a careful evaluation is made.

While we think of overtraining as being only sports-related, other lifestyle factors may contribute to the cause. Increased work, family or job stress, social obligations, raising children, poor sleep habits, and other factors can significantly and indirectly contribute to overtraining.

## Functional Conditions

The earliest onset of overtraining can be very elusive. This is an example of a functional problem, often with few, if any, obvious signs or symptoms to let you know something is wrong. Understanding functional conditions is very important especially in relation to understanding the first stage of the overtraining syndrome.

Functional conditions in athletes are common. While some have serious symptoms, such as debilitating pain, even these problems are usually not accompanied by serious conditions, such as a torn tendon or broken bone. Functional problems are sometimes called "subclinical." This state of dysfunction makes up the majority of complaints by athletes. For example, a cyclist may have low back pain, whether mild or severe, but show no positive neurological, X-ray, or MRI findings. Another person may experience significant fatigue but show normal values in all blood, urine, and other tests. Yet another person has acute diminishing athletic performance but by all standard medical assessments continues to be in the so-called normal ranges. This contributes to serious frustration in the athlete, who as a result often goes from one health-care professional to another looking for a traditional diagnosis. However, a standard diagnosis—a ruptured disc in the case of back pain, pernicious anemia in those very fatigued—is not appropriate for these functional problems. Moreover, there are no common names that can be attached to functional problems. Unfortunately, many patients expect and want a fancy medical name for their problem; when they have one, accurate or not, misdiagnosed or not, they embrace it.

In my own practice, some patients even listed conditions on the forms they initially filled out before meeting with me that included fancy diagnoses such as Osgood Slaughter's disease (a childhood condition of the shinbone below the knee). When I asked them about it, they would say that the diagnosis was given to them twenty years earlier; they've been holding on to this "condition" for two decades!

Lateral knee pain in an endurance athlete is another example, typically the result of simple muscle imbalance, no matter how serious the pain. But explaining that to some patients is not as reassuring or comforting as calling it "iliotibial band syndrome." Worse is that western medical practice and health-care insurance companies demand a standard diagnosis, one from a long list of possibilities they provide, for each condition. But explaining the real condition to an insurance company and not playing the name game results in less or, more often, no coverage. This has resulted in doctors coming up with the closest named condition regardless of the accuracy of the diagnosis. I often made fun of this dilemma by saying to athletes, after they didn't get an expected named condition, that I could make up a name if it would make them feel better. That often produced a nervous laugh. I would then explain my findings, mentioning significant factors such as muscle imbalance and inflammation; how the injury could have occurred (improper bike form); how it could be corrected (through biofeedback and dietary changes); and how soon they'd be free from pain and begin to train again.

Another type of functional problem can occur in many athletes who possess various signs and symptoms not related to an injury or disease. Examples include an elevated resting heart rate, low body temperature, irregular gait, and other abnormal findings. In many cases, these functional problems are not only manifestations of the pre-injury state, but contribute to a lack of endurance progress. They're much easier to observe in an athlete, rather than for an athlete himself to feel it. Watching an athlete run, bike, or swim, for example, often shows these physical irregularities. This is known as "body language"—observing how the body portrays some imbalance. If left unchecked, it may result in an overtraining related injury, or eventually even disease.

Functional problems make it easier to understand that an injury is not always synonymous with pain, trauma, or obvious debilitation. It is possible for an injury to be an asymptomatic dysfunction, producing no symptoms.

A functional injury is a dysfunction in the body's structural, chemical, or mental and emotional process. It is somewhere between the state of optimal health or excellent function and specific injury or disease. A common functional problem in an endurance athlete marks the first stage of the overtraining syndrome.

## Stage 1: Functional Overtraining

The first stage of overtraining is not usually accompanied by obvious problems, but rather, by very subtle or subclinical ones. The most obvious may be an abnormal plateau or regression in your MAF Test, indicating an imbalance between aerobic and anaerobic function. In addition, changes in such measurements as heart rate variability begin to appear, and resting heart rate may start to rise.

Interestingly, this first stage of overtraining is sometimes accompanied by a sudden, short-lived improvement in competitive performance that may convince one that training is progressing well. This temporary improvement, which often exists in one race, for example, may be caused by the autonomic nervous system imbalance resulting in overactivity of the sympathetic part, temporarily improving muscle function and strength. This is accompanied by an imbalance between the aerobic and anaerobic systems.

The aerobic and anaerobic imbalance may be determined by various tests, some of which are not readily accessible to many athletes. These include an evaluation of respiratory quotient (RQ), salivary cortisol measurements, and others. However, the easiest evaluations for all athletes are the MAF Test and testing the resting heart rate. In addition, comparing max

aerobic training performance, such as the first mile of an MAF Test, with competitive performance, such as the average pace per mile in a 10K race, could demonstrate this imbalance. Runners, for example, will have a relatively slower aerobic pace, as per their MAF Test, compared to a faster race pace. This occurs because, in this first stage of overtraining, the aerobic system is deficient, while the anaerobic system is overactive.

Stage 1 overtraining develops out of the phenomenon of *overreaching*, the normal state in which athletes train slightly beyond their ability. This slight stress on the body's physical, chemical, and mental state is an important aspect of becoming a better athlete, so it's necessary. In fact, studies show this gray area between easy training and overtraining—overreaching—can boost performance. But without backing off, many athletes continue pushing down the road to overtraining. Exactly when you go from overreaching to overtraining is difficult to assess. But if the MAF Test shows a slowing of pace, you've passed the normal state of overreaching into the first stage of overtraining. You may even have one last good performance in you, although in some cases you're already injured and can't race. In the overreaching state, more time is needed for recovery, and when this is not done, the onset of overtraining amplifies minor functional imbalances, often progressing to symptoms of pain or fatigue, along with signs of higher resting heart rates and slowing MAF Tests.

## HEART RATE VARIABILITY (HRV)

In addition to resting heart rate and the MAF Test, heart rate variability also reflects autonomic imbalance and can be used to monitor training, stress, and other relationships including heart health. HRV is a measurement of the time between each heart beat while resting and provides much more information than just knowing the resting rate. The heart, in fact, speeds up when you inhale, and slows down when you exhale. A healthy, well-rested body will produce a larger gap and higher HRV than a stressed-out, overtrained body.

While more detailed measurements of HRV (along with other factors) is best achieved by an ECG (electrocardiogram) evaluation by a cardiologist, any athlete can measure HRV at home using a simple, practical, and useful method.

During my years in practice, in addition to resting heart rate and the MAF Test, I used a modified master's two-step test to help assess autonomic function. As you would expect, autonomic balance, as measured by HRV, is main-

---

The first stage of overtraining is usually accompanied by two other functional problems. The first is adrenal gland dysfunction and, typically, aerobic deficiency is also part of the overtraining syndrome at this early period. Fatigue, physical injury, sleeping irregularities, abnormal hunger, or cravings, especially for sweets and refined carbohydrates, and other complaints related to adrenal and aerobic problems mark a more obvious Stage 1 overtraining. Some athletes may be unable to lose that extra body fat, get sleepy after meals, and have an uncanny craving for caffeine, or other signs and symptoms.

Other complaints common in the first stage of overtraining include:

- Increasing vulnerability to back, knee, ankle, and foot injuries
- Abnormal adrenal hormone levels—typically, elevations in cortisol only at certain times of the day or evening, with secondary lowering of testosterone, estrogen, and/or DHEA levels
- Amenorrhea in women, or secondarily, premenstrual syndrome or menopausal symptoms
- Reduced sexual desire, with infertility in some cases

tained following an aerobic workout; however, after an anaerobic workout, autonomic balance is slightly disturbed until the body recovers. In addition, athletes who maintain a good balance of autonomic function, as indicated by HRV, perform better.

Today, new technology allows athletes to more accurately monitor their HRV. A device called the "ithlete" is compatible with iPhones and touch-screen iPods, allowing you to record your resting heart rate for one minute using a standard chest strap heart monitor and accurately calculate your HRV. The device provides great animation of the heart and lungs in action, graphs of your results, stores your personal information, and allows for daily testing comparing your weekly and monthly results. As such, it warns you if HRV worsens, indicating an autonomic imbalance and the need for additional rest that day, or an easy rather than hard workout. For more information on HRV and the ithlete, go to www.ithlete.net.

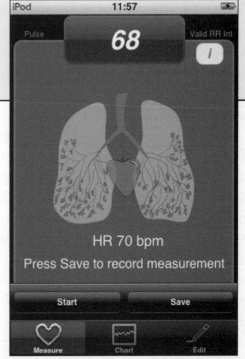

- Mental and emotional stress, including mild depression and anxiety

When the first stage of functional overtraining is not corrected by making the appropriate training, stress, diet, or other changes, all these signs, symptoms, and functional problems worsen, and the athlete enters into the second stage of the overtraining syndrome.

### Stage 2: Sympathetic Overtraining

Many health-care professionals and athletes recognize the start of overtraining in Stage 2. But by this point, as overtraining

*Monochrome image of ithlete screen at end of 60-second test showing heart rate variability value at the top and resting heart rate beneath the lungs.*

progresses, imbalances of various systems worsen and become more difficult to remedy easily. Specifically, the sympathetic part of the nervous system becomes even more overactive than in Stage 1, with further worsening of the aerobic system. There is a more significant elevation in the resting heart rate and training heart rate, which further worsens the MAF Test. Many athletes become aware of this if they regularly measure their morning heart rate and train with a heart-rate monitor. Often associated with this elevated heart rate is restlessness and over-excitability.

Stage 2 overtraining is more common in athletes with anaerobic training as a significant part of their workout schedules, including those with too much training volume, those with too much lifestyle stress, and most often those athletes who have a combination of these factors.

Adrenal gland dysfunction and aerobic deficiency more noticeably worsen during sympathetic overtraining. Cortisol output may rise to abnormal levels at various points throughout the day and night. The keen awareness and fine eye-hand coordination required in some sports are adversely affected by these hormone problems. High cortisol levels also have a harmful effect on the physical, chemical, and mental state, much like that produced by exhaustive, prolonged training, including the development of more significant muscle imbalances.

High cortisol also can increase insulin levels, which reduces fat burning and increases fat storage. While aerobic training usually suppresses insulin production during exercise, studies show that maximal training intensities can increase the insulin response significantly. This problem also further raises sympathetic system activity, increases carbohydrate intolerance with more carbohydrate foods converting to fat, and worsens the overtraining syndrome. In addition, elevated cortisol lowers testosterone and DHEA, both important for muscle recovery. Those who frequently wake in the middle of the night and don't easily fall back asleep typically have high cortisol levels, which is another sign of overtraining.

Fortunately, this hormone imbalance is relatively easy to correct through diet and lifestyle changes, including one's training and competition schedules. Those who don't listen to their body and continue overtraining can have worsening signs and symptoms, including reduction in performance and development of chronic injuries. Many athletes remain stuck in this stage of overtraining for months and even years; some "progress" into a more serious and third stage of overtraining.

### Stage 3: Parasympathetic Overtraining

Chronic overtraining can lead to more serious brain, muscle, and metabolic imbalances. These continue to parallel chronic adrenal dysfunction and aerobic deficiency. Eventually, the body becomes exhausted, and many hormones are significantly reduced. In the adrenal glands, for example, the ability to produce normal levels of cortisol, DHEA, testosterone, and other hormones is lost; the result is just the opposite from Stages 1 and 2—low cortisol. This contributes to a worsening physical, chemical, and mental condition.

Stage 3 is typically accompanied by the lack of desire to compete and sometimes train, depression, significant injury, and most notably severe exhaustion. Performance may diminish considerably and many athletes in this state consider themselves "sidelined" or even retire from competitive sports. They are chronically fatigued, can't keep up their normal training or racing paces, and typically have serious physical injuries. The MAF Test has usually regressed dramatically as the training heart rate is high, even though there is an abnormally low resting heart rate (the now overactive parasympathetic system lowers the resting heart rate). The chronic hormonal problems can result in increased sodium loss due to reduced aldosterone (the adrenal hormone that regulates minerals and water) and may increase the athlete's vulnerability to hyponatremia—a serious condition of low sodium (although this condition can also appear in Stage 2). Athletes who are in the third stage of overtraining are seriously unwell, with some heading to chronic diseases of the heart, blood vessels, and other areas. Recovery and return to previous optimal levels of performance is a very difficult task.

∽

I've treated many athletes who came to my clinic in all the stages of overtraining. In addition, I've also watched too many athletes go through all three stages. One of the great American distance runners, Alberto Salazar, is a prime example. He wasn't a patient of mine but his story has been told in countless magazine articles. In a span of three years, his performances were nothing short of amazing. He made the U.S. Olympic team in 1980 during the boycott. In his marathon debut later that same year, Salazar won his first marathon in New York. Just three months later, he set an American indoor 5K record (13:22). He also won the New York City Marathon the next two years and won the Boston Marathon in 1982. Along the way that year, he set an American 5K (12:11) and 10K (27:25) record.

Media reports about Salazar's gruesome workout schedule made anyone wince with awe. I could not help thinking these incredible efforts could not last. And, seeing him a number of times at various races, I noticed his gait worsening. Around that time I met Salazar's coach, Bill Dellinger, also the University of Oregon's track coach, who himself was a three-time Olympian. We were both lecturing at a running camp. Dellinger had invited me to Oregon to see the school's program and facilities.

Soon afterward, I spent time at the university with Dellinger, at his home, and at Salazar's home. I witnessed Salazar's training and diet routine firsthand. At the track, I watched

Salazar run five one-mile repeats at 4:20 pace with a ninety-second one-lap recovery. There was no warm-up or cool-down; afterward Salazar drank two cans of soda and had lunch from Burger King.

Neither Dellinger nor Salazar were interested in making changes to a training routine that produced incredible victories in distances from 5K to the marathon. Salazar's training routine included not only hard running but also extremely high mileage; he was running 200-mile weeks at one point, thinking that more was better. In addition he raced often. By 1983, Salazar's times started to fall, beginning with a last-place finish in the 10K at the World Track and Field Championships, and two fifth-place finishes in the Rotterdam and Fukuoka marathons that year. He made the U.S. Olympic marathon team in 1984, but finished in fifteenth place at the Olympic race in Los Angeles.

## QA

**Question:** Long before I sensibly incorporated the MAF program into my running, every few months I would get to a certain level of conditioning—say, like ninety minutes—then my body would seem to start falling apart. Not a specific injury, but more like general fatigue and heavy-legs syndrome. That was then. Now, after six months of MAF training, that type of fatigue is thankfully gone. Last week, I went on a five-hour trail run, and all went reasonably well. My quads were a bit trashed from all the downhills, but I was in good shape and rested for the following four days, except for an easy one-hour bike ride. My first run was a forty-five-minute hilly run, at a slow pace. My legs still felt a little tired—but what I noticed was that there wasn't fatigue or heavy legs like I'd had before MAF. Can you explain the difference between normal "soreness" and abnormal "soreness" caused by overtraining?

**Answer:** One difference is having built a good aerobic base. This will help with recovery in a dramatic way. For example, improved circulation brings in more nutrients and removes waste products, and improved aerobic muscle function better supports joints and muscles. Essentially, what you were experiencing in the past was an injury, albeit not your typical injury but one from which you could not recover quickly, like your body today can. Poor recovery is sometimes a chemical type of injury along with deficiencies in the aerobic system. Congratulations on remedying this problem. Being sore from some injury is usually more painful and longer lasting than being sore from a hard effort or a long hilly race, from which you can recover much faster.

Illness and injury became a chronic problem, and Salazar was always looking for a diagnosis of the cause of his declining performances. After the 1984 Olympics, Salazar attempted various comebacks, but his body and brain never allowed him to race seriously again. He reportedly even took Prozac for motivation to train. Salazar turned to coach other runners for Nike. In 2007, Salazar had a serious heart attack, and in 2008 was hospitalized again for severe high blood pressure and dehydration.

∽

There are two important responses regarding the overtraining syndrome. The first, and most important, is to prevent it from occurring by learning how to get the most out of your training without going over the line. The second is recovering from overtraining if you're already there.

### Prevent Overtraining

One key to avoiding the overtraining syndrome is biofeedback, including measuring the resting heart rate, training at your maximum aerobic heart rate, and the MAF Test.

Overtraining is a reflection of an imbalance of the autonomic nervous system's two components—the sympathetic and parasympathetic mechanisms. With imbalance, overtraining in Stages 1 and 2 is a demonstration of excess sympathetic and diminished parasympathetic activity, while Stage 3 is the loss of sympathetic function with too much parasympathetic.

An example of how the body responds to autonomic dysfunction—the imbalance of sympathetic and parasympathetic—can be seen with resting heart rate. Most athletes are aware that if the morning resting heart rate is higher than usual, it may signal some problem such as an oncoming illness, excess stress, or overtraining. This is due to an increase in sympathetic activity, which raises the heart rate. The higher resting rate also accompanies a higher training heart rate as reflected by a slower MAF Test. The interesting phenomenon of a sudden increased performance being associated with the early stage of overtraining is due to the fact that overactivity of the sympathetic system temporarily improves muscle strength and raises blood sugar, but it's done at the expense of overall fitness and health.

Likewise, chronic overtraining in the third stage is associated with a lower resting heart rate due to the parasympathetic effects accompanied by the loss of normal sympathetic function. However, in the case of an MAF Test, this won't make you run or bike faster because your training heart rate is still higher.

Balance of the autonomic system is key. Both sympathetic and parasympathetic are working all the time in some type of balance depending on whether you're working out, resting, or racing. For example, before a big event you generally feel a bit anxious and tense, some athletes more than others. This is normal, and an example of the sympathetic

# WOMEN AND OVERTRAINING

Physician, athlete, and holistic family practitioner Coralee Thompson, MD, says that "over-trained female athletes often have serious metabolic problems, particularly with hormone imbalance. The most common sign of this problem is amenorrhea, the absence of a menstrual period." A recent published study (Archives of Physical Medicine and Rehabilitation) showed that 40 percent of a group of female triathletes had a history of amenorrhea. Other common menstrual abnormalities include oligomenorrhea (a menstrual cycle between thirty-five and ninety days), and, in young athletes, delayed menarche (onset of first period).

Amenorrhea is a sign of a potentially serious problem for athletes, now and for their future health. The hormonal imbalance causing menstrual dysfunction can also adversely affect sports performance. Dr. Thompson states, "The long-term risks of such hormonal imbalance include infertility, osteoporosis, and sexual and adrenal dysfunction."

Overtraining and its associated lifestyle factors, especially dietary imbalance, contribute to amenorrhea. Endurance athletes, those focused on aesthetics, and those involved with high-intensity training and competition are at greatest risk.

In the study cited above, 60 percent of the group had diets deficient in calories and nutrients, especially protein, healthy fats, and calcium. Excessively low body weight and body fat frequently accompany this deficiency. Femoral fat stores—those around the hips, buttocks, and thighs—are important for female health. While some amenorrheic athletes consume an energy-deficient diet, others consume the same total calories as those with normal menstrual cycles but eat much less protein and fat (up to 50 percent less) and more refined carbohydrates (which alone can contribute to amenorrhea). Reduced fat intake can interfere with calcium absorption, resulting in lower total bone calcium. This is typically aggravated by concurrent low dietary calcium intake. In spite of this, blood levels of calcium most often remain normal.

Dr. Thompson also says, "Disordered eating itself is a complex issue, involving a full spectrum of problems from poor eating, dieting, and preoccupation with low fat consumption to clinically diagnosed anorexia nervosa and bulimia. The hormonal equilibrium that regulates reproductive function can also be affected by other psychological factors, the stress associated with athletic competition being a significant variable."

Bone loss is one of the most serious problems associated with amenorrhea and is secondary to hormone imbalance. This includes reduction in growth hormone which results in reduced training benefits and poor recovery. Overtraining and competition elevate the body's stress hormone cortisol. This overproduction of cortisol "steals" from female hormone production, resulting in lower estrogen, testosterone, and progesterone levels. This hormonal imbalance is very similar to the postmenopausal state. When this occurs at a younger age, the body has more time to lose bone and muscle. Decreased bone density increases the risk of stress fractures, muscle problems, and physical fatigue—serious conditions for the athlete now and later in life. Bone loss most commonly occurs in the spine, hip, wrist, and foot. Scoliosis (abnormal curvature of the spine) is an additional risk of bone and muscle problems.

Further structural problems in the skeleton occur later in life due to osteoporosis. Similar hormonal balances may be seen in men, specifically associated with reduced testosterone, which also causes bone loss and increased risk of fractures. Despite outdoor training, the lack of proper sun exposure and reduced levels of vitamin D, not uncommon in female athletes, places women at further risk of bone loss, muscle imbalance, and other health problems.

As more women of all ages aspire to strenuous athletics and competition, preventing the overtraining syndrome is most important. Young girls under the influence of coaches, teachers, and famous athletes need to understand that consuming an abundance of healthy nutrients and avoiding junk food and drinks is critical to their success as athletes and their health. Coaches and trainers have a responsibility to help prevent the overtraining mentality that grips budding young athletes. When one recognizes the overtraining syndrome, a comprehensive approach to treatment—including diet and nutrition, balanced training and competition, and stress management—can successfully reestablish normal hormonal profiles and menstrual activity in athletes. A healthier athlete will also compete better, without injury, and for longer periods.

system preparing you for the event. When your race is done, and you finally settle in for a nice relaxing dinner—now your sympathetic system can quiet down—and your parasympathetic system is dominating. Imagine if that pre-race tension was always with you. Your sympathetic system would be stuck in the "on" position—you'd be unable to relax and have continuous anxiety and tension. That's what the first two stages of overtraining are like.

# Recovery from Overtraining

Even in the early Stage 1 functional over-training, the significant imbalance should be corrected as the first step to a better approach to endurance training. In order to remedy this problem, it must first be properly assessed so that treatment and improvement can also be monitored. In addition to the MAF Test and HRV, other evaluations are very important. Questions that pertain to mood, energy levels, sleep quality, performance, and infections are also important to answer and monitor. Proper diet and stress management are often key components of proper recovery from overtraining.

Correcting overtraining often begins by immediately restructuring the training schedule, modifying lifestyle factors including diet and nutrition, and addressing all levels of stress. Here are some other suggestions that will get you and your body back in sync:

### Training

- Decrease training time by 50 to 70 percent, or more if necessary.
- Immediately cease all anaerobic training and competition.
- A helpful remedy for an overtrained athlete is walking, which can gently stimulate circulation and aerobic muscles and offers mental benefits much like those of meditation. Walking also helps redevelop

the aerobic system—the first phase of retraining.

- Building (or rebuilding) the aerobic base may take three to six months and does not include any anaerobic training or competition. This time period should be sufficient for most athletes in Stages 1 and 2 to recover well. Stage 3 may take much longer.

### Diet and Nutrition

- Reduce (or eliminate) all high-glycemic foods, which are mostly processed grains such as most breads and products made from flour, and all sugar and sugar-containing foods. Moderating carbohydrate intake overall can also be helpful as high-carbohydrate diets may further elevate cortisol levels.
- Consume smaller, more frequent meals to help control blood sugar and cortisol, especially for those with symptoms of depression, fatigue, hunger, and restless sleep.
- Adequate caloric intake is very important—never get hungry. Include moderate amounts of protein (especially eggs and meats) and healthy fats such as olive and coconut oils, avocados, and nuts and seeds.
- Overtraining may disrupt the normal balance of fats in the body, causing inflammatory-related injuries. Eliminate the intake of vegetable oils (soy, peanut, safflower, corn), which can promote inflammation. EPA (fish oil) supplements can help reduce

inflammation. (If serious inflammation exists, avoid all dairy fats too, including milk, cream, butter, and cheese.)

- Caffeine consumption may aggravate the overtrained state for many athletes. Avoid stimulants such as coffee, tea, soda, and chocolate (beware of caffeine-containing over-the-counter and prescription drugs). Some athletes can tolerate small amounts of caffeine, but many should avoid it completely.

- Malabsorption of nutrients is common in overtrained athletes due to the high stress levels causing poor intestinal function. This is especially common in those over the age of forty years. Dietary supplements such as betaine hydrochloride may improve digestion, and L-glutamine can improve nutrient absorption.

When committed, athletes can often recover rapidly from overtraining. This is especially true in Stage 1, where modifying the training schedule and making appropriate nutritional and dietary adjustments often provide improvements of symptoms and even the MAF Test within two weeks.

Athletes in the first and second stages of overtraining can respond quickly to proper recovery. However, those with upcoming competitions may be required to modify or cancel those events to allow for a more complete recovery from overtraining.

Athletes who are chronically overtrained—those in the third stage—generally respond much slower, even when the best care is available. They may need to cancel their next competitive season (as though they had a physical injury that prevented competing) and spend time building the aerobic system, reducing stress, and improving their nutrition. These athletes will require six months or more, and sometimes a year or two, before resuming effective competition.

# CHAPTER 9

# "PERSONALIZE" YOUR TRAINING—
## Less Often Means Success

**W**hile most professional athletes get paid to train and compete, the vast majority of endurance athletes are age-groupers who follow very similar training and are just as dedicated to their sport. As such, they must fit training and competition into a year filled with career, family, and other obligations.

If you're a serious recreational or amateur athlete, or even a professional without the luxury of a big sponsorship contract, you still need to carefully piece together the best possible training schedule that will help you achieve optimal performance in endurance events. The most important aspect of training, the one most neglected, and the real "secret" in endurance sports, is to individualize your workout and recovery schedules. And by individualize I mean make it personalized.

The main goal of training is to develop the ability to compete successfully and without injury or ill health. Then, your day-to-day schedule becomes a secondary feature—exactly how many minutes per day you train is no longer the main focus.

### Training Diary

Each of us have important stories to tell. And if you keep a training diary, part of your story is written in it. Like any story, you often have a good idea what may happen next. Is it time to add anaerobic training? Are you ready for competition? Are you getting stale? Your diary should include everything from total time and heart rates of each workout to which course you trained on that day and how far you went. It may mention the weather, how you felt, along with your fears and dreams. Most importantly, your diary should include a chart of all your MAF Tests. Neatly plot them out so a quick glance will give you the last few months of progress. Looking back over the past few months in your diary, you can more objectively assess your progress. Check for consistency and gradual increases in total time of each workout, indicating increased fitness. Write down your goals

Traditionally, most athletes record the distance and pace of the workout. For example, five miles at an 8:20 average pace or a thirty mile ride averaging 22 mph. However, it's better to emphasize total time and heart rate, for two reasons:

1. When measuring only distance, total training volume will diminish over time as aerobic speed improves. This results in the completion of the same course in less time.
2. When measuring only distance, some athletes feel pressured to complete a certain weekly mileage. This is a way to compare themselves to other athletes, training partners, or younger versions of themselves, or even compare to some

article written in a sports magazine that "recommends" a certain mileage. Heart rate is a more useful parameter than distance because it relates to the quality, rather than the quantity, of the activity.

### Training Volume

Perhaps a better title for this chapter is "Less Is More." Meaning that for the average athlete with other responsibilities, less training usually produces better athletic performance than trying to accumulate many miles and hours of training.

While I have worked with many professional athletes in virtually all sports during my career, the majority of the athletes I've helped are not professionals. I've learned that if you work a full-time job and have a family, a house, and other responsibilities, you can still train and perform at very high levels. But don't expect to be able to put in the same amount of time and mileage as professional athletes. Nor do you need to for success. In fact, many of these pros put in much less time training than you'd think.

Most of the time, I find that less rather than more total training hours per week allows for better recovery and less stress. This helps the aerobic system build itself much more efficiently. When your competitive season comes, you're more refreshed and ready to race.

I had one patient by the name of Carla who was a middle-of-the-pack triathlete in her late thirties with hopes of improving her times. But after her fourth year of diminishing returns, she searched for a better approach. After reading one of my earlier books, she strictly followed the program, except for one thing: her training schedule averaged eighteen hours per week. Unfortunately, Carla really didn't have the time for that amount of training, but she tried to squeeze in the workouts. She worked part-time and had a family with two young children. As a result, she woke earlier in the morning and stayed up later in the evening to catch up on other work. For Carla, this meant less sleep and inadequate recovery. After some improvements in her MAF during the first few months, she became very fatigued and began feeling physical discomfort in her lower back and knees.

In late fall, Carla came to my clinic for help. My first recommendation was that she reduce her schedule to about twelve hours per week—it was the only training schedule change necessary. Carla was doing everything else right. By next summer's racing season, eight out of nine races were personal bests for Carla, and she placed in the top five of her age-group in four of those events.

## Training Cycles

The importance of planning your training and competition, including racing goals, cannot be overemphasized. This means considering the twelve-month year as a cycle, with one or two base periods, and one or two competitive "seasons." In North America, for

**Q&A**

**Question:** On one wet, Sunday afternoon, I was plodding along in the heavy rain, all by myself, pleased with myself for going outside in the soup and running for forty-five minutes, when common sense might have said, "Stay indoors." Then, another runner appeared out of the mist and blazed right past. My initial instinct was to pick up the pace and not let him get ahead. Then I realized, "What's the point?" So I remained at my current (slow, aerobic) pace and watched him run off. Which leads me to the following questions: Is there a competitive gene in the brain? And why are some people so much more competitive than others? Can one be taught or trained to think or feel this way as an endurance athlete? Or is it something innate that we carry from birth? In fact, I have a training buddy who will not let anyone—strangers or friends—pass him on a bike training ride; he will practically kill himself to ensure that he always finishes first.

**Answer:** I think there are two forms of competition. One is healthy competition, which is based on a logical approach; first there's a great training routine, where we don't compete with anyone but ourselves in getting most fit. Next is the race, where we also compete with ourselves but can feed off others in a positive way. Healthy example, the weather dictates much of this pattern as competitive events occur mostly from spring to fall. For example, winter is generally a time to build an aerobic base, leading up to spring races. Summer is a stressful time with hot temperatures, making it a good period for recovery from competition and easier training again—and a time to build a bit more aerobic function. This leads to more competition in the fall, ending the season in December when your long aerobic base period starts again.

The training cycle can always be modified as various factors present themselves. For example, if an unexpected busy work schedule suddenly affects your training, or if an unfortunate bike crash slows your aerobic base building period, modifications are easily made. Or, if your MAF Tests are exceptionally good, or not progressing as well due to poor diet, adjustments can easily be made.

An important part of your diary can be the early winter, when you plan your training cycle for the next twelve months. You can also highlight specific races.

### Less Means Success

For many years, researchers have known that there is a limit to how much an athlete can train before it adversely affects performance. Many studies have shown that, compared to athletes who train with much more volume, lower-volume trained athletes can perform as well, if not better. The majority of your physical benefits received from training may occur

competition relies on the brain to balance the physical, chemical, and mental efforts used during training and racing.

Unhealthy competition is much more common. This is based on a "no pain, no gain" approach, where emotions can overshadow logic and common sense. With unhealthy competition, we can't face the fact that someone out there is more fit than we are, and, as if we can just turn on a switch to go faster than anyone else, we work ourselves into a rage to beat that person. It's more than a game, it's an obsession. It's like the bully we all knew in grade school, always looking for a fight. As mature adults, we should know better. Likewise, as intelligent endurance athletes, we want the best out of our bodies, and a well-planned strategy helps provide that, with a brain that also balances emotions.

Humans are naturally not only competitive, but very successful competitors. It's how we evolved so successfully as a species. So in a sense, we all have that built-in competitiveness. Those most successful can control it. In training and racing, like all other aspects of life, harnessing that attribute can make us better athletes.

# MY PERSPECTIVE—BY DR. CORALEE THOMPSON

*Dr. Coralee Thompson lectures worldwide and is known for her work with neurologically delayed children, and is author of the book* Healthy Brains, Healthy Children.

✳ ✳ ✳

Growing up on a small farm in Idaho, I was no stranger to hard physical work: changing sprinkler pipes, bucking alfalfa bales, tilling soil by hand, riding bareback, and swimming in the irrigation canals. I complied with the compulsory physical education classes, never enjoying the feeling of competition with my peers. I felt lanky, awkward, and slow with almost every sport. Not until college did I discover my natural grace and speed in the water. With a six-foot-plus arm span, I soon realized how effortless swimming could be and how fast I could move through the water.

Except on two occasions, competition did not appeal to me. The first "race" was during an intercollegiate event. I was eighteen years old. I entered six events in swimming and won them all: 100-free, 100-breast, 100-back, 100-butterfly, 500-free, and 500-back. The second "race" was during a masters swimming event in Cairo, Egypt. I was thirty-three years old. Once again, I won all the events that I entered. For a brief moment, I considered what a thrill athletic competition might be for me. Instead, I chose to continue a variety of physical activities while allowing myself to focus on the health and fitness of my developing children.

---

in the first ten weeks or so of the training cycle. For example, if your competitive season ends in November, then go on to build an aerobic base from December through mid-April, since the training benefits obtained in those early months, including those in the brain, muscles, and metabolism, can be maintained very easily. Afterward, you can then reduce your total workout time to make room in your schedule for anaerobic training as well as racing. By early July, you can slowly raise your aerobic training during the remaining summer months again—without the stress of anaerobic workouts or racing—before cutting back again in mid September for more anaerobic training and competition.

All this, of course, should be based on one's individual needs and conditioning. Some athletes won't use anaerobic training but instead add a couple of short races at the end of their base building, then begin a racing season. Others will not increase outdoor training time in the summer months if the weather is too hot.

As a mother and physician, I never pushed organized sports on my sons, although we exercised together every day. By age six and every fall until age thirteen, they would participate in their grade school–sponsored triathlon, which included 400 meters of swimming, ten kilometers of biking, and five kilometers of running. Throughout the year, we would swim two or three times a week and run at least four days a week. These workouts were always slow and easy. While running, the boys would wear heart-rate monitors to make sure their heart rates did not exceed 165 beats per minute. We had fun being together and feeling the positive effects of exercise. As soon as school finished, we would start biking together on park trails while gradually increasing the distance of successive rides. Two months before the triathlon, we would start putting two different exercises together, for example, run then swim. The most difficult transition was always biking followed by running. No matter how easily we would bike, our legs felt like jelly in the beginning of the run. By one month before the triathlon, every day included two exercises together. Two weeks before the event, we would do a mock trial. Every triathlon was a joyful experience among their classmates, teachers, and parents. When finished with their own triathlon, each kid would continue running with younger classmates until everyone had finished. Years following grade school, my sons would go back to coach, run with, and encourage the young triathletes. As a parent, my greatest satisfaction was not the result of the triathlons, but rather our consistent exercising together.

Despite the evidence that less training offers more benefits, overtraining due to high volume is still common. If you are training for a single sport, your schedule is usually easier than if you are a multisport athlete. Single-sport athletes will usually have one workout a day. The best time to do this is based more on your daily non-training schedule rather than on the latest ever-changing research. When do you work? What other obligations exist? Many runners, for example, find a morning workout most suitable. Athletes in other sports may have limits; swimmers usually have pool hours to consider, cyclists and skiers the weather. I frequently recommend single-sport athletes perform some other activity one to three times per week. As previously noted throughout this book, cross-training has a positive benefit, especially for the brain and nervous system, as long as it is aerobic and fits into your schedule.

If you are a multisport athlete, you may have a busier schedule. But this does not mean you have to perform each sport every

For one school year, we had an exchange student from Japan. Morokazu, thirteen, had amazing self-discipline in three distinct behaviors: he played the violin in the basement from two to four hours a day, he never ate processed foods, and he faithfully ran six days a week. I observed his running routine with curiosity. He would slowly walk out the front door, looking at his watch, taking small steps with increasing speed and breadth. While checking his watch several times, he would begin a slight jog down the block. About fifteen minutes later, he would round the corner and pass the house running at an easy pace. Each time he would pass the house, he would be running faster, but still looking comfortable and relaxed. After about five passes or so (just over five miles), he would begin walking again while periodically checking his watch. On the weekends, he would be out running for up to two hours and return to the house as if he'd simply walked around the block. From time to time and with quiet pride, he would tell me about his best mile times—6:30, for example. I admired his method. One day, he showed me his exercise "bible," a book written in Japanese called *The Maffetone Method*. From then on, I followed Phil's recommendations, too. One is never too old to learn from a child.

Both of my sons are grown now, but every time they visit me, we still take the time for long hikes. It's just a way of life.

day. However, many endurance athletes still attempt this, and often to their detriment. Let me use the example of Jay. He loved triathlon but was stuck in an overtraining cycle for three years. He would train in each of his three events as many days as possible. He would run at 5 AM, swim at noon, and ride late in the day. The problem: Jay had his own business and worked from 7 AM until 9 PM He also had a family. Maintaining that schedule for five days, with Tuesday and Thursday reserved for his long bike ride and run

respectively, was quite a chore. Jay was often exhausted, and about every couple of months, he'd have to take about a week off completely due to illness. As he started feeling better, he would pick up his "normal" schedule again. But as this vicious cycle would not end, Jay consulted me for help. I gave Jay my version of a program tailored to his needs, explaining how he would race better and get healthier. However, he could not understand how one could improve without the very high-volume weeks, noting that the pro triathletes all trained that way. I assured him this was not the case. Unfortunately, Jay was not compatible with my approach, and I never saw him again in my office. But occasionally we would meet at a race, where year after year he showed no improvement and often had an injury.

If you're a multisport athlete with at least three days a week of each activity, your schedule can be very effective, although even this much volume is not always necessary. If possible, spread these workouts through the week so they are not on consecutive days. For example:

- Swim—Monday, Wednesday, Saturday
- Bike—Tuesday, Thursday, Saturday, Sunday
- Run—Monday, Thursday, Sunday

### Rest Days

Notice the above schedule has nothing planned for Friday. It may be the end of a workweek, and the beginning of a busy training weekend, making Friday a perfect "off" day. If you feel better calling this a "rest" or "recovery" day, that's perfectly okay. Sometimes the word "off" refers to not doing anything. But these days provide a most important part of the training formula that I like to keep repeating in this book due to its overpowering significance:

**Training = Work + Rest**

For most athletes, the weekend can be a time for longer workouts, including one on the bike on Saturday and a long run Sunday. Or, you can combine two events and make one longer workout such as a two-hour bike followed by a forty-five-minute run. A favorite cold weather workout is a swim immediately followed by an hour of indoor biking on rollers or a trainer. These combined sessions provide not only a longer workout but also help mimic race transitions, where your body has to adjust to the stress of changing from one event to another.

I often recommend at least one rest day per week to help with recovery. During the racing season, you will more easily maintain your fitness level with less training but require more recovery; in fact, two rest days are even better since anaerobic stimulation (from training or racing) will be added. Off days are best taken going into a weekend, if that is your busiest training time or if there is a race. Another appropriate time is Monday, which is a day when a lot of your energy is needed for recovery. Or make Monday an easy day if Friday is an off day and the weekend includes a lot of training.

When planning rest days (and easy ones), consider job stress too. If Mondays are always busy at work, don't train that day.

Seasonal stress may also be a factor. If you own a retail business and your busiest time is the fall holiday season, end racing before that time.

Another important time to take it easy is at the end of your training and competitive season. For some athletes, this may be

November or December. At this time, I recommend taking up to two or three weeks off, or more if you need it. While periods of rest are helpful for the body, a mental break is just as important. During this time just let your body do what it wants: easy running, hiking, or walking. Some athletes seem to benefit from doing nothing for a week or so. Or, train short and easy every other day instead of doing it daily.

CHAPTER 10

# COMPETITION—
## Getting Ready for Race Day

For a majority of endurance athletes, it all comes down to one word: competition. Racing should not only be rewarding and fun, but serve as a valuable learning process that will help you in future events. Competition is the culmination of all your workout ethic and self-discipline; it is the end result of all your labors. Yet for many athletes, competition can also turn into a time of disappointment. Why is that? Let's examine the possible reasons.

My first rule for competition is planning. This should be a part of your twelve-month calendar. Many athletes have a variety of options for specific events, and as the endurance sports scene has grown, races are everywhere all year long. Just because it's April (or whatever the month) doesn't mean you have to compete, unless, of course, you're in a sport with required events, or you're under contract to perform at certain races. Don't let the calendar dictate your competitive schedule unless it's a necessity; it may not correlate with your body's readiness. If you want to compete at a certain time of year, make sure you're prepared by allowing enough time to build an aerobic base. If you compete too early in your training calendar, or too frequently throughout your racing season, it can frequently be a frustrating and depressing experience. For competitive success, three important actions must be effectively executed: preparation, implementation, and recovery.

## Preparation

The most important aspect of competition is in understanding of when your body is ready to race. This also involves planning for your competitive season as a whole, and in particular each race. The most effective way to determine the ideal time to start competing is to assess your body with the MAF Test, which guides your aerobic development. Building your aerobic base is the most important aspect of training, and the most significant factor in competition. So before your base period begins, be sure to plan for ample time to allow your body to build as much aerobic function as possible. An improvement in your aerobic speed and a natural plateau may indicate you've reached your maximum aerobic benefits for that base period. This may be a good time to start competing, or a time when shorter competitions can serve as anaerobic workouts. For many endurance athletes, the ideal approach is to build a significant aerobic base, then start competing. Let the early events satisfy any need for anaerobic stimulation.

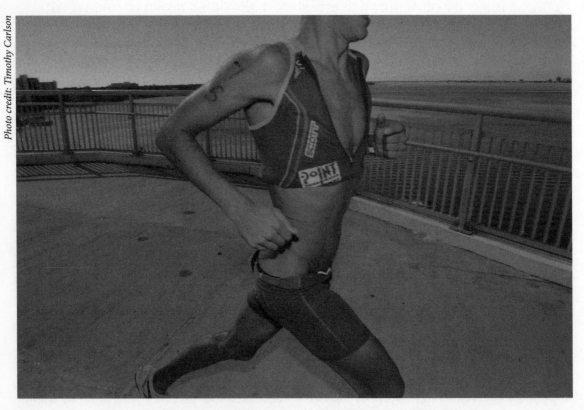

*Photo credit: Timothy Carlson*

**The most important aspect of competition is understanding when your body is ready to race.**

## Tapering

Reduction in training volume and intensity, or both, for a specific period of time previous to competition is called tapering. The most important benefit of *tapering* is increased recovery, which can improve the function of your brain, muscles, and metabolism. The ultimate goal of tapering is improved performance.

An optimum taper depends on the individual athlete, the training volume and intensity, and overall health. It's possible that athletes who are healthier may not require as much taper because they recover better from day-to-day training.

Tapering is traditionally considered before a big event, such as an Ironman triathlon or a marathon. But a taper is also very useful at the start of the competitive season. The period of time that encompasses the taper is typically from two to four weeks, depending on the event and how you feel. If you feel more tired than normal, have had a recent cold, flu, or other infection, or sustained some other type of injury, a longer taper can help assure better recovery, allowing the body to correct imbalances. This includes balancing muscles that may be a problem.

A taper can also be short, such as a day or two off before a shorter race. During this time, many athletes are a bit anxious, especially before the first race of the season or an important event. In this case, going for a relaxing walk during the two-day taper is ideal.

During a longer taper period, reduce your training in a stepwise fashion by 50 to 70 percent with less training as you get closer to your event. Add some off days during this period. For example, in a two-week taper, take one or two days off each week, including a day or two before the race. Walking can also be used during these off days. In addition, reduce or avoid all anaerobic training during the taper period. Each week, one or two downhill runs or spinning on your bike, for example, can help the brain and muscles maintain quickness.

When tapering, you won't lose fitness; in fact, your muscle strength can actually increase and there should be no reduction in your MAF Test. Another benefit of tapering is that resting significantly improves leg power; some studies have even noted improved arm strength in swimmers. Other benefits include improved lactate metabolism once competition begins.

Many athletes fear they'll lose fitness by taking days off. *But tapering is not the same as detraining,* which is the complete cessation of training. With no training, endurance is adversely affected within a two-week period. Even though the taper period is 50 to 70 percent less training, it not only maintains fitness but usually improves it because it allows better recovery, and thus the body can improve its function.

# Other Factors to Watch Before Racing

In addition to preparation and tapering, other factors should be considered.

## *Heart Rate*

The resting heart rate is one of the standby traditional biofeedback readings used for decades to help assess fitness. In the course of training, the resting heart rate normally lowers, the result of increased cardiac efficiency. If you have a cold or other stress looming over you, your resting heart rate increases a few or more beats reflecting that stress. As you approach your competitive season, your resting heart rate should be at or near its lowest level. However, the resting heart rate is not meant to be used exclusively as an indicator for anything, as doing that can mislead you. A case in point is during the third stage of overtraining, when the resting rate may actually diminish, making it appear like you're doing well. Without other indicators, such as how you feel, injuries, and especially your MAF Test, you can easily be misled.

## *Weight and Body Fat*

Both are a common concern for athletes, and an important part of race preparation. Many gain weight during the "off" season, due either to training less, eating the wrong foods, or both.

There are three important reasons weight and body fat are important for competition. First, if your body weight is too high for your frame, it can slow you down. That's due to more gravity stress, not to mention that more oxygen is required. But it does not mean the thinner you are, the faster you'll be. Like everything else in life, both extremes are dangerous.

A second potential problem is if you're too thin and have lost too much lean body mass, you'll have less muscle for competing. And, if you have too little fat stored, your metabolism as well as protective padding may be jeopardized, adversely affecting performance and health. That cushioning prevents damage to the bones in your feet when running, the pelvis when riding, and even organs and glands, which rely on fat padding for support.

A third factor is that those who have too much or too little body fat usually have muscle imbalance. In other words, if you're less fit and less healthy—a cause of too much or too little body fat—there is usually more muscle imbalance. Obviously, muscle imbalance will adversely affect race performance, but it also predisposes you to injury.

The ideal, of course, is not to gain weight or excess body fat in the winter. So, if your program is effective, your weight and fat content will come down to "normal" healthy levels.

## *Mental Readiness*

As your diary pages fill up, your training enjoyment should too. Note how you've felt along the way. For example, as your rides become longer, are they still playful? Is your long run leaving you with a more positive feeling about training? With this type of analysis, you'll more easily see your readiness to compete.

Also, and even more subjective, is your intuition. Brain fitness—your mental emotional state as it pertains to the brain-body connection and overall health—is a powerful preparation for competition. As you derive benefits from training, you should not only get more fit, but more healthy.

### Pre-Event Practices and Mistakes to Avoid

An important component to any individual competition is your pre-event routine—the habits you adopt the few days before your race. It's Thursday, and you're getting ready for Sunday's marathon. Your habits

over the next few days can make a dramatic difference in your race performance, and how well you recover.

Sometimes even subtle stresses can have significant effects on your race performance. Being aware of the most important ones, and making the appropriate adjustments, can help you have a more efficient and enjoyable race day:

1. Perhaps the most common nutritional deficiency in athletes before racing is water. Dehydration may increase with pre-race stress and especially during hot, dry weather. Athletes are too often dehydrated, with the problem more prevalent in the days before an event. The best way to remain hydrated is to drink small amounts of water—perhaps four to six

**Q&A**

**Question:** Why are some endurance athletes—I am thinking specifically of Mark Allen during his Ironman Hawaii heyday—so much better able to handle stress than their peers? Pre-race day, they seem so relaxed and calm. Or are they just better able to hide pre-competition jitters? Others, however, seem like basket cases—tense, stressed out, and nervous.

**Answer:** Part of an athlete's ability to handle stress better is associated with their confidence. They know the training has gone well, they feel good, and the discipline carries over to race day. Some have previously experienced the stress of race day in a negative way and have made a conscious effort to find a way to deal with it. But even Mark Allen had pre-race tension—it didn't show because of his powerful focus on the event at hand. Others have trouble controlling their stress, not just at a race but in all other facets of life. They get to the start on race day and it's as if they've already raced but now have to do another one.

ounces each time—throughout the day and evening, rather than a couple of high-volume loads here and there. Carry a water bottle around with you at all times.

2. Keep workouts to a minimum, if at all, in both duration and intensity. The best rule regarding training before a race, especially the few days before, is "less is best." You'll receive no race benefits by training during these last few days, but only potential stress that adversely affects your race. However, you want to keep loose and relaxed, as too little activity can make you stiff and jittery. Walking is the best option when you're feeling this way. And the day or two before the race you should consider taking off completely, using walking in order to stay loose.

3. While most athletes ponder the power behind their muscles, they usually underestimate the power of the mind. But you can train it just like your muscles. You have control over some potentially stressful activity before you race, namely how you think. Negative thoughts about the race can and should be turned into a positive outlook with realistic aspirations. You are in charge of your mind, but traditions, past experiences (yours and those of other people), and other memories have major influences. So remember, you're there to have fun and perform the best you can.

4. Continue to eat the same kinds of healthy food you're used to. Also, try to stay on the same time schedule. Late-night dinners with foods and alcoholic beverages you don't usually consume can potentially be dangerous to your performance. Remember, the body doesn't like too much change.

5. Follow the same race routine that has proven to work for you, assuming it's a healthy one. If you're not sure what works, pay more attention to your body. Don't just blindly copy what others do. Avoid trying new equipment, shoes, drinks, and food before and during your event. Experiment during training, not on the day of competition.

6. Warm-up on race morning. Depending on the distance and the event layout, you can walk or perform the particular activity you'll be competing in, but with very little intensity. If you have an adequate aerobic base, a good warm-up should total at least about twenty to thirty minutes for shorter races and at least fifteen minutes for any event.

7. Eating on the morning of an event is very individual. Experiment during a hard training workout or a low-key event to determine what works best. Avoid high-sugar foods and drinks since these can adversely affect fat burning during the race, reducing endurance.

## Implementation

Whether you're competing in a 5K road race or in a triathlon, the first rule of most competition is to not start too fast. That would push your body to burn more sugar, running the risk of depleting your glycogen stores early, which would cause your fat burning to diminish too. Starting some races at a comfortable pace, perhaps just slightly faster than your average speed for the race, is the most practical solution. It may take discipline to avoid getting caught up with the pack—most of whom will go out too hard. But don't worry; you'll pass them later in the race. This may not always work in events such as cycling and is more of a reason to warm up well. For some events, like ultramarathons, going slower for the first part of the race works even better. You'll build your speed throughout and finish very strong.

Another important component of competition is learning how to relax. The start of any event can leave you anxious and gripped with tension. Just think about standing there waiting for the start. Your heart rate is high, you're tense, and your breathing is fast and shallow. While some of this energy is important for the race, too much of it is an overstatement by the mind and an unnecessary drain of energy.

From the moments before the race starts, focus on your breathing and relaxation. If you're successful at this, your form will be better, your muscles more balanced, you'll have a lower heart rate, and your overall performance can improve—all from being more efficient. Perhaps you require a physical focus on race day; write the word *breathe* or *relax* on your hand or arm where you can easily see it.

Another successful and important strategy is to avoid high peaks in your heart rate during the event. This can only be done if you're using a heart-rate monitor, unless you're very experienced or well in sync with your body. The

**Q&A**

**Question:** I always have difficulty falling asleep the night before a triathlon. In fact, it's the same whether it's a full Ironman or sprint race. I am lucky to get three solid hours of sleep. I am waking up constantly, or tossing and turning. What strategies or tips can you recommend for a good night's sleep?

**Answer:** This is not unusual, as pre-race tension can keep you awake long after you've gotten into bed. In addition to dealing with stress better, sticking to your usual routine can be very helpful. This means keeping the same eating habits and other daily activities, and avoiding getting caught up in the many pre-race festivities—these are for all the non-competitors but not for you. These activities are where you'll find many other stressed competitors. An easy walk after dinner may be very helpful in relaxing, and a hot tub or shower right before getting into bed can help with falling asleep.

heart rate normally increases when you are ascending a hill or speeding up, sometimes dramatically. For example, you may be riding along on the road with an average heart rate of 150, when suddenly you begin to climb a steep grade. Your heart rate might climb to 170, 180, or to its maximum level if you're on the right grade. In a shorter event, this poses less of a problem. But in longer races it can have devastating effects on your energy, using up too much sugar and glycogen. If this is done too early in a long event—even one lasting only an hour or two—you may risk running out of fuel later in the race. That doesn't mean you should let the pack out of your sight or slow to a crawl at every hill. If you've built enough aerobic speed, you'll be able to ascend hills at a good pace without the heart rate rising to maximum levels. In some events, such as running or a triathlon, you'll allow the athletes near you to get ahead, only to catch them soon afterward by having used less energy to get to that same point. However, in some long events, like an Ironman-distance triathlon, riding at your maximum aerobic heart rate and never higher during the bike portion is essential to maintain sufficient energy and still have enough left for an effective marathon.

For runners, in particular, a potential loss of energy during a race comes from overstriding. For some reason, as fatigue increases, many athletes want to reach out with their legs, as if they'll go farther with the same energy. Instead, as you stride longer your body uses more energy, indicated by a higher heart rate. The best recommendation is to allow your stride length to be governed by your brain and the body's energy levels rather than by your image of what you should look like.

Another common problem encountered by competitors during or just prior to an event is last-minute experimentation. Some athletes even decide to change their routine right in the middle of a race. For example, knowing which "energy" drinks are provided on the course is important, especially if you don't tolerate that particular product. But the most important issue during a race is hydration. Consider the fact that by the end of a long endurance event, most athletes are dehydrated to the point where it adversely affects performance. So the simple action of drinking water is vital for a good race.

### Recovery

Successful competition does not end at the finish line, even for winners. The final step—an optimal recovery—enables your body to "heal" from the race and prepare you for the resumption of training. Recovery is also the first step in preparing for your next race.

Recovery involves changes in the physical, chemical, and mental aspects of your body. Of the two forms—active and passive recovery—the active type is preferred for the endurance athlete and is discussed here. Passive recovery is reserved for more severe or first-aid situations, often with recovery including lying down on a cot with an IV stuck in your arm.

The first phase of recovery is your cool-down. Walking, easy jogging, spinning on your bike, or swimming are very effective ways to aid recovery. Fifteen to twenty minutes is usually enough for most events, less for very long races. Intensity should be very low; do not exceed about 70 percent of your maximum aerobic heart rate. For example, if your maximum aerobic rate is 140, your recovery heart rate should not exceed about 100 but can be below this level. This can be done immediately following the event, or you can wait until you hydrate and consume some nutrients. Be sure to wear your heart-rate monitor to ensure you're not overdoing it while cooling down. It's often more difficult to gauge body intensity following a hard effort. In some long events, such as an Ironman-distance triathlon, even a few minutes of walking—especially in cool water—can be very therapeutic and can speed recovery. In the evening after the race, another short walk or easy swim can also greatly speed recovery.

Walking is especially helpful if you have a long trip home following the race—when you may be sitting for some time. If you're on a plane, walk at the airport and in the aisles on the plane. If you have an extended drive, stop to take a walking break. Sitting is a stressful position anytime, but more so after a race, when muscle imbalance can quickly develop.

Getting part or much of your body in cold water is also a very good therapy to help speed recovery. It assists in the healing of overtaxed muscles and other soft tissues by increasing circulation and cooling otherwise overheated areas. A local stream, lake, or even bath can work wonders, even if only for five minutes.

Post-race food and drink that will provide much-needed nutrients for energy and glycogen repletion are also important for recovery, as discussed in the next section.

No matter how much you consumed during the race, you're probably still dehydrated, and will remain so for twenty-four hours or more. Avoid alcohol, which increases dehydration, until you have consumed lots of water and eaten a meal. Salty foods or drinks with sodium are also important for most athletes and will help replace the large volume of sodium lost in sweat, especially following long events.

Getting a good night's sleep following a race is a key part of recovery. It's best to plan on sleeping in the next morning if possible. The day after your race is also especially important: perhaps an easy swim or walk in the morning, or an easy spin or swim later in the day for most situations. Obviously avoid any hard or long workouts. If you recover well by the end of Monday after a Sunday race, for example, you can resume normal training on Tuesday. In the case of a long event like an Ironman, a long bike ride, or a marathon, it will take many more days to recover. Allow your body all the time it needs.

### Individualize Your Racing Season

In many endurance sports, competition has become a year-round season. Runners can find a race within a short drive of home virtually all year long. For other sports, seasons are

## SAMPLE TRAINING AND RACING SCHEDULES

Example of four athletes' twelve-month endurance training and racing schedules beginning in November (this is only an example as regional, national, and international racing is so diverse today).

|  | Athlete #1 | Athlete #2 | Athlete #3 | Athlete #4 |
|---|---|---|---|---|
| Location: | Arizona, USA | Calgary, Canada | New York City, USA | Sydney, Australia |
| November | taper for final race; short rest period; start aerobic base | taper for final races; start aerobic base | last race of season; short rest period; start aerobic base | end of aerobic base mid-month; start anaerobic work |
| December | aerobic base | aerobic intervals/ downhill work | aerobic base | start racing |
| January | aerobic intervals; downhill work | continue above | aerobic intervals; downhill work | reduce overall training; continue racing |
| February | start race season | continue above | continue above | continue racing |
| March | reduce overall training; continue racing | anaerobic work | start anaerobic work mid-month | taper for final race; short rest period; start aerobic base |
| April | continue racing | start race season | reduce overall training; start race season | aerobic base |
| May | taper for final races | reduce overall training; continue racing | continue racing | aerobic intervals; downhill work |
| June | short rest period; start of aerobic base | continue racing | taper for final races | continue aerobic work |

| | Athlete #1 | Athlete #2 | Athlete #3 | Athlete #4 |
|---|---|---|---|---|
| July | continue aerobic base | taper for final races | short rest period; start aerobic base | start anaerobic work mid-month |
| August | add aerobic intervals and downhill work | short rest period; begin aerobic base | continue aerobic base | reduce overall training; begin racing |
| September | start racing mid-month | add aerobic intervals and downhill work | anaerobic work; start racing | continue racing |
| October | reduce training; continue racing | start anaerobic work and racing | reduce overall training; continue racing | continue racing |

restricted, mostly due to the weather. But even in this case, the race season is often a long one, as sporting events have become big business. For a triathlete living in Minnesota, a race is just a plane ride away to, say, Florida. And still other situations exist; if you're a pro, you may just pack up your gear and head south or north when the weather changes, and suddenly you're in a different environment and often a new competitive season.

Whatever your situation, at some point you'll need to make your own racing schedule. All it takes is a little planning and discipline. If you live in cooler areas, where autumn is the end of your season, the weather does half your job of scheduling. In the northeast United States, for example, most key running races begin with the onset of nice weather—usually April or May. The competitions continue until the cold temperatures begin, usually around the end of November or December. This season, from mid-spring to mid-autumn, can be up to eight months. That's too long for any endurance athlete to maintain health and compete well, so breaking up this long season into two shorter ones is a consideration. The best and simplest way to do this is to take a break from competition in the middle of the season. For example, your first season may be from April or May through June or mid-July, and your second season may begin late August or early September into November or mid-December. Adjust this to your specific race dates, overall training and racing calendar, and your various individual needs, such as seasonal work hours or other family

## MY PERSPECTIVE—BY BOB BROYLES

*Bob Broyles, forty-one, is the warehouse manager for TriSports.com—one of the nation's largest online stores for multisport athletes. He lives outside Tucson on a small farm with his family.*

✷✷✷

I began my life as a triathlete in 1988. Since that time, I have witnessed great changes as triathlon has grown by leaps and bounds. Back in 1988 there was very little information available for training. Even the gadgets and gear were very minimal by today's standards. Companies such as PowerBar and Clif Bar were still a few years away. In fact, I bought my first heart-rate monitor in 1990. At that time, I knew enough that training with a heart-rate monitor could enhance my training, yet I knew very little about what was a good training zone, as there was not a lot of information available back then.

Over the years, I improved by persistence and by looking for new ways to enhance my training. It wasn't until around 1994 that, through Mike Pigg, I started learning about Phil Maffetone. Mike was having a lot of success, and I knew that he was onto something good. The thought of going slower to get faster was intriguing but was almost a scary proposition at the time. I thought to myself, "Can this actually work? Or will this just turn me into a back-of-the-pack age-grouper with slower finishing times?"

At the same time, I was questioning my carbohydrate intake. I was eating a huge amount of carbohydrates every day, yet it puzzled me that two and a half hours into a training ride I was out of gas. How was this possible? I was eating pre-ride meals that were often 1,200+ calories, which were primarily carbohydrates, yet consistently hitting the wall. At this time, I actually shied away from anything with protein or fat in it. Honestly, I felt hungry for several years.

Then I finally decided that I needed to make some changes to my training and nutrition. This was really a leap of faith for me. To begin a training program in which I would be going slow, and to start eating foods with a higher amount of protein and fats in them, was a personal revolution for me. This was not simply a change in pace and diet; it was a total makeover in my training plans, which included a social aspect as well. Among my training partners, I was known as someone that would always insist on hammer training sessions. Often times on training rides and runs, I would have to slow down or stop and wait for others to catch up. Yet I made the decision to change to the Maffetone Method of training at the end of the season in 1994. My thought was that I would give this a serious try for a few months, and if I wasn't seeing results that I would revert back to my old training methods.

I realized that I would have to train at my own pace, which meant much slower than what I was accustomed to. I will always remember my first few weeks of this "new" training method. I was "slow." So slow that if I was running uphill, I would often end up walking. Psychologically, this took a lot of inner discipline. After all, I had been a triathlete for about six years at this point; I was "fit," I had all the cool gear, yet I was running and walking at a pace that is usually reserved for the elderly, not someone in their mid-twenties.

To top it off, a good friend and training partner of mine read me the riot act for doing something as crazy as this. He made his case very clear that I was ruining everything I had built up over the years and that when the spring races came, I would be totally out of race shape; in fact I would probably be so slow that I would get discouraged from racing and probably give up the triathlon altogether. In addition, he made no bones about it that no one would want to train with me because "no one" trains that slowly.

Faced with all of this, I knew deep down that I had to do what I believed in, and so I continued following the Maffetone Method. A few weeks went by, and there was little improvement. Then around the six-to-eight-week mark, my times began dropping, while my heart rate was staying low. Was the program working? It was. Soon after that, I was running as fast as I was before I made the change. I even surpassed my old run times, and my heart rate was staying low the whole time. After a while, I really had to run (and bike) fast to keep my heart at the MAF target. What a great feeling that was, to be training in the spring at times faster than I had in the fall, except with a much lower heart rate. So, yes, training slower does make you faster. In addition, by keeping your heart rate in a true aerobic zone, the chance of injury is much lower. So much for the "no pain, no gain" theory.

Once the spring races came about, I was turning in times that I had only dreamt about in previous years. Also, I found that when I was in a race situation and I had to dig deep, I had what it took to succeed. This ability came from truly developing my aerobic capacity, and my confidence that I did the "right" changes in my training program.

Had I not made these changes, or had I followed my friend's advice, I would never have been able to take my racing to the next level. I would have stayed like him and wallowed in doing the same thing and expecting different results. Sometimes, you just have to think outside of the box.

In 1996, I really began to have a lot of success, winning a few small races and qualifying for the 1997 Long Course World Championships in Nice, France. The Nice race was quite possibly the most memorable race of my life. I really focused on keeping my training and diet within Maffetone's principles. I was getting stronger and fitter at all three disciplines. Days before the actual race, I did a last minute bike-shoe change that proved disastrous. In fact, when I finished the bike course, I was in so much pain that I literally thought there was no way that I could finish the race. At that point, running 18.6 miles seemed impossible, certainly a long struggle at best. While in the second transition, the light bulb went on, and I was reminded of just how much time, effort, money, and pride I had put into doing my best at this event. At that time, Nice was raced at the following distance; 4K (2.49 miles) swim, 120K (74.6 miles) bike, and 30K (18.6 miles) for the run. Due to both my mental strength and my great physical condition, I went on and ran 1:53, only two minutes slower than the race leader, Luc Van Lierde. I only mention this because if I had not followed Maffetone's training advice, a run like this would never have been possible for me. To be within two minutes of one of the greatest long distance triathletes in one of his best years was a real breakthrough for me.

Over time, I became an elite triathlete, progressed up the ranks, moved to San Diego, worked with John Howard, and was scheduled to go to Italy for the World's Duathlon Championship in September of 2001. But just days before the race, I had a serious accident and broke my clavicle and scapula in three places, fractured two ribs, one vertebra, and popped my right lung.

After the accident, it became my goal to recover as fast as possible. I got in shape enough to head to Tucson with John Howard at the end of November to complete the El Tour Bike Race in a time that barely put me in the event's Platinum status. After that, I pretty much hung things up and moved on with life. I felt that it was time to "move on" and focus on other areas of life. I relocated from the shores of North County, San Diego, to the desert of Tucson, Arizona. I was offered a great management position with a sister company to one I'd worked at for years in the Northwest. Once I settled into my new life in Tucson, it was easy to immerse myself in work. I still trained, but it was very occasionally, leading to no training whatsoever. As strange as this might seem to anyone who knew just how serious I had been involved in the triathlon life, the distance from the sport actually felt good.

I think I was enjoying my new "freedom" of eating whatever tasted good and doing whatever I felt like doing. During this time, I still thought I was young enough that "nature" would keep me in shape for years or a lifetime, yet too old to continue to race competitively.

Fast-forward to 2009: I have now been married five years, and recently turned forty-one. I have a two-year-old boy and a six-month-old son. We live on four acres made into a small farm, and there's plenty to do to keep me busy, but not necessarily healthy and fit. Since I entered fatherhood fairly late in life, I want to be around long enough to see my kids grow up and settle into their own lives. I am 5'8" and when I was in my racing prime, I weighed between 145 and 150 pounds. But in 2009, I tipped the scale at 180. The new me was a lot different from the old, single me, living in a condo half a block off the Pacific coast in Solana Beach.

The company that I help manage, TriSports.com, recently expo'ed at the Vineman Triathlon in Santa Rosa, California, and I had to drive our truck and trailer to the event. Even though I am involved in the multisport industry, I had escaped (for the most part) the lure of getting back into training. But Vineman got me hooked again. Now that I am older and (hopefully) wiser, I decided that this was the perfect opportunity to find my own road back to health and fitness. I knew that my life is just too busy to really tackle triathlons again (at least while our children are small), but then it dawned on me that I could somewhat "easily" get fit by running. Running is very simple: not a lot of gadgets, just some clothes, the right pair of shoes, sunglasses, a hat, and of course a heart-rate monitor.

Knowing that my time was precious, I needed to be effective with my training. Fearing that I could easily fall into the trap of overtraining due to the fact that I was a former elite athlete, I needed ways to keep a healthy perspective on things. I started looking at some of the current running books on the market. I found that with my background, experience, and my current life situation, everything was either too simple or way too regimented for me. Going back into my own library of books, I instantly knew that Maffetone's books were just what I needed. He offers good practical advice that I had used with great success before, and I knew that this would also aid me in what I wanted to do now.

Fortunately for me, when I looked up Dr. Maffetone online, I was happily surprised that he was still out there, doing what he had been doing for years: offering great advice that is simple, yet very comprehensive, and more importantly, I knew it made sense. His principles are completely founded, almost so simple that some people may not understand them in the same regard that some people cannot see the forest for the trees. Primarily there is the message to look at yourself holistically, adjust your diet to a more natural selection, and keep your stress levels in check. This is where many other "coaches" fall short. Today, I see plenty of people out there that offer coaching services for endurance athletes. While most of these coaches have good intentions, most do not have the ability to offer athletes the full, holistic package that Maffetone presents. In addition as athletes, we have become very comfortable in wanting others to tell us step-by-step what we need to do to achieve our goals. This is a very formidable challenge, given that cookie-cutter plans cannot possibly be optimal for everyone. These strict step-by-step plans also fail to look at things such as the stresses (which accumulate) in your life, and how that will affect an "off the shelf" training plan.

My fitness goal was to run the Tucson Half-Marathon on December 13, 2009, under 1:30, and to reduce my weight from 180 to 155. And while I was training, I actually kept this quiet around the people I worked with. I believe we all have our own "things" that inspire us. My "things" come from inside, and having the added pressure of others wanting me to train with them and ask me questions about my progress was something I could live without.

I ran the half-marathon in 1:38, not as fast as I had wanted to but still a good performance considering that a few short months before, I could not complete this distance. I later got my weight down to 140, which is actually at or below my old racing weight of years ago. This was accomplished by following Maffetone's sound nutritional and training advice. I have continued to see improvements in my training times, which is very exciting and motivating. With more races on the horizon, the future looks bright!

In addition to my weight and fitness improvements, I have all but eliminated caffeine, and I find that I don't miss it a bit. My diet has changed from processed foods to a diet filled with fruits, veggies, nuts, seeds, and whole protein sources, including plenty of eggs. Prior to this change, I have always had allergies, primarily hay fever and pollens. Due to proper nutrition, I have actually eliminated my allergies. Prior to this, I have taken multiple over-the-counter and prescription medications to mask the symptoms, but never to rid them from my body. As a horse owner who is around hay every day, this is something that has made a world of difference.

obligations, like children's school schedules. But the most important aspect in this example is your midsummer, or midseason, break.

This midseason period is a time to build another small aerobic base. It's short but sufficient to develop more aerobic function while providing you with rest and recovery from anaerobic activity. By taking this break after the first season, you will often have better second season performances. And in many sports, the more important events are scheduled in late summer or autumn.

The midseason aerobic base should be no less than about four weeks, with up to six or eight weeks in some locations and for some individuals. The more events in the first season, the more time you need to recover. And, the more important the second season is to you, the more additional aerobic base you'll need before it.

Whether you live in Australia or New Zealand, the Caribbean or Hawaii, or even Alaska, you can make your own schedule to match the local weather, the events taking place, and your own lifestyle. And if you're fortunate enough to move with the seasons, you can still do the same. But don't try to do what I've seen many endurance athlete attempt, and that is race too much in the United States from spring through fall, and then race even more in Australia during that hemisphere's racing season. This is a quick way to develop the overtraining syndrome.

In general, if you rely on racing to get your anaerobic stimulation, you can race a little more. In other words, if you perform anaerobic workouts, you can't race as often without creating additional stress.

One important consideration regarding your race schedule is extremes in the weather. In Arizona, for example, there may not be as many races or you may not want to compete as much in the summer. During this time, even morning temperatures can be in the 100°F range in some areas like Phoenix. If you're racing locally, you may want to use the summer as your long base period. In this case, break your winter into two seasons. One problem with this is the case where you may want to travel north for one or two big races. These are usually held in the summer, and if that's your base time you may not want to race then. Planning your twelve-month schedule ahead of time enables you to resolve these issues.

## Racing During Your Next Base Buildup—An Exception

If you've built at least one good long base (e.g., December through March), had a good competitive season, and stayed healthy, you may want to consider some added races in the off-season. This is an exception to the rules discussed earlier. Only consider this if your fitness and health is high, and never if you're injured, not feeling full of energy, your MAF Tests are down, or if your work, family, or other schedules are busy.

During your next long base period you can race occasionally—perhaps once or twice—without ill effects. Let me repeat the criteria:

1. You've already built at least one long base period.
2. You had a good race season.
3. You were healthy throughout both base and race season. This means you performed well and did not get injured or ill.

If this is the case, competing once or twice during your long winter base (as opposed to the short summer one) should not take away from your health or fitness. And you should be able to race extremely well.

If you're ready to compete, successfully following proper preparation, implementation, and recovery procedures will ensure you of success. But what if you're not ready to race? Don't. You'll have to sacrifice at least part of the season and get back on track by improving your aerobic system and other aspects of fitness and health. Modify and correct your training, diet or whatever needs improvement, until you are ready.

Steve, a competitive runner, came to see me at age forty-nine, complaining of chronic injuries in the knee and calf, accompanied by a variety of other overtraining symptoms such as extreme fatigue, sleep irregularities, asthma, and feelings of muscle weakness. His running schedule was often over 100 miles a week when not injured, and included track work from spring through fall. In addition, when running at his normal training pace with the heart monitor, his rate was in the high 150s. Steve also went to the company gym two to three times a week for weight training.

Since it was now early May, his main concern was to eliminate his injuries so he could start his racing season. But my consideration was for Steve's current health and future training and racing. So this particular season, I explained to him, had to be modified. We had to correct his injuries and start building an aerobic base, which would take at least three months. If all went well, the plan was to make a new season starting in July. This was a difficult concept for Steve to accept.

But he had been to a number of health-care professionals over the past two years without success and finally decided to give in and try this approach, citing his worsening performances and diminishing health.

Steve's physical injuries were corrected by balancing the muscles that caused the knee and calf problem. Changing to a properly fitting running shoe was also important. His first month showed good improvement in his aerobic pace, from 9:20 to 8:40. By the next month, Steve's energy was very good, with sleeping and breathing problems resolved. By mid-June, I helped Steve plan his race season that would start in late July with an 8K cross-country event, a race he had run each year for the past five. Steve had some of his best racing ever from July through early October, including a personal best in his first 8K event.

# CHAPTER 11

# TRAINING AT ALTITUDE—
## Outdoor and "Indoor" Benefits

**F**or many years, training at altitude has achieved a certain mystique. Cities like Boulder and Flagstaff have blossomed into endurance meccas. But their appeal, like any other high-altitude locale, is not the magic ingredient for the improved endurance many seek. In fact, having personally spent time in these locations with many athletes during my coaching career, and observing firsthand how many others train, it's clear that the risk of overtraining is very high.

Even the moderate elevations of 3,000 feet in altitude can increase the training heart rate by several beats or more for several days or even weeks, depending on the individual. If training is based on pace rather than heart rate, most athletes end up working out too hard, too often. This is mostly due to the "thinner" air, which really means the lower barometric pressure at higher altitudes reduces the ability

of the body to take oxygen out of the air into the capillaries of the lungs, so it's now in the bloodstream. In addition to higher resting and training heart rates, recovery can be significantly reduced.

Just being in a pressurized cabin of a commercial airliner is the same as being at 6,000 to 8,000 feet (1830 to 2440 meters) even though the plane may be flying at 30,000 feet. As soon as you step off the plane and arrive at a high-altitude location, your body is exposed to significant stress; in addition to thinner air, your training performance is also reduced dramatically. Furthermore, reduced food intake is common, which may not match your energy expenditure needs—a form of nutritional stress. Moreover, there is much less moisture in the air, and the risk of dehydration must be avoided. Ascending to higher altitudes can be such a stress that a condition called acute mountain sickness can follow in some athletes, resulting in headache, nausea, insomnia, and malaise. You don't have to be that high above sea level either, as even skiers, for example, visiting resorts at 6,000 feet can have this condition

Your body will compensate for the stress of altitude, at least the oxygen-debt aspect, partly by increasing your heart rate and breathing rate, enabling you to carry more oxygen. Over time, the kidney makes more of the hormone EPO (erythropoietin), which stimulates the bone marrow to make more red blood cells, and larger ones, for further compensation. This increases the body's ability to bring oxygen to the muscles. After about three weeks at altitude, these and other adaptations result in better oxygenation, perhaps closer to sea-level conditions.

Eventually, after several weeks and depending on your body, because everyone responds differently, all this compensation enables you to train without the stress encountered when you first arrived at alti-tude. However, there are benefits to being at altitude. "Thinner" air means less physical resistance during a workout or race. This is due to reduced moisture in the air. So cycling and skiing performance, for example, can improve only after—not before—you have adapted to the altitude. Once these changes take place, and the athlete returns to lower altitudes, such as sea level, the increases in red blood cells and associated increased oxygen carrying potential may increase performance.

With sufficient time, higher altitude training comes with other benefits. But the real advantage is in living there long enough—such as three or four months—and not neces-sarily in the training. The worse scenario is visiting the mountains for only a couple of weeks thinking it will help your training—but that's not sufficient time for your body to make the necessary adjustments. One result of spending adequate time at altitude is that you produce more oxygen-carrying red blood cells and higher hemoglobin from increased EPO. While these benefits are good for your health, they only significantly improve your fitness when you return to lower altitudes to compete.

Returning to sea level three weeks before a major race offers the best of both altitudes. First, when descending to a lower altitude your oxygen uptake is greater. And second, you maintain the improved oxygen-carrying capacity developed during your time at alti-tude, which helps you in competition. These changes disappear quickly after a month or so at lower altitudes, but the approach is very effective. This was one of Mark Allen's strategies when he won six Ironman Hawaii races. Each summer he would spend several months living and training in Boulder.

All these potential changes and responses by the body are also individual. Some respond better to altitude while other have a difficult time. The overall levels of fitness and health may be the most important factors, with a

variety of specific dietary, nutritional, and stress factors being necessary to obtain benefits at altitude. For example, if your ability to make red blood cells is impaired due to low folic acid or iron levels, being at altitude won't help. This does not mean you should take an iron supplement if you're going to train at altitude. Consuming a healthy diet, sufficient in iron, will provide your body with the amount of iron needed to make appropriate

*Photo credit: Timothy Carlson*

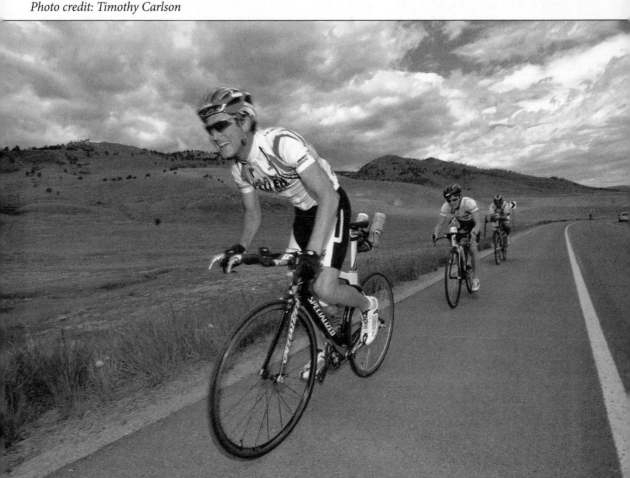

*Biking outside Boulder—a high-altitude mecca for endurance athletes*

levels of red cells. And when going to altitude, the body automatically adjusts by absorbing three to four times more iron from your diet (like with most nutrients, the brain and body know just how much you need to take from your food as it passes through the intestines). Taking iron supplements when you're not anemic can be dangerous as it can cause significant chemical stress and even physical stress on the intestines.

For many athletes, going to altitude for some period of time often results in extra stress while the body is adapting to the changes induced by altitude. This is shown by an increase in the stress hormone cortisol, which is produced as a result of any stress—including an environmental one like altitude. Adrenal stress not only can raise cortisol to unhealthy levels but also reduce other adrenal hormones, notably aldosterone, which can result in poor electrolyte and water regulation. One requirement of training at a higher altitude is wearing a heart-rate monitor and remaining aerobic for the first few weeks. This will help you obtain the potential benefits of altitude training while diminishing the risks.

In addition to improved changes in blood chemistry, other potentially healthy changes may occur in aerobic muscles while living and training long enough at altitude. These include increased circulation in aerobic muscles, increases in myoglobin (the red pigment in aerobic fibers) and aerobic enzymes to help with fat burning, and improvements in lactate metabolism.

The particular altitude effects vary with the ascent, with higher altitudes producing better results. It's difficult to say what that magic altitude is because of individual variation and positive and negative effects of various altitudes. For example, red blood cell responses may be better at an 8,000-foot altitude compared to 5,000 feet, but other stresses exist at the higher levels, such as the increased risk of dehydration and even lower oxygen uptake slowing your training pace. Altitudes between 4,000 and 7,000 feet may be the best general range for potential improvement in fitness and health, if you're already fit and healthy, you train with a heart-rate monitor adhering to the maximum aerobic heart rate based on the 180 Formula, and you carefully assess your progress and avoid entering the first stage of overtraining.

The benefits of training at altitude are not just physiological. The enjoyment of being in most moderate-level mountainous regions is socially and psychologically rewarding. Whether in the Rocky Mountains, for example, or many other areas around the world, these locations offer a healthy, low-stress place to train and live compared to hurried, tension-ridden areas around New York, Los Angeles, and similar locales. Moreover, the summer weather in these mountain areas offers the additional benefit of being cooler without very high humidity. This social and psychological enjoyment may help offset some of the other stresses.

## Specific Changes

Let's look at the details of the changes that occur when training at altitude. The more you understand them, the better you can compensate with appropriate lifestyle changes while there and the better your strategy for competing afterwards:

- The air you breathe at higher altitudes contains the same mix of oxygen and other gases as the air at sea level—about 20.9 percent oxygen. The barometric pressure, however, is lower as you ascend in altitude, and this difference reduces your lungs' ability to get oxygen out of the air.

- As you ascend, air temperature drops quickly. For example, going from 4,000 feet at a temperature of 45ºF to 6,000 feet will bring the temperature to 38ºF. This can be significant when cycling, more so at even greater altitude changes, especially when considering the wind chill.

- Humidity is much lower at higher altitudes, since cooler air holds less water. In addition to increasing your need to consume water to stay hydrated, higher altitudes can dry out your sinuses and thus increase your vulnerability to colds and flu.

- You should also be aware that the increased solar danger at higher altitudes significantly raises your risk of sunburn. The decreased water in the air, which normally absorbs light, also increases the amount of sunlight that hits your body. Midday summer training outdoors is probably best avoided.

- The muscles can be affected at altitudes of 5,248 feet (1,600 meters) and above. Overall muscle performance is diminished due to the reduced oxygen, resulting in a slower pace. (Mountain climbers above 20,000 feet feel like they are moving in slow motion.) In addition, muscle enzymes, which regulate energy production, decline, and total surface area of the muscle is diminished.

- While there are a lot of factors to consider when training at altitude, wearing your heart-rate monitor and following your max aerobic heart rate will allow you to compensate quite well, reduce the potential training stress, and continue building your aerobic system.

- After weighing the positive and negative factors of spending time at altitude, some athletes will invariably decide it's worth it. My strongest recommendation is this: Altitude training should be a strategy implemented only after you have improved your overall health and built a great aerobic base—but it should not be used as a way to get more fit or healthy.

Below are additional recommendations for those planning a high-altitude period of endurance training:

- If you can't spend two to four months at altitude, it may not make much sense as a training strategy. However, it makes a wonderful vacation, and training during this period should be reduced and always done with a heart-rate monitor.

- The altitude for endurance training benefits begins at lower levels, but significant effects start around 5,000 feet (just under 1,600 meters) after adequate time there and for a short period when you return to sea level.
- Your training should be diminished for the first two weeks of arriving at altitude. For the first two or three days, training should be restricted to easy walking.

- Anaerobic workouts should be minimized at altitude—it's a great time to build an aerobic base. If you do perform anaerobic work, keep it to short intervals, emphasize recovery, and use your heart-rate monitor.

If competing at altitude, train aerobically for at least two weeks at that altitude in order to better adapt. If you are not able to stay at altitude for two weeks before competition, arrive at your race the night before. Many of the negative physiological changes become

*Using a mild hyperbaric chamber is easy.*

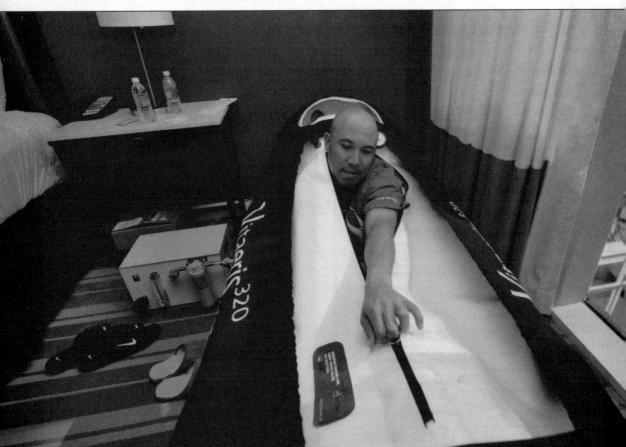

significant after the first twenty-four hours at altitude.

The optimal situation is to live at higher altitudes, and train at lower ones—for example, living at 5,000 to 6,000 feet, then driving down the mountain for your training sessions. This is not very practical for most athletes. But technology has changed all this. You could live year-round in Florida and still receive the benefits of high-altitude training. This is made possible with two types of portable indoor chambers.

You can simulate low altitude with a mild hyperbaric chamber and high altitude with a hypobaric chamber. The hyperbaric chamber can have an altitude range of about 5,000 feet or lower relative to your current altitude. The hypobaric chamber can have an altitude range above 5,000 and even up to 18,000 feet. In other words, the hyperbaric chamber mimics lower altitude/higher barometric pressure; the hypobaric chamber mimics higher altitude/lower pressure.

## Mild Hyperbaric Chambers

In the late 1980s, while lecturing in Boulder, Colorado, I met with Professor R. Igor Gamow, who was interested in human performance at various altitudes. He invited me to his lab in the chemical engineering department of the University of Colorado, where he was working on a portable mild hyperbaric chamber for use in mountaineering. Climbers who experience mountain sickness at very high altitudes risk death if not carried down to safer altitudes, which is

often a difficult task, and this new portable chamber, operated with a foot pump, would soon save lives. Gamow's portable hyperbaric chamber compresses the air inside a lightweight nylon inflatable "bag," creating a high-pressure environment that mimics low altitude. Even without adding additional oxygen, the body's ability to get more oxygen out of the compressed air inside increases significantly, just like at lower altitudes.

I immediately saw two benefits beyond those for the mountaineering community. One was to help endurance athletes recover more quickly and effectively, because the chamber would simulate lower altitude and increased oxygen uptake. Another was for the improvement of overall wellness and the treatment of various health problems.

## Athletic Use of Hyperbaric Chambers

For athletes who lived at higher altitudes, the use of the Gamow Bag, as it was first called, was significant. Athletes could spend forty-five minutes to an hour each day in this small plastic inflatable chamber with pressures similar to those about 5,000 feet lower and recover better from their daily training; it was especially helpful immediately before competition. This was important for athletes living or training at higher altitudes, as well as for those traveling to higher altitudes for a race.

The additional benefit was obvious: Athletes at any altitude could obtain the same relative benefits because the difference in pressure at lower altitudes made significant beneficial changes in the body. While at sea level, a short forty-five-minute stay in the hyperbaric chamber would still increase barometric pressure as if the athlete were much lower in altitude. This significantly increases the body's oxygen uptake, even without adding additional oxygen to the chamber. And the effect lasts for hours and sometimes days after the athlete comes out of the chamber.

The original study on the body's response to altitude changes appeared in the *Journal of Applied Physiology* in 1971. The researchers showed that oxygen uptake would increase 11 to 12 percent immediately after ascending in a deep mine of 5,784 feet (1,763 meters).

This was dramatic and just what the mild hyperbaric chambers offered. For athletes, it was an incredible "therapy" and training aid. Within a couple of months, I began using the new hyperbaric chamber with many of the endurance athletes I was coaching. Since the chamber was portable—it was like a lightweight plastic bag with a small pump that all fit into a backpack—it was easy to bring to many endurance events around the world.

The athletic protocol I developed included using the chamber for forty-five-minute sessions (at a pressure of four pounds per square inch) to help recover from training

**QA**

**Question:** I'm a young athlete hoping to turn professional in the sport of cycling. Before I spend thousands of dollars on a hyperbaric or hypobaric chamber, is there any certainty of benefits? I know a certain pedal system will help me ride faster, and certain drinks will give me energy for my long events. What about these chambers?

**Answer:** There's no guarantee that certain pedals, energy drinks, or any other items will help you as an athlete during competition. The same is true for hyperbaric and hypobaric chambers. We do know that being inside a mild hyperbaric chamber will increase your oxygen uptake substantially. And we know that even with short-term use, a hypobaric chamber can increase EPO. However, the real question is, will these activities, and the potential benefits they provide, help your performance? Because so many factors affect how well you race, it's difficult to say. For example, if your folic acid or vitamin B12 levels are low, higher EPO may not significantly increase red blood cells. Large controlled studies have not been done on endurance athletes using either hypobaric or hyperbaric chambers. Most importantly, it's best to see these devices as part of a training program that includes other valuable components, such as building a great aerobic base, monitoring MAF Tests, optimizing nutrition, and other key factors.

## MY PERSPECTIVE—BY DR. IGOR GAMOW

*Rustem Igor Gamow's father, George, developed the big bang theory of the creation of the universe; scientific curiosity was in Igor's DNA. Following a stint as a dancer with the National Ballet Company and as a motorcycle courier for CBS News at the White House, the younger Gamow became a professor of chemical engineering at the University of Colorado at Boulder. His best-known patented inventions include an inflatable pressure chamber used to treat mountain climbers for altitude sickness and a shallow underwater breathing apparatus.*

✳✳✳

In the early eighties, I was convinced by my research in Boulder that one should train under conditions where one's performance is maximum—train at or below sea level while living higher in elevation. I was in the midst of trying to figure out how these high-low experiments could be tested when I read in our local newspaper that Dr. Phil Maffetone was giving a clinic in downtown Boulder, Colorado that afternoon. I had never been in a health gym, but I decided to attend to see if I could pick up some ideas. His lecture was very well attended and I stood back in the crowd with my hands in my pockets. Phil asked for volunteers and I stood perfectly still without moving. Sure enough he picked me and asked me to be a guinea pig to demonstrate the use of a heart-rate monitor while riding a stationary bike.

After the talk, we spent some time discussing the pros and cons of high-altitude training. Phil visited my lab the next day, and I demonstrated a large fabric hyperbaric bubble, which you could inflate, here in Boulder, a mile high city, and be immediately transported to sea level. I also demonstrated a smaller version of our bubble, the Gamow Bag, that could be used to treat climbers suffering from mountain sickness. Phil became very excited about the prospect of using our portable hyperbaric chambers not only to train athletes but to treat other aliments that included brain injury in children, obesity, and cardiac problems. It has been my pleasure and delight for these past twenty-five or so years to exchange ideas on and anecdotes of the various benefits provided by portable both hypobaric and hyperbaric chambers.

and competition, and to use it several times the week of competition.

In addition to improved oxygen uptake, which by itself is a significant benefit of the chamber, spending time in the device relaxed many of the athletes I used it with on the days leading up to a race. Some would even fall asleep while inside. They also experienced improvements in muscle function, ranges of motion, posture, and gait. These athletes always said they felt better overall, and many looked forward to their turn in the chamber.

In my New York clinic, the hyperbaric chamber was often in use, with athletes who lived in the area scheduling sessions throughout the week. They would use it during periods of a busy training schedule, before important events, after a race, and when they were feeling fatigue, were training hard, or were late in their long racing season.

I would often bring my mild hyperbaric chamber to the more important races, such as the Ironman Hawaii, the Seoul Olympics, or the big triathlon race in Nice, France. Athletes would be scheduled every day for a forty-five-minute hyperbaric session. Post-race, these same athletes would use the chamber to help speed recovery.

In a real sense, I used the hyperbaric chamber as another therapeutic tool in my health-care arsenal. Tom was a patient of mine. He was twenty-nine years old and

## HYPERBARIA VERSUS HYPEROXIA

Increasing the pressure of ambient air, such as inside the mild hyperbaric chamber, is called hyperbaria. While this increases oxygen uptake, it's not the same as breathing pure oxygen, which is called hyperoxia. While I've worked with hyperbaric chambers with and without added oxygen, I don't think, in most situations, that additional oxygen is necessary. Some still contend that there is no difference between increased oxygen utilization from room air while in a hyperbaric chamber, and breathing pure oxygen without hyperbaria. But many professionals who have worked in this area agree that hyperbaria (increased pressure) and hyperoxia (increased oxygen) don't have the same clinical effects. One important difference is the oxygen and carbon dioxide levels of the blood flow to the brain. Hyperoxia, breathing pure oxygen, actually lowers brain blood flow, and can even reduce oxygen utilization—not a healthy thing for any brain. In general, breathing high concentrations of oxygen can even lower oxygen levels throughout the rest of the body, and can create an oxygen toxicity, not to mention the dangers of free radical damage. Unlike breathing oxygen, the positive effects of mild hyperbaria can last several hours to days after one forty-five-minute period in a chamber, without the risk of breathing pure oxygen.

very active with cycling, running, and swimming. He came to my office one morning the day after a bicycle accident that put him in the hospital emergency room. His range of motion in both shoulders was very restricted due to pain. He was also antalgic—a term that describes a severe distorted postural position of people with serious physical injuries. After an extensive examination, which was difficult to perform due to his pain, I had him lie in the hyperbaric chamber for forty-five minutes. His vital (lung) capacity significantly increased after being in the chamber—from 5,100 to 5,900 cubic centers. His temperature was a low 96.8°F before getting in the chamber, and was elevated to a near normal 98.0°F after. Also, several muscles in his lower back, shoulders, and legs that had tested very weak due to the accident were normal and without pain following his time in the chamber. This improved muscle function also resulted in a dramatic change in posture, with an almost normal stance and gait. And his shoulders improved significantly, with normal ranges of motion. Most remarkably, Tom successfully competed in a local three-mile open-water swimming race the following morning, finishing second in his age-group. All evaluations one week and again two weeks later showed continued improvement.

Mild hyperbaric chambers range in price considerably, from a few thousand to $10,000 or more for the newest devices. The fancy ones have more pressure and gadgets for additional comfort. But the low-end devices work quite well for athletes—those that go up to a pressure of 4 psi (pounds per square inch) are the ones I've used. Those with higher pressures increase oxygen uptake further, but not significantly more. As with other sports equipment, used chambers can be found by searching online.

### Use of Hyperbaric Chambers for Improving Health

The second benefit that immediately became evident was the use of mild hyperbaria for improvements in health and in the treatment of various conditions. In my clinic I was able to use the chamber as a therapy and see how different patients responded. In addition to improved oxygenation, I observed many other healthy changes, from greater vital capacity (improved lung function) and improved pH to muscle balance and increased range of motion. As such, I began using the mild hyperbaric chamber on patients with a variety of problems, including those seeking to lose weight (the increased oxygenation improved fat burning), children and adults with brain injury, those with muscle problems, patients with sleep apnea, and many others.

Traditionally, large metal hyperbaric chambers of very high pressure and added oxygen have been used for decades as first aid. The most common applications include treatment of scuba divers and pilots for decompression sickness resulting from too rapid or extreme a change in pressure exerted on the body. In addition, patients with heart problems, chronic infections, severe burns, and many other aliments have also been treated successfully in these types of hyperbaric chambers.

### Hypobaric Chambers

While mild hyperbaric chambers simulate low altitude and high barometric pressure, another type of device does the opposite. Hypobaric chambers simulate higher altitude and low pressure. The hypobaric chamber offers individuals exposure to a high-altitude environment while at rest—while napping, reading, and relaxing, or sleeping through the night—with normal training taking place at the level of altitude where they live. This provides the convenience of "living high and training low." In most cases, athletes sleep in the hypobaric chambers, and each night they obtain a variety of high-altitude benefits. Others spend a shorter time in the chamber during the day reading, working, or napping.

Hypobaric chambers are not as portable as the small inflatable mild hyperbaric chambers. But my use of these high-altitude simulators, both personally and with athletes, has also been very positive. The most dramatic benefit of hypobaric exposure is the increase in your body's natural production of EPO (erythropoietin), which begins almost immediately with hypobaric exposure. EPO stimulates the production of more red blood cells, which increase the body's oxygen-carrying capacity, or ability to get oxygen to working muscles,

by as much as 150 percent. In addition, more blood vessels are developed and a significant overall improvement in sports performance can be attained. It's obviously more healthy and natural to increase your EPO this way than to inject synthetic EPO (which is illegal for most people and dangerous) or use other blood-doping methods (also illegal and dangerous). The result is improved oxygen-carrying capacity and dramatic performance enhancements—all obtained legally and healthfully.

The time necessary to obtain these benefits depends on the individual and the elevation used in the chamber, which can be adjusted to simulate various altitudes. One study showed significant benefits could begin in as little as thirty minutes. The effects of shorter periods of exposure are well substantiated by other research as well. Another study showed a three-fold increase in EPO production after only eighty-four minutes in a hypobaric environment equal to about 13,000 feet elevation. The dramatic effectiveness of hypobaric therapy in athletes might be best exemplified by a group that used a chamber in preparation for an ascent on Mount Everest. The climbers used hypobaric chambers for four days, averaging nine and a half hours per night, before their climb. On Mount Everest, the speed of ascent was much quicker (5,600 meters of altitude gain in six days), whereas in conventional expeditions, twelve to thirty-two days are generally necessary to safely reach the same altitude.

Other fitness and health benefits of using a hypobaric chamber include increases in total blood volume, hematocrit, capillaries, mitochondria volume, and oxygen utilization. These benefits also translate directly into performance increases. One study demonstrated a nearly 4 percent improvement in running speed after only nine days of using the chamber. For a person who runs a 35:00 10K race, that would be an improvement of 1:24, improving the time to 33:36. For a three-hour marathoner, this would equate to more than a seven-minute improvement. For someone who goes ten hours in an Ironman event, this would equate to shaving off thirty minutes—and give him a 9:30 time!

Once again, it's important to emphasize that the use of a hypobaric chamber should be done only when you are already fit and healthy. Care should be taken to avoid entering the first stage of overtraining, and using a heart-rate monitor becomes even more important if you're using a hypobaric chamber. And, its use may be best started during a base period. This is because both overtraining and anaerobic workouts increase the risk of inflammation, which can reduce EPO production.

Precisely how long higher levels of EPO, red blood cells, hematocrit, and other measurable factors can be maintained is not known due to individual variation, as well as time and consistency of exposure. One study showed that regular hypobaric chamber use maintained elevated EPO levels for up to twenty days of not using the chamber. The more fit and healthy you are, the better response you will most likely achieve.

The ideal option for an athlete is to monitor progression through blood tests. This may be done using a simple finger prick for some evaluations. More extensive testing, during and after a period of hypobaric therapy, and may include the following:

- A complete blood count (CBC) to monitor red-cell count, hemoglobin, and hematocrit gives a more complete picture of physiological benefits.
- Testing levels of iron, ferritin, folic acid, vitamin B12, and other nutrients provides information to ensure athletes have the raw materials to obtain optimal benefits from hypobaric exposure.
- The C-reactive protein (CRP) and erythrocyte sedimentation rate (ESR) are important tests to help rule out inflammation.

Both diet and nutrition can have a significant influence on the effectiveness of hypobaric therapy in an athlete's program. The topic of diet is discussed in more detail later, but there are some important factors related to hypobaric therapy that apply here:

- Because chronic inflammation can inhibit EPO production, when using an altitude chamber it's important to consider the powerful dietary aspects that regulate inflammation, including balancing dietary fats, and making sure you get certain vitamins and minerals and adequate protein. It is also important to assess your iron, B12, and folic acid status, and your antioxidant intake as well when using any device that increases EPO.

- Some nutrients have obvious potential impact on the athlete's physiology, and this impact becomes even more acute with hypobaric exposure. A variety of specific nutritional factors may further help athletes who use hypobaric chambers to improve health and performance. Below is a list of some:

  - Iron deficiency could decrease oxygen-carrying capability.
  - Inadequate protein intake could negatively influence EPO production.
  - Zinc may be required at levels higher than normal.
  - Those undergoing hypobaric therapy may have an increased need for antioxidant nutrients.
  - Folic acid could have a significant effect on the production of EPO and red blood cells.
  - Omega-3 fatty acids from fish oil may impact the quality of red blood cells produced, and help reduce inflammation.

Hypobaric chambers are much larger and heavier than the mild hyperbaric devices, with a bed inside. The price range is also considerably higher, into the $10,000 and higher range. Today, the market has more used devices for less, and older units without the fancy components and comfort can be even cheaper.

The hypobaric chamber can be used regularly and for as long as is practical during each session. The athlete must balance the practicality, availability, and improvement potentials. All this may depend on whether several athletes share a chamber or have their own. Here are some options to consider:

- Ease yourself up. When using the hypobaric chamber, begin with an 8,000-foot equivalent (likened to airline travel) and increase proportionately to 15,000 feet over several days. This altitude simulation can then be maintained, and may be the ideal level.
- Some athletes may choose to sleep in the chamber for three weeks each night just before key competitions or their season. This may ensure optimal performance benefits in a relatively short period.
- Build long-term benefits. An easier choice is to use the chamber for shorter periods but regularly over a longer period of time. This can provide very similar benefits, but with the added benefit of training for weeks and months with higher red-blood counts and oxygen utilization. This can provide the athlete with potentially more benefits from training with improved recovery.

**QA**

**Question:** Have you personally used or slept in a hyperbaric or hypobaric chamber? What specific changes did you experience? And for how long?

**Answer:** I have used both a mild hyperbaric chamber and a hypobaric chamber from the early days when they were first developed. These came into existence after I stopped competing, so my use was both experimental—I wanted to use it before having athletes use it—and for general health reasons. I still own a hyperbaric chamber. When I use it, I feel more relaxed, energized, and more balanced overall. I find it especially useful after long flights through several time zones in helping to recover from jet lag. They are just roomy enough to be comfortable for the forty-five-minutes you're inside. Despite the noise of the compressed air coming in, you can dose off, meditate, or read without any trouble.

I no longer have a hypobaric chamber, but sleeping in one is much like being at high altitude with a higher heart rate, and benefits are not felt for at least a few days or more. Most of these have more room inside and are made for an all-night sleep, although the compressor noise is more than obvious, especially if you're used to a very quiet environment.

- Short exposures can also be effective, although the time spent in the chamber may be proportionate to the benefits obtained. While sleeping in the chamber every night may be optimal, significant benefits can be achieved with much less exposure—beginning with sixty to ninety minutes five days a week, for example.

- Share your hypoxia with friends. Since shorter periods of exposure can be effective, a number of athletes can benefit by sharing one chamber. In this way a group of athletes can cost-effectively schedule individual chamber times throughout the day and evening, for varying amounts of time. In addition, one athlete may also sleep in the chamber during the night. In this scenario, ten or more athletes could easily obtain benefits from one chamber.

- Maintaining the benefits obtained with previous hypobaric exposure can be accomplished with less exposure. It is important for athletes to monitor their performance improvements through use of the MAF Test.

- Monitor the results. Blood tests allow more objective monitoring of physiological changes. Due to biochemical individuality, responses to the use of hypobaric chambers may vary. However, if significant measurable improvements are not seen following sufficient hypobaric use, it usually means there is some nutritional, dietary, or other lifestyle factor interfering. It would be optimal for individual athletes to monitor specific indices, such as hematocrit, to assess these improvements. Only then can each athlete determine optimal time requirements in the chamber and how long optimal benefits can be maintained during periods when the hypobaric chamber is not used.

While the use of EPO is banned in sports by the World Anti-Doping Agency, the use of hypo- and hyperbaric chamsbers is not. However, athletes who are found to have unusually high levels of EPO must demonstrate that the concentration is due to physiological conditions, such as a chamber or living at high altitude.

# PERSONAL NOTES

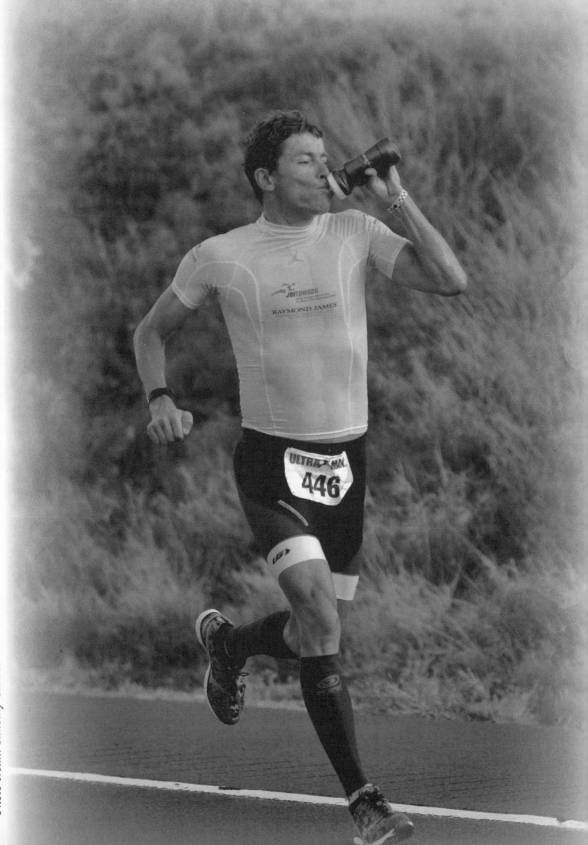

Section

TWO

# Diet and Nutrition

# CHAPTER 12

# DIET, NUTRITION, AND ENERGY— An Introduction

In the first section, I discussed various ways to improve aerobic function, including increasing speed, burning more body fat for energy, and various approaches to training and racing for optimal endurance performance without injury. But unless you also pay attention to diet and nutrition, many of these positive changes will be negated.

The body is like a machine—one accustomed to running on a certain kind of fuel. It's only been in the past several decades that our culture has embraced a dietary lifestyle that is harmful to overall health—a diet rich in white sugar and other bad carbohydrates, bad fats, and other processed, unnatural foods. While endurance athletes are often very discerning in deciding what to put on their plates, they may overlook some considerations critical to training and racing.

This second section of the book examines how diet and nutrition contribute to the vital role in improving fitness and health. Diet pertains to the foods we eat, while nutrition refers to specific nutrients—vitamins and minerals, carbohydrates, fats and proteins, and thousands of plant compounds called phytonutrients.

Let's kick off this discussion with a brief history of one of my patients. Rick was in his late twenties and, after a successful college career as a cross-country runner, began cross-training. A year later, with his road racing improving, he wanted additional help with a training schedule for triathlons. Rick was eager to learn more about individualizing his training and especially liked the notion of self-assessments including the MAF Test. However, I could not help noticing his lack of enthusiasm when I asked about his food intake, which consisted of highly processed meals and high-sugar snacks. Despite his diet, Rick progressed well in his training, and once or twice yearly he would consult with me for training purposes. On one of these visits, it was apparent that his MAF Tests were no longer progressing as well as the previous ones, and for the first time he talked about some physical pains that would come and go and some general fatigue. Rick said that hitting age thirty was the cause, but I assured him that progress should not cease, nor symptoms begin at such an early age. Yet no matter what I said to him, I could not convince him to improve his diet.

Soon after one of our talks, Rick's wife, Kathleen, made an appointment with me. Several months earlier, she'd had a bike crash that still caused knee and hip pain. The problem became chronic with lingering inflammation. Fortunately, it was easily remedied with biofeedback on the muscles that were physically traumatized, and within a week Kathleen was out of pain and riding again. I explained how balancing her dietary fats would help assure the elimination of chronic inflammation to avoid potential problems in the coming months.

A month later, both Kathleen and Rick came to see me. At long last, Rick wanted a plan to improve his diet. His wife also wanted to be involved. The first thing I did was evaluate their current food habits, using a computerized diet analysis program. This diet assessment showed that they were not even consuming RDA levels of various nutrients and that other imbalances existed, including essential fats and high-quality protein. I provided each with specific foods to add—more fresh vegetables, olive oil, and whole eggs daily. I listed foods to avoid, including processed flour products such as bread, rolls, and cereal, and vegetable oils and margarine.

Two months later they returned for a follow-up visit. Both had improved their diet significantly and were on their way to optimizing their overall food and nutrition. Kathleen had improved her fat burning as indicated by improved energy, a better MAF Test, and a loss of over an inch on her waist. Rick had finally broken out of his endurance rut, improving his MAF Test, and no longer had physical aches and pains. Both were now convinced of the power of food and were full of questions about additional ways to eat better.

## Fueling Aerobic Function

Now that you're on your way to developing maximum aerobic function through proper training—the fine-tuning of your body's fat-burning engine—it's important to get the right fuel for this task. This fuel comes from the nutrients in many of the foods we should eat. In addition to increased fat burning, these nutrients are needed for our brain, muscles, metabolism, and all bodily function.

There are three groups of nutrients in our diet:

- *Macronutrients* include carbohydrates, fats, and proteins. Most of our energy comes predominantly from carbohydrates and fats, but protein also plays an important role. Other macronutrients include water and fiber.
- *Micronutrients*—the vitamins and minerals—are equally valuable in helping carbohydrates and fats convert to energy. They also help prevent muscle damage, improve recovery, and many other important features.
- *Phytonutrients* include thousands of plant compounds that may be just as important as micronutrients in helping to control inflammation, improve immunity, and assist in repair, recovery, and other healthy functions.

There are no magic formulas or special diet plans unique to endurance athletes, except eating a balance of real foods. This will improve your endurance better than anything.

And, *it's most important to rely on your food intake to provide all three categories of nutrients.* Only after making your food intake as optimal as possible should the use of dietary supplements be added if necessary. If you match the body's needs with the appropriate foods, your endurance will improve dramatically, as will your health. In addition, the rest of your body will function optimally, perhaps like it did when you were younger—or even better. Or if you're a youngster, you'll avoid the injuries, ill health, and poor performances that many athletes experience at alarming rates in their twenties, thirties, and later in life. With proper nutrition and training, your endurance could—and should—actually improve with age.

Once you find the proper dietary balance, this will result in nearly unlimited levels of energy and endurance for sports as well as other areas of your life. *Ergogenic nourishment* refers to the consumption of food to obtain nutrients for optimal human performance.

Athletes, scientists, and clinicians have long agreed that eating habits directly affect endurance in general and, specifically, training and competition. In many cases, it's not a question of the latest research but rather an understanding of basic physiology and biochemistry. For example, it's well known that water is the most important ergogenic aid in sports. Even minor deficiencies cause dehydration and can be devastating to your performance results. This same principle applies to electrolytes—reduced sodium content in the body, for example, will usually have major adverse effects on training and competition. But just consuming these nutrients may not help if your adrenal gland system, which helps regulate water and electrolytes, is not properly functioning.

## Fat Burning

If you want to achieve optimal endurance, then you need to burn more fat. It's that simple. Your body has plenty of fat stores, where most of the fat you eat is first deposited. This stored fat, even the small amounts in super-lean athletes, represents a tremendous reserve of potential energy. For example, an endurance runner who is six feet tall and weighs 150 pounds has enough potential energy stores from his fat stores to power a run for over 100 hours. Trying to obtain more energy from sugar won't come close to that feat.

During rest, fat may contribute significant amounts of energy, up to 60 to 80 percent, or more. The same is true during light to moderate workouts, where fat may provide well over half of the necessary energy; likewise during longer training periods and competitions. In well-trained athletes, up to 80 percent or more of their energy needs can come from fat during training. From a standpoint of athletic performance, eating enough fat helps a well-trained aerobic engine burn more fat for energy. And an increased consumption of dietary fat spares stored glycogen during exercise, an important function for endurance and competition.

To maintain efficient fat burning, we also must burn some sugar in the form of glucose. Both fat and sugar are almost always being used for energy at all times. Right now, you may be getting half of your energy from fat and half from sugar. When you improve your aerobic system and fat-burning capabilities, you may be able to obtain 70 percent of your energy from fat and 30 percent from sugar. But many people can only get 10 percent of their energy from fat, forcing a full 90 percent to come from sugar. That's a very inefficient way to get energy and it could lead to fatigue, increased body-fat stores, and other problems. In fact, it became evident to me decades ago that those who burn more fat for energy are healthier, more fit, recover better, and have less illness and injury.

## Measuring Fat and Sugar Burning

This mix of fuels can be easily measured in a person with a gas analyzer, which measures the amount of oxygen a person takes into his or her body and the amount of carbon dioxide eliminated. The ratio of carbon dioxide to oxygen is called the respiratory quotient (RQ), and from it is determined the percentage of fat and sugar used for energy. A lower RQ number corresponds to greater fat burning and a higher level of aerobic function. I do not necessarily recommend most people have an RQ test because it is not readily available and many coaches and healthcare professionals don't relate the findings to endurance training. And the protocol used by most people is the same one used to measure $VO_2$max, which is an unnatural test. However, it is useful for you to understand the RQ concept in order to better understand the physiology of how all the information in this book will improve your endurance.

In addition to increased fat burning and better aerobic function for significant improvement in fitness, it's common to see better health associated with more utilization of fat as a fuel. Following is a list of some of my patient's RQ numbers at rest and their symptoms. Take away the patient initials and the chart could really be one person who progresses on the program outlined in this book. In general, the less sugar and more fat burning

at any level of intensity, the more healthy and fit the individual.

Dietary carbohydrates are also important nutrients for our endurance and overall health. But just like the need to consume high-quality fat, the same is true for carbohydrates. We should consume them in their natural form and avoid processed/refined carbohydrates, which can impair our endurance because it can reduce fat burning.

Perhaps just as important as the food we eat is the ability to properly digest and absorb these nutrients. Without proper digestion of macronutrients to make glucose, fat, and amino acids available for absorption, and the breakdown of foods so micronutrients and phytonutrients are available for absorption, imbalances can occur even with the ideal diet.

| Sugar and Fat Burning Percentages in Various Patients | | |
| --- | --- | --- |
| Patient | Approx Sugar/Fat Burning | Signs/Symptoms |
| JC | 88% sugar, 12% fat | extreme fatigue, insomnia, 45 pounds overweight |
| BK | 74% sugar, 26% fat | afternoon and evening fatigue, asthma, headaches |
| JO | 62% sugar, 38% fat | afternoon fatigue, seasonal allergies, 10 pounds overweight |
| PS | 55% sugar, 45% fat | chronic, mild knee pain, indigestion |
| MK | 42% sugar, 58% fat | occasional low-back pain |
| BE | 37% sugar, 63% fat | none |

# CHAPTER 13

# THE GUT—
## Intestinal Digestion and Absorption of Nutrients

**N**apoleon once famously declared that an army marches on its stomach. The same can be said of endurance athletes—but the marching is replaced by running, biking, swimming, and other physical activities.

Complaints of intestinal distress probably affect more than half of all endurance athletes. In my experience, another 25 percent have functional intestinal problems that produce little or no overt signs or symptoms. Any of these problems can affect training and especially competition, and often occur at rest as well, influencing a person's nutritional state. This problem is not only one of comfort, but an indication that the intestines—also called the gut—may not be functioning properly. If this is the case, one may be unable to obtain all the nutrients from one's diet. A faulty gut can also have a negative impact on immune, muscle, and brain function.

A better understanding about the gut will help correct many intestinal problems and provide more nutrients—and energy—for endurance. The main function of the gut is digestion of food and absorption of nutrients.

Most people are well aware of these activities, but the gut is also home to most of the adult immune system: it assists the liver by eliminating toxins, it produces vitamins and hormones, and it has an extensive nervous system of its own. The gut is also in constant communication with the brain. All these areas can become disturbed when the gut is under stress, such as from poor digestion. For example, even if you eat the right foods, if they're not properly digested and the small intestine does not absorb the nutrients, nutritional imbalances can occur due to malabsorption. This could create a problem identical to those associated with *not* eating the right foods. Or, a poor functioning gut can reduce immune function, leading to more colds, flu, and other illness.

## Gut Problems in Athletes

Signs and symptoms of gut dysfunction are common in athletes. They include nausea, vomiting, and diarrhea, and various other complaints of symptoms similar to indigestion. Often, these problems affect the outcome of competition. Among the biggest sellers of drugs, both over-the-counter and prescription, are those that cover the symptoms of an improperly functioning gut. Most don't treat or correct the causes of the problems.

Running seems to bring out more of these problems, probably because of its higher physical stress, although cycling, swimming, and other activities are also associated with gut problems. More than half the runners in a race will have some type of intestinal distress, with some published studies showing that number to be as high as 80 percent. Many runners report that these problems affect their running performance. It appears that athletes who don't properly regulate water balance, often due to poor adrenal function, have more gut symptoms during training and competition.

Causes for many gut problems depend on the athlete. They range from poor diet or nervous system stress to hormone imbalance and dehydration. A healthy athlete has much less gut trouble, not only during training and competition but at all other times, making the focus of overall health important to prevent these common problems.

Taking non-steroidal anti-inflammatory drugs (NSAIDs) before running can significantly increase nausea and vomiting and cause injury to the gut. Consuming certain types of carbohydrates (such as sucrose, maltose-based sugars, and corn sugars) can also cause intestinal bloating and nausea. Eating solid food that requires digestion can also cause vomiting during or after training or competition. These problems can occur especially if food is not chewed or liquids not mixed with saliva to assist in digestion. Starting your race too fast or not warming up can also contribute to intestinal stress.

Upper gut symptoms are those that come from the stomach, including cramping, vomiting, and "gastric" problems. Those specifically associated with lower intestinal stress are also very common and include lower abdominal cramping and diarrhea.

In general, intestinal problems incurred during training and competition may represent an expression of existing gut problems. Some of these may also be evident during rest, while others may not have obvious signs or symptoms.

The good news is that the majority of gut problems can be significantly improved or eliminated by making some relatively simple changes in your food intake and other factors that influence the gut, such as stress. This includes problems in the mouth, such as tooth problems and indigestion, ulcers, reflux, and other chronic diseases such as Crohn's and ulcerative colitis. Let's consider each major area of the gut, its purpose, and how one can help it function better.

## The Mouth

We use it for talking, singing, screaming, kissing, and even making odd noises. The mouth, however, serves another important function that many people neglect—helping us get more nutrients from our food and keeping the gut working well. Many gut problems begin in the mouth, and many can be significantly improved by using the mouth more.

Gut problems often come from not properly chewing food or rushing our meals. Gut problems can sometimes be due to teeth issues, such as loose teeth or other neglected problems. The jaw joint (TMJ) can also be a problem, such as when it is not balanced,

causing the bite to be out of alignment and resulting in a poor chewing mechanism. The chemistry of the mouth can also be a problem, such as low salivary pH, which can contribute to poor use of digestive enzymes.

The mouth, and its connection to the brain, can help athletes in other ways too. The taste buds on our tongue are important for sending messages to the brain, informing it about the nutrients coming into the body. For example, studies show that during physical activity, just the taste of sugar in the mouth can improve performance. Beginning very early in my career, I instructed my athletes who were competing in long events to suck on salt tablets, which often made them feel better and stronger almost instantly. Today, scientists know the important connections between the taste buds in the mouth and the brain, which can even help improve muscle activity.

## Chewing

Russian physiologist Ivan Pavlov's groundbreaking research into the importance of chewing and human digestion won him a Nobel Prize in 1904. After more than a century, physiologists continue building on that understanding.

The taste receptors on the tongue detect extremely small concentrations of substances within a fraction of a second of tasting it—one reason we love the taste of food. This stimulation elicits a variety of immediate responses throughout the body, including stimulating heat production and fat burning and improving digestion, absorption, and even the use of nutrients from foods. Chewing our food, called the "cephalic phase" of digestion because the brain immediately senses and responds to what's being consumed, can also help control blood sugar and control fluid and mineral balance. Most of us have experienced being ravenously hungry after a long workout and even feeling weak, only to perk up the moment we started chewing on some food.

All food should be chewed for better digestion. But those that require the most chewing include concentrated carbohydrates—bread and other starchy grain products, including pasta, rice and beans, all cereals, starchy vegetables such as potatoes and corn, and most sugars. The exceptions are fruit and honey, which don't require chemical digestion to obtain the important sugars. However, fruit needs to be chewed into smaller pieces to help the intestine obtain the nutrients within.

An important enzyme in saliva, amylase, starts digestion of carbohydrate foods, and without it normal digestion of this food group may not occur, with the risk of producing gas, indigestion, and other common intestinal problems. The use of sugars—fruit and honey—that don't require digestion are best for many athletes before, during, and after long training and competitive events. All other carbohydrates should be chewed sufficiently or mixed with saliva for better digestion; otherwise, you may not get as many nutrients—including sugar during your training or race—from them.

Most significant in relation to eating is to chew your food well. Keep it simple: rather than counting each mouthful, just chew and enjoy the tastes and textures of the food you're eating. Once it has turned into very small pieces and is well moistened, swallow it and enjoy another bite. Rushing meals, eating while working at your desk, and other poor habits make it almost impossible to chew and digest well. Listening to music during meals can help all phases of digestion.

### Oral pH

The environment of the mouth is a critical part of its overall health, especially the acid-alkaline balance—the pH—of the saliva. The pH can be measured with pH paper, available at a pharmacy, health store, or online. The pH of the mouth should be slightly alkaline, in the range of about 7.4 to 7.6 (slightly higher in children). You may hear or read that the mouth should be an acid pH, but this is confused with the fact that many people have a mouth with a pH in the acid range—6.0, 6.5, 6.8, and so forth. (A pH of 7.0 is neutral; above is alkaline and below is acid.)

One key relationship with oral pH is fat burning. Those with lower pH levels typically have higher RQ (respiratory quotient) numbers, indicating reduced fat burning. As you improve your diet, build your aerobic system, and develop more endurance, your oral pH, among other things, will improve.

Here's the procedure to test your pH:

- Wait about fifteen minutes after eating or drinking, or rinse your mouth well with water and wait about five minutes.
- Use a small strip of pH paper and thoroughly moisten it in your mouth for about five seconds.
- Immediately compare the color on your test strip with the color on the pH paper container to determine the approximate pH.

Initially, perform this test two or three times in one day, then again a few days later to establish your average pH level—although it should not vary by much if you follow the above procedure properly. If your pH is consistently too high (above 7.6), it may indicate a need to increase natural carbohydrates—such as fruits and whole grains. But if your pH is too low, it may indicate two things: you're eating too many carbohydrates, most likely the refined types, and you need to add more protein and fat to your diet. After making the appropriate dietary changes, check the pH twice a week to follow progress; improvements in pH could take up to a month or more.

In children and adults, low pH—less than 7.0—promotes tooth decay. While in practice I noticed those individuals with proper pH did not get cavities, but those who had tooth decay almost always had low pH.

## Stomach

From the mouth, food is swallowed down a long muscular tube, the esophagus, into the stomach. The two most important aspects of digestion here are the physical mixing of food and the chemical action of hydrochloric acid, which is produced in certain cells in the stomach. Food is mixed with the help of three layers of smooth muscle that make up the stomach. This is the reason you may feel and hear normal noises from your gut—there's a lot of churning going on there, especially after a meal. It's much like your washing machine.

When food enters the stomach, hydrochloric acid is normally secreted and is vital to proper digestion, helping to make nutrients from foods available for absorption. This natural acid stimulates other digestive enzymes, such as pepsin for the breakdown of protein. Hydrochloric acid helps make vitamins, minerals, and other nutrients more absorbable. It also kills bacteria, viruses, parasites, and other potentially harmful invaders that commonly enter through almost all foods. Reducing your hydrochloric acid with antacids can be detrimental for many reasons. First, protein digestion may be impaired and you may not absorb the much-needed amino acids. It can trigger immune reactions if undigested (whole proteins) are absorbed, one common cause of allergies. Hydrochloric acid also triggers digestive enzymes in the small intestines and pancreas, areas that complete the digestive process and prepare nutrients for absorption.

Taking antacids is not the only way to reduce levels of hydrochloric acid. As we age, there is often a lowering level of normal stomach acid, and stress can do the same. Excess stress typically reduces the stomach's acid, despite the common notion that stress overproduces acid—much of this myth comes from the marketing of very popular antacids. Fewer people than one might think over-produce hydrochloric acid under stress. This usually happens between meals, where most have learned that eating a small amount of food reduces or eliminates the discomfort caused by too much acid.

Drinking liquids with meals may also dilute stomach acid and enzymes resulting in less-efficient digestion. Drink all your water between meals, avoiding it about twenty minutes before and an hour or more after eating. Soda, milk, sports drinks, fruit juice, and other liquids are not part of a healthy diet and as such should be avoided. An exception to drinking liquids with meals is wine, which may be consumed with meals as it can help digestion.

For those with inadequate hydrochloric acid production, supplements containing betaine hydrochloride (a solid which turns to hydrochloric acid when swallowed) can be very helpful. Common symptoms in people with low levels of normal stomach acid include belching and bloating after meals (especially with protein), bad breath, loss of appetite, and large amounts of foul-smelling gas. Those with reduced acid can develop abnormal fermentation in the stomach that produces other acids that are irritating, especially if they go upward into the esophagus, causing a burning feeling.

A common condition called GERD—gastroesophageal reflux—has become a frequently diagnosed problem. Drugs to treat the symptoms are among the biggest sellers, yet people still have the symptoms. In true cases of GERD, stomach contents back up into the esophagus, causing irritation, with symptoms occurring mostly after meals, or when lying down or bending over with the head below the waist. In severe cases, ulceration can occur in the esophagus. Most people have less serious but sometimes very uncomfortable symptoms associated with bloating due to gas. This often comes from eating starchy or processed carbohydrates, especially at the same time as eating dense proteins, overeating, and other causes of gas. Reducing or eliminating refined carbohydrates often eliminates the symptoms of GERD. In some individuals, eliminating lactose from dairy can do the same (lactose is a sugar that requires digestion). In other cases, poor stomach digestion, often from not enough stomach acid, causes GERD.

### Small Intestine

Following digestion in the stomach, food passes into the small intestines for the completion of digestion and the absorption of nutrients. The small intestine, with its finger-like projections called *villi*, is capable of pulling nutrients from the now well-digested foods. Certain portions of the small intestine

# INTESTINAL GAS

When too much gas accumulates in the intestine, it can cause more than discomfort. Pockets of gas anywhere in the gut can trigger a sympathetic nervous system response—a stress reaction. Small amounts of gas in the gut are normal. But larger volumes of gas are not, and usually indicate something is wrong with your diet or even the way you're eating. Here are the four most common causes of intestinal gas:

The most common causes are starchy carbohydrates—bread, cereal, the many products made from wheat flour—and sugar. This includes milk sugar (lactose) from dairy products.

Another common cause of intestinal gas is swallowing air. This occurs during eating and drinking liquids, especially water, as people tend to drink several ounces or more at one time. Drink liquids slowly to avoid swallowing air and, most importantly, keep your head tilted forward—not backward—to avoid swallowing air. In addition, chewing food and not rushing meals will help you avoid swallowing large amounts of air. Once air is swallowed, if it doesn't come back up soon as a burp, most of it must travel through the gut and come out the other end.

Stomach dysfunction is a common cause of gas. This is typically due to low levels of hydrochloric acid, as discussed above.

Large intestine dysfunction—often due to the wrong bacteria residing in the gut (discussed below) may cause excess gas. This can also cause bad breath as some of this gas is absorbed into the blood and released through the lungs.

Other foods that promote gas include chewing gum, especially the "sugar-free" products containing sorbitol and other alcohol sugars. In addition, some individuals are sensitive to the natural fruit sugar fructose found in fruits, and especially high in fruit juice.

Drugs to reduce gas don't work. The American College of Gastroenterology states, "Despite the many commercials and advertisements for medications which reduce gas pains and bloating, very few have any proven scientific value." If you have excess gas, addressing the causes as discussed here can usually significantly reduce the problem.

absorb specific nutrients as they pass. Once nutrients are made available through the action of digestion, they can now be absorbed into the bloodstream for transport to the liver and throughout the body.

The *villis'* function is vital for good nutrient absorption. Stress, poor digestion, and not eating (dieting, fasting, hospitalization) can significantly impair their function. In addition, the *villi* use an important amino acid, L-glutamine, as their energy source for the absorptive mechanism to function. Without adequate glutamine, absorption of nutrients can be impaired. Glutamine is a common amino acid found in meats and other proteins, but it is easily destroyed by heat.

Once absorbed into the blood, nutrients are carried to the liver for processing. The liver acts like a manufacturing plant and distribution center. Some nutrients rely on others for their utilization. For example, calcium requires certain fats to be carried into bones and muscles. Other nutrients, such as thiamin, can go directly into cells to help generate energy.

Digestion of macronutrients—carbohydrates, fats, and proteins—into their basic components of glucose, small fat particles, and amino acids, respectively, provides the raw materials for our energy needs. Once absorbed, glucose is acted upon by insulin and either used immediately for energy, stored as fat, or stored as glycogen. Fats are sent to storage until called for by the aerobic muscles for use as energy, and even amino acids are used to produce small amounts of energy.

### Large Intestine

After digestion and absorption of nutrients in the small intestines, the remainder of the food material passes into the large intestine or colon. Here, it is acted upon by healthy bacteria, microorganisms that humans have hosted for millions of years. An assortment of bacterial strains is normally present and varies with an individual's diet and lifestyle. These bacteria produce some very important nutrients, including vitamin K, some B vitamins, and biotin. Important end products produced by the bacteria are fatty acids, which help regulate the acid-alkaline balance in the large intestine and in turn control the type of bacteria that thrives there. Some fatty acids also serve as an important energy source for the cells in the lower intestine. These microorganisms ferment some of the fiber from the diet, also improving the health of our intestine. Optimal large intestine function also impacts immune function.

Antibiotics, the lack of adequate dietary fiber, and excess carbohydrates are some reasons why bacteria in the large intestine change to a less friendly and often harmful type. These harmful bacteria and other microorganisms can produce metabolites that are absorbed into the bloodstream and can adversely affect brain and body function.

For those athletes who have taken antibiotics, which quickly kill the natural gut bacteria, a dietary supplement containing live, freeze-dried friendly bacteria may be useful. Care must be taken when purchasing these products as many no longer contain live cultures. The best products are those that are refrigerated, contain six, eight, or even ten or more different strains of bacteria, and have bacterial counts in the *billions*, not millions. In addition, cultured foods, such as yogurt and kefir, may help accomplish the same task. However, avoid products containing added sugar and starch.

The bulk of the waste leaving the body is greatly influenced by gut bacteria. In some cases, up to 40 percent of waste volume can be attributed to bacteria. Reduced stool volume may be an indication of poor microorganism population. Foul odor is another common sign. Likewise, reduction of odor and increased stool bulk would indicate an improved gut environment.

Constipation and diarrhea are two of the most common gut complaints, not only in athletes but in all individuals. Most people can avoid or resolve these problems by being fit and healthy. Constipation technically refers to excess straining with bowel movements and the passage of small hard stools. It can occur when the waste (stool) moves too slowly through the lower gut. The most common causes include dehydration, changes in diet (this may occur initially, even when improving your diet), physical inactivity, and a variety of drugs. Treatment and prevention measures include sufficient water between meals, ten servings of vegetables and fruits (prunes are very effective; one to three per day with a large glass of water), psyllium (taken with a large glass of water), and easy physical activity (such as regular walking). In almost all cases, these habits will result in normal gut function (having at least one to three bowel movements a day). However, if more remedies are needed to treat constipation, it's best to see your doctor. The use of laxatives is usually not needed in those who follow a good diet and are healthy.

Diarrhea is an abnormal looseness of the stools, usually with increased frequency. Acute watery diarrhea is usually associated with some illness, with symptoms of gas, cramping, and intestinal pain. When severe, it can lead to dehydration and dangerous losses of electrolytes (including sodium, potassium, calcium, and magnesium). Acute diarrhea is often caused by a viral infection and sometimes by drugs (especially antibiotics). Bacterial infections are sometimes the cause, especially when blood is present. Artificial sweeteners can also cause acute diarrhea (especially the alcohol sugars sorbitol, xylitol, and others). Athletes, in particular, can have diarrhea associated with competition, typically when adrenal dysfunction exists as previously discussed.

If you have acute diarrhea lasting more than ten days to two weeks, see your doctor. When acute diarrhea becomes chronic, it may be associated with more serious problems. NSAIDs, antibiotics, and antacids can also cause chronic diarrhea, as can dairy foods and gluten-containing grains—especially wheat. Finding and eliminating the cause of the problem is the best remedy. In the meantime, keeping well hydrated is important, and pectin, best consumed from fresh apples or applesauce, can be effective as well.

The gut plays a vital role for athletes seeking optimal endurance and overall health. Perhaps the most common problem affecting gut function is the intake of certain types of carbohydrates. And as endurance athletes know all too well, carbs are critical for sustained performance.

# CHAPTER 14

# CARBOHYDRATES AND TAKING THE TWO-WEEK TEST

**E**ndurance athletes thrive and survive on glucose, which comes from dietary carbohydrates. The body can also obtain glucose from both fat and protein. For most athletes, carbohydrates are the majority macronutrient in their diet, providing the body with energy. Carbohydrate foods include fruits, whole grains, vegetables, brown rice, lentils, beans, and honey; they also provide vitamins, minerals, fiber, water, and many phytonutrients.

Unfortunately, most of the carbohydrate foods athletes eat are highly processed, such as refined wheat flour—which is made into bread, rolls, bagels, and cereal. Other carb no-nos include white rice, fruit juice, and sugar or sugar-containing products, such as desserts. These foods can be very unhealthy for athletes because they don't provide the full spectrum of nutrients compared to their natural counterparts, and they can cause increased production of the hormone insulin, which reduces fat burning.

## Types of Carbohydrates

All carbohydrates are composed of single sugar molecules that exist in three forms—glucose, fructose, and galactose:

- Complex carbohydrates, also called starches (polysaccharides), contain many single sugars attached together: for example, many glucose molecules held together (glucose + glucose + glucose). These carbs can be found in potatoes, corn, all grains, and beans.
- Double sugars (disaccharides) are made up of two sugars attached to each other. They include sucrose (glucose + fructose), lactose (glucose + galactose), and maltose (glucose + glucose). These are found in table sugar (sucrose), milk sugar (lactose), maple syrup (maltose), and other "malt" sugars, such as maltodextrin.
- Simple sugars (monosaccharides) contain single, unattached sugars. These are found in ripe fruits and vegetables and honey, all of which have various amounts of glucose and fructose.

Unripe fruits and vegetables contain higher amounts of starch and double sugars. During the ripening process, these complex carbs and double sugars are converted to simple sugars, making ripe fruit taste sweeter. As an example, green bananas turn yellow (with black spots) when ripe. Even vegetables are sweeter when ripe: green peppers are unripe and turn red (or yellow) when ripe. Because most of the sugars contained in these plant foods are broken down to simple sugars, no further digestion of these carbohydrates is needed. For some people, eating unripe fruit or vegetables is the reason they get indigestion.

It's most important to understand this aspect of carbohydrates: Both complex carbs and double sugars require digestion in order to break apart the simple sugars that are attached to each other. This must occur in order for sugar to be absorbed and made available for energy. Complex carbohydrates require the most digestion. Simple sugars don't require digestion; they are immediately available for absorption.

During the process of digestion, both complex and double-sugar carbohydrates are chemically broken down to their simple sugars (monosaccharide). Digestion occurs primarily in the mouth and small intestine. Once digested, the sugars are absorbed into the blood and are then referred to as "blood sugar."

Complex carbohydrates and double sugars often don't completely digest into their simple sugars. This may be due to insufficient chewing of food in order to mix it with the enzymes in saliva, common during the stress of competition or long training. Those incompletely digested carbohydrates can cause significant amounts of intestinal gas, causing discomfort or often pain. We've all experienced this type of stress in our intestines during physical activity.

One problem with a high amount of refined carbohydrates in the diet is that they take the

**Types of Carbohydrates**

## The Building Blocks of Carbohydrates

### Monosaccharides
**one simple sugar molecule**
Examples: Glucose and fructose (and small amounts of galactose), found predominantly in fruit and fruit juice, honey, and vegetables.

### Disaccharides
**Two simple sugar molecules**
Examples: Sucrose (glucose + fructose), lactose (glucose + galactose), and maltose (glucose + glucose). These are found in table sugar (sucrose), milk sugar (lactose), maple syrup (maltose), and others.

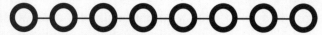

### Polysaccharides
**Several sugar molecules**
Examples: Starch (glucose + glucose + glucose, etc.). These are predominantly found in potatoes. corn, all grains, and beans.

place of other healthy foods—fats, proteins, and vegetables. For endurance athletes, this can produce inadequate nutrition as well as reduce fat burning and aerobic function.

While many scientists believe that humans have no true requirement for carbohydrates (because fat and protein can be converted to glucose), many people consume refined carbs as a staple of their diet—and in very high amounts. In fact, most athletes consume the majority of their carbohydrates as the refined, processed type.

## Carbohydrates and Insulin

When we consume carbohydrates, most are broken down to glucose and absorbed into the blood. The rise in blood sugar immediately triggers the release of the hormone insulin from the pancreas. Insulin is a very important hormone but too much adversely affects one's endurance and health, especially by reducing the ability to burn body fat.

Insulin allows us to use and store glucose, and as this happens, blood sugar is lowered. Insulin works through three different mechanisms:

About 50 percent of the blood sugar (about half the carbohydrates you eat) is quickly used throughout the body for energy, especially in muscles and the brain.

Up to about 10 percent of the carbohydrates you eat are converted to glycogen, a storage form of sugar. The glycogen is stored in the muscles and liver. The amount depends on the level of your glycogen stores. (Muscle glycogen, for example, is converted back to glucose for energy, and liver glycogen helps maintain blood sugar levels between meals and during nighttime sleep.)

About 40 percent or more of the carbohydrates you eat is converted to fat and stored as body fat. This is the source of fat used by the aerobic muscles for energy, but if the fat-burning mechanisms are not working well, or if too much carbohydrate is consumed, fat stores can get larger.

Insulin is produced whenever you eat carbohydrates, except when you consume them during training or competition. Insulin levels are reduced during physical activity, helping the body burn more fat for energy. Smaller amounts of insulin may also be produced if you consume a protein-only meal, and in some people, a high-protein meal can stimulate significant amounts of insulin. But for most people, it's predominantly carbohydrates that trigger the insulin mechanism. As noted, too much insulin causes problems for endurance athletes, as can too little (a problem for diabetics).

In the past several decades, the high consumption of highly refined carbohydrates has contributed significantly to the obesity epidemic and other chronic illness such as diabetes and heart disease. In addition, there is an "overfat" (as opposed to "overweight") problem, even among athletes. The trend in carbohydrate over-consumption continues today, propelled by companies selling refined carbohydrates and sugar. This is quite prevalent in the endurance sports market.

During most of our evolutionary history, humans lived near the sea and consumed significant amounts of fish, seafood, and other land-animal proteins. More importantly, large amounts of plant foods were also part of our diet. These included vegetables, fruits, nuts, and seeds. In addition, our ancestors were very active physically, even more than most endurance athletes today. Only in the last five-thousand years has this changed. The agricultural revolution brought a dramatic increase in carbohydrate foods and the industrial revolution brought highly refined carbohydrates to the table. The intake of refined carbohydrates by humans has never been as dramatically high as in just the last one hundred years. This relatively short period of significant dietary change has contributed to the overfat problem, and to many problems leading to heart disease, cancer, obesity, and other diseases. This is due, in part, to the over-consumption of refined carbohydrates, higher levels of insulin production, higher fat stores, and chronic inflammation.

The more carbohydrates consumed, the more insulin produced by the pancreas. Even healthy people can overproduce insulin by eating excessive amounts of carbohydrates. While this problem is thought to occur in those who are overfat, it can also occur in lean people as well.

This potentially leads to a condition referred to as "insulin resistance," associated with the inability of insulin to efficiently fuel the muscles with glucose. As a result, energy is reduced, along with fat burning. Hunger is another result—because the cells don't get enough energy, each time these people eat carbohydrates, the brain gets the message that the cells don't have enough sugar and the brain tells the pancreas to make more insulin. Finally, insulin is produced beyond normal limits, a condition referred to as "hyperinsulinism." While it takes more insulin to get glucose into the insulin-resistant cells efficiently, this hormone continues to perform its other tasks, including turning carbohydrates into fat for storage.

In addition to causing even more carbohydrates to convert and store as fat, excess insulin can continue lowering the blood sugar—because that's one of its functions, including converting glucose to fat. Since the brain exclusively relies on glucose for fuel, periods of reduced blood sugar can result in impaired mental function, including loss of memory, reduced concentration, and other cognitive impairments. Low blood sugar also results in hunger, sometimes only a couple of hours or less after the meal. Cravings for sweets are typically part of this cycle and resorting to snacking on more carbohydrates maintains the vicious cycle. And if you don't eat, you just feel worse. Eventually, the fat-storage deposits get bigger. While this problem can be relatively minor, in some athletes it can cause a more serious condition, such as higher body fat or even diabetes, the full spectrum of this carbohydrate problem is a condition I term *carbohydrate intolerance*, discussed below.

High insulin levels also suppress two important hormones: glucagon and growth hormone. Glucagon has the opposite effect of insulin and is produced following protein consumption. While insulin promotes fat storage, glucagon promotes the use of fat and sugar for energy. Growth hormone helps provide many of the endurance benefits we obtain through training, including muscle development, sugar and fat burning, and the regulation of minerals and amino acids.

### Glycemic Index

The general measure of how much your blood sugar increases after eating specific carbohydrates is called the glycemic index (GI). This is associated with the amount of insulin produced. The GI is a general measure of individual responses to particular carbohydrate foods; however, individual variation is not considered in studies of foods and their glycemic effects.

High-GI foods, which produce the greatest glucose response (and highest insulin), include bagels, breads, potatoes, sweets, and other foods that contain refined flour and sugar. Many processed cereals, especially those containing malt sugars (maple syrup, maltose, maltodextrin, etc.), have a very high GI. Even foods you may think are good for you can trigger high amounts of insulin, including fruit juice and large bananas, especially when unripe. The biggest problems in most diets may be wheat products, potatoes, fruit juice, and sugar or sugar-containing products. Most sports drinks, energy bars, and other carbohydrate-based products are very high glycemic; they can be useful *during* training or competition when insulin levels are much lower but not as a regular part of an athlete's diet.

Carbohydrates with a moderate and low GI include many fruits, such as apples, peaches, pears, grapefruits, and cherries, as well as legumes such as lentils. Non-carbohydrate foods—proteins and fats—usually don't cause a glycemic problem, although in some people even meals high in protein can trigger an abnormal insulin response.

Eating smaller and more frequent moderate- and low-glycemic meals often reduces high insulin production, as discussed later under healthy snacking. Most vegetables contain only small amounts of carbohydrates—except very starchy ones like potatoes and corn. Carrots were at one time believed to be a high-glycemic food, but studies have shown the glycemic effect of this root vegetable to be much lower than previously thought.

In practical terms, this means that eating refined foods like a large cookie or piece of cake will cause more problems than eating a piece of fruit or whole-grain cracker with the same amount of carbohydrates and calories.

Low-fat foods or low-fat meals containing carbohydrates have a relatively higher glycemic index because digestion and absorption of sugar are quicker when less fat is present. Eating carbohydrate foods in combination with some fats, such as olive oil or butter, slows digestion and absorption, thus moderating the insulin response. Moderate protein levels in a meal also can lower the glycemic index of the meal, as can fiber.

By moderating carbohydrate intake to control insulin production, you can increase your ability to burn fat as an optimal and efficient source of almost unlimited energy. Rather than using the glycemic index as a guide, which has become common, it may be best for athletes to learn which foods and food combinations work best for their individual needs.

### Carbohydrate Intolerance

With generations of people over-consuming refined carbohydrates, many now have a health problem I have termed "carbohydrate intolerance," or CI. It's a widespread phenomenon. Though most people are unaware such a condition even exists in its early stages, a high percentage of the population suffers from CI in all stages. The symptoms of early CI are very common and include sleepiness after meals, intestinal bloating, increased body fat, fatigue, and many others as shown in the survey below. The middle stages of CI are often accompanied by higher blood fats—especially triglycerides but also

| Some Examples of Higher and Lower Glycemic Foods |
| --- |
| **Higher Glycemic Foods** |
| Refined flour products: bread, chips, bagels, cereals |
| Sugar and sugar-containing foods: candy, cookies, soda |
| Sweet fruits: pineapple, watermelon, grapes, bananas, all fruit juice |
| Starchy vegetables: potatoes, corn |
| **Lower Glycemic Foods** |
| Unrefined grains: whole rye, wheat germ, high fiber products |
| Low sugar fruits: apples, peaches, pears, berries, melon |
| Lentils, beans |
| All other vegetables |

full spectrum of carbohydrate (glucose) function in the body, from the normal, healthy condition to the other extreme of diabetes. In between are many abnormal states, some more mild and others more serious. Many people go through life progressing through part of or the entire spectrum. Rather than getting confused about defining the different stages (an important task for researchers and clinicians), it's best to just call this full spectrum carbohydrate intolerance.

Many clinicians discuss this full spectrum of CI from a standpoint of glucose: there's normal glucose and impaired glucose. Depending on test results and their interpretations, a concoction of names has resulted, which has continued to confuse healthcare professionals and lay people alike. For example, common classifications of early stages CI include *impaired glucose metabolism*, *impaired blood sugar*, *glucose intolerance*, and others. *Insulin resistance* and *hyperinsulinemia* are names applied in later, more chronic conditions.

Even the term *hypoglycemia*, originally only discussed in relation to diabetics, is a condition now known to occur in individuals who are free of measurable disease. Further confusion exists because some hypoglycemic reactions are normal; it's the abnormal form that exists as a result of excess insulin production.

CI can also affect endurance performance in several ways, including reduction of fat burning, promotion of chronic inflammation, and injuries.

cholesterol—and hypertension. Later stages include diabetes, obesity, cancer, and heart disease.

The early stages of CI can be vague, often unrecognized by health-care professionals and lay people alike. A variety of names and changing definitions have been used by organizations like the ADA (American Diabetes Association) and WHO (World Health Organization) in relation to these abnormal carbohydrate and glucose problems. All this is an attempt to better understand the issues, although more comprehensive standardized definitions are still lacking. We know there's a

Like most problems, CI is an individual one, affecting different people in different ways. Only you can determine how intolerant you are to carbohydrates and to what degree. Blood tests will diagnose the problem only in the middle and later stages, but the signs and symptoms may have begun years earlier. The key to avoiding the full spectrum of CI is to be aware of it in its earliest stage and to make the appropriate diet and lifestyle changes. This can improve athletic performance and quality of life immediately, and prevent the onset of disease later.

Following is a list of some common signs and symptoms of various stages of CI. Many complaints occur immediately following a meal heavy in carbohydrates. Keeping in mind that these signs and symptoms may be related to other causes, ask yourself if you have any of these problems:

*Physical fatigue.* Whether you call it fatigue or exhaustion, the most common feature of CI is that it wears people out. Some are tired just in the morning or afternoon; others are exhausted all day.

*Mental fatigue.* Sometimes the fatigue of CI is physical, but often it's mental (as opposed to psychological); the inability to concentrate is the most evident symptom. Poor memory, failing or poor grades in school, and loss of creativity often accompany CI, as do various forms of "learning disabilities." This is much more pronounced immediately after a meal, or if a meal is delayed or missed. The worker who returns to his or her job site after lunch,

only to be unable to concentrate due to mental fatigue, is a very common example. Some actually fall asleep at their desk after lunch.

*Blood sugar problems.* The blood sugar may be normal until a carbohydrate meal is consumed, or if meals are not eaten on a regular schedule. Periods of erratic blood sugar, including abnormal hypoglycemia, accompanied by many of the symptoms listed here, are not normal. Feeling jittery, agitated, and moody is common with CI and is relieved almost immediately once food is eaten. Dizziness is also common, as is the craving for sweets, chocolate, or caffeine. These symptoms are not necessarily associated with abnormal blood sugar levels but may be related to neurological stress, possibly due to the rapid changes in blood sugar and insulin.

*Intestinal bloating.* Foods that produce the most intestinal gas are complex carbohydrates, specifically starches, such as wheat products and potatoes, and other non-starch carbohydrates such as sugar. People with CI often suffer from excessive gas production. Antacids, or other remedies for symptomatic relief, are not very successful in dealing with the problem. The gas tends to build and is worse later in the day and at night.

*Sleepiness.* Many people with CI get sleepy immediately after meals containing more than their limit of carbohydrates. This occurs typically after a pasta meal, or even a meat meal that includes bread, potatoes, or dessert.

*Increased body fat.* For most people, too much weight is also too much fat. Often, the location of this excess body fat is unique between the sexes. In males, an increase in abdominal fat is more evident and an early sign of CI; this leads to a "carbo belly." In females, fat storage is often more prominent in the upper body; in a woman's face, "chipmunk cheeks" may be a telltale sign.

*Increased triglycerides.* High triglycerides in the blood are often seen in people with CI. These triglycerides are the direct result of carbohydrates from the diet being converted by insulin into fat. In my experience, fasting triglyceride levels over 100 mg/dl may be an indication of a carbohydrate-intolerance problem (even though 150 and above is considered abnormal).

*High blood pressure.* Most people with hypertension have CI. There is often a direct relationship between insulin levels and blood pressure—as average insulin levels elevate, so does blood pressure. For some, regardless of whether the blood pressure is elevated, sodium sensitivity is common and eating too much sodium causes water retention along with elevated blood pressure.

*Depression.* Because carbohydrates can be a natural "downer," depression is common among people who have CI. Carbohydrates do this by adversely affecting levels of neurotransmitters made in the brain, producing feelings of depression. Many people have been taught that sugar is stimulating, but actually the opposite can be true. Some people have a short, initial burst of energy after eating sugar, but it does not last.

Furthermore, the medical history of you or your immediate family may indicate a vulnerability to CI. This includes a personal or family history of diabetes, kidney or gall stones, gout, high blood pressure, high cholesterol/low HDL, high triglycerides, heart disease, stroke, or breast cancer.

Certain types of people are more vulnerable to CI, including those who are under more stress, taking estrogen, dark skinned, and those with a family history of diabetes or other metabolic syndrome diseases. In addition, aging is frequently accompanied by increased carbohydrate intolerance.

## The Two-Week Test: Taking It Will Improve Your Diet and Endurance

In the mid-1980s I developed an effective method to help people find their optimal level of carbohydrate intake. It's called the Two-Week Test. Tens of thousands of athletes have used it as a necessary platform to get healthy, lose body fat, and significantly improve aerobic function and overall endurance.

The Two-Week Test is also the best way to jump-start your metabolism because it quickly shifts the body into a higher fat-burning state. It has turned many people's lives around, sometimes helping people reduce or eliminate medications. Of all the tools I've used throughout my professional career, the Two-Week Test surprised me the most in terms of its overall effectiveness. I repeatedly saw how it was possible that someone could go from one extreme of poor health to great health in a short time.

I had one patient named Rose. She was in her early thirties and a runner. She had improved her performances in the previous year by building a good aerobic base and following a better diet. Her MAF Test also improved from its original time of 9:35 to about 8:05 for her first test mile. But Rose still had a high level of body fat for her level of training and caloric intake. She also suffered from frequent fatigue, sleepiness, and bloating after meals. Her overall intake of refined carbohydrates was down from earlier years, but about half her caloric intake still included these "bad" foods, and at almost each meal. She was resistant about giving up her refined carbohydrates, but I finally convinced Rose to take the Two-Week Test.

Here's what happened: After two weeks of no refined carbohydrates, virtually all her lingering symptoms disappeared. And her MAF Test improved to 7:40 for the same first test mile—a drop of twenty-five seconds. After adjusting her diet, a month later Rose had to buy smaller clothes because of weight loss, going from 134 to 123 pounds. Several weeks later, she began her racing season with a personal best in the 10K.

The Two-Week Test marks a period of time in which your insulin levels are moderated because your carbohydrate intake is decreased. It is not the purpose of the test to restrict calories or fat. It merely restricts moderate- and high-glycemic carbohydrates. Nor is its purpose to avoid all carbohydrates, or go into *ketosis* (a metabolic state where chemicals called ketones are produced in the body due to an extremely low carbohydrate intake) like other low-carb diet regimes. And there's no need to weigh food or count grams or calories. Most importantly, this is not a diet. Just eat what you're allowed and avoid what should be avoided, properly snack, and don't get hungry, all for two weeks.

The Two-Week Test is best performed during your aerobic base period, and periods when you're not competing or involved with anaerobic training. However, many athletes have successfully completed the test during these phases of training without problems.

Before you start the test, ask yourself about the signs and symptoms of carbohydrate intolerance described above. Write down the problems that you have from this list, along with any and all other complaints you might have. This may take you a few days as many people are so used to certain problems they can't recall them all at once. This is very important because after the test, you will review these complaints to see which ones have improved.

Next, weigh yourself before starting the test. During the test you may lose some excess water your body is holding, but you'll also go into a high fat-burning state and lose body fat. I've seen some people lose only a few pounds during the test, and others twenty or more pounds. This is not a weight-loss regimen, and the main purpose of weighing yourself

# ARE CARBS ADDICTIVE?

Carbohydrates, especially sugar, can be addictive. Some people have trouble accepting this notion because, surprisingly, there are no clear scientific studies to demonstrate that claim. Many health-care professionals have struggled to help patients who could not reduce or eliminate sugar despite its unhealthy hold on them.

While we don't have a clear scientific study that shows addictive properties of sugar or other refined carbohydrate foods, studies do show that sugar and high-glycemic foods can trigger the brain's reward centers. These are the same brain areas stimulated by cocaine, nicotine, and other widely accepted addictive substances.

The fact that sweet-tasting and so-called comfort foods can be addictive is well accepted—and even proven—by the very companies who employ marketing as a powerful tool to sell these products. Food advertisers who spend billions of dollars each year know very well about addiction and how to tease and tempt you with foods that can end up killing you. These ad campaigns are especially successful with teens and children, and they are not unlike those used by the tobacco industry for so many decades. Just look at the beverage giants like Coca-Cola and Pepsi. Each twelve-ounce can may contain forty grams of carbohydrates, or about nine teaspoons of sugar. In late 2009, Coke came out with a smaller-size can, marketing it as a "healthier alternative" since it has fewer calories!

If society truly recognized the real harm caused by refined carbohydrates, especially sugar, much like what has happened with cigarettes in recent years, there would be a revolution by consumers. State, city, and even federal government agencies would place a huge tax or outright ban on sugar and refined carbohydrate foods due to the astronomical cost of health care associated with their use. Companies that make cereals, candies, cookies, and sugar itself would be sued, much like the tobacco class-action lawsuits. I can imagine the secret after-school cookie deals, or sugar by prescription only, and the growth of sugar addiction clinics where the treatment of choice would be artificial sweeteners. Well, things may be heading that way.

Some European countries are already banning sugary food ads during children's television shows, and California is prohibiting the sale of soda in schools. Restaurants are now required to post the calories of their meals. So yes, the food war has already begun. Science is catching up too. But let's not rely on the government, science, or society—or anything or anyone else—to get us to act. As with other addictions, we are the responsible party. There is help if we need it, but after spending a long time in clinical practice, it's clear to me that each of us holds the key to control or eliminate addiction despite the ongoing propaganda from big corporations who continue to peddle their deadly foods.

Not only can carbohydrates be addictive, but CI is a prevalent problem in persons addicted to alcohol, caffeine, cigarettes, or other drugs. Often, the drug is the secondary problem, with CI being the primary one. Treating this primary problem should obviously be a major focus of any addiction therapy, which can make recovery from other drugs more successful.

is to have another sign of how your body is working, especially after the test.

Before starting the test, perform an MAF Test. Then perform it again soon after the test for comparison.

Plan your shopping list. Before you start the test, make sure you have enough of the foods you'll be eating during the test—these are listed below. Go shopping and stock up on these items. Make a list of the foods you want to eat and the meals and snacks you want to have available. In addition, go through your cabinets and refrigerator and get rid of any sweets in your house, or you'll be tempted. Remember, many people are addicted to sugar and other carbohydrates, and for the first few days you may crave these foods even more.

Make sure you do not go hungry during the test; this is best accomplished by eating frequently, even every two hours if necessary. Schedule the test during a two-week period when you are relatively unlikely to have festive distractions such as the holidays or times when social engagements are planned; these can make it too easy to stray from the plan. As noted, avoid athletic competition during this period.

Following the diet for less than two weeks will probably not give you a valid result. So, if after five days, for example, you eat a bowl of pasta or a box of cookies, you will need to restart the test from the very beginning.

### Foods to Eat During the Test

You may eat as much of these foods as you like during the Two-Week Test:

- Eggs (whites and yolk), unprocessed (real) cheeses, heavy (whipping) cream, sour cream
- Unprocessed meats including beef, turkey, chicken, lamb, fish, shellfish, and others

# METABOLIC SYNDROME—LATE STAGE OF CARBOHYDRATE INTOLERANCE

If CI is not corrected in the early stages of the spectrum, your signs and symptoms and your overall health can easily worsen and even lead to disease. In recent years, a whole complex of related diseases, all preventable, have been identified as related to CI, including some of the biggest killers of today: heart disease, cancer, stroke, and diabetes. These diseases kill more people in the United States each year than the number of people who died in all of the U.S. wars combined. This disease complex is referred to as "metabolic syndrome." The specific disorders include:

- Diabetes (type 2)
- Hypertension
- Obesity
- Polycystic ovary
- Stroke
- Breast cancer
- Coronary heart disease
- Hyperlipidemia (high blood cholesterol and triglycerides)

These problems don't necessarily all develop according to a precise sequence. But all are related to CI. Unfortunately, once some of these diseases develop, they are more difficult to treat conservatively, and more extreme care may be needed. However, even these conditions can improve with the right dietary control, which includes solving the problem of excess carbohydrate intake.

Athletes are not immune to disease and dysfunction, nor are they protected from excess fat storage, especially in their arteries, as many athletic deaths show. How can athletes best determine the level and type of dietary carbohydrates that best suits their needs? The first step may be to take the Two-Week Test.

- Tomato, V-8, or other vegetable juices such as carrot juice
- Water
- Cooked or raw vegetables except potatoes and corn
- Nuts, seeds, nut butters
- Oils, vinegar, mayonnaise, salsa, mustard, and spices
- Sea salt, unless you are sodium sensitive
- All coffee and tea (if you normally drink it)

Be sure to read the ingredients for many of these foods if they are packaged, as some form of sugar is commonly added.

## Foods to Avoid During the Test

You may not eat any of the following foods during the Two-Week Test:

- Bread, rolls, pasta, pancakes, cereal, muffins, chips, crackers, rice cakes, and similar carbohydrate foods
- Sweets, including products that contain sugar such as ketchup, honey, and many other prepared foods (read the labels)
- Fruits and fruit juice
- Highly processed meats such as cold cuts, which often contain sugar
- Potatoes (all types), corn, rice, and beans
- Milk, half-and-half, and yogurt
- So-called healthy snacks, including all energy bars and drinks
- All soda, including so-called diet types

## A Note on Alcohol

If you normally drink small to moderate amounts of alcohol, some forms are allowed during the test. Alcohol allowed: dry wines and pure distilled spirits (gin, vodka, whiskey, etc.) mixed with plain carbonated water, including seltzer. Alcohol not allowed: sweet wines, all beer, champagne, alcohol containing sugar (rum, liqueurs, etc.), or alcohol mixed with sweet ingredients such as tonic, soda, or other sugary liquids. If in doubt, avoid it.

## Meal Suggestions

Below are some other suggestions for eating, food preparation, and dining out, which may be helpful during or after the Two-Week Test:

### Breakfast

- Omelets with any combination of vegetables, meats, and cheeses
- Scrambled eggs with guacamole, sour cream, and salsa
- Scrambled eggs with a scoop of ricotta cheese and tomato sauce
- Boiled or poached eggs with spinach or asparagus and hollandaise or cheese sauce
- Eggs with bacon or other meats
- Soufflés

### Salads

- Chef—leaf lettuce, meats, cheeses, eggs
- Spinach—with bacon, eggs, anchovies
- Caesar—Romaine lettuce, eggs, Parmesan cheese, anchovies
- Any salad with chicken, tuna, shrimp, or other meat or cheese

### Salad Dressings

- Extra virgin olive oil and vinegar (balsamic, wine, apple cider) with or without sea salt and spices.
- Creamy—made with heavy cream, mayonnaise, garlic, and spices

## Fish and Meats

- Pot roast cooked with onions, carrots, and celery
- Roasted chicken stuffed with a bulb of anise, celery, and carrots
- Chili-type dish made with fresh, chopped meat and a variety of vegetables such as diced eggplant, onions, celery, peppers, zucchini, tomatoes, and spices (no beans)
- Steak and eggs
- Any meat with a vegetable and a mixed salad
- Chicken parmigiana (not breaded or deep-fried) with a mixed salad
- Fish (not breaded or deep-fried) with any variety of sauces and vegetables
- Tuna melt on a bed of broccoli or asparagus

## Sauces

- Plain melted butter
- A quick cream sauce can be made by simmering heavy cream with mustard or curry powder and cayenne pepper, or any flavor of choice. It's delicious over eggs, poultry, and vegetables.
- Italian-style tomato sauce helps makes a quick parmigiana out of any fish, meat, or vegetables. Put this over spaghetti squash for a pasta-like dish. Or make lasagna with sliced grilled eggplant or zucchini instead of pasta.

## Snacks

- Hard-boiled eggs

- Rolled slices of fresh meat or cheese wrapped in lettuce
- Vegetable juices
- Almonds, cashews, pecans
- Celery stuffed with nut butter or cream cheese
- Guacamole with vegetable sticks for dipping
- Leftovers from a previous meal

## Dining Out

- Let the waiter know you do not want any bread, to avoid temptation
- Ask for an extra vegetable instead of rice or potato
- Chinese: steamed meat, fish, or vegetables (no rice or sweet sauce)
- Continental: steak, roast, duck, fish, or seafood
- French: coquilles Saint-Jacques, bœuf à la Bourguignonne
- Italian: veal parmigiana (not breaded or deep-fried), seafood marinara
- Avoid all fried food as it usually has breading or is coated in flour

### *After the Two-Week Test*

Reevaluate your original list of complaints after the Two-Week Test is completed. Is your energy better? Do you have less fatigue? Are you less sleepy after meals? Are you sleeping better at night? Do you feel less depressed? Is your MAF Test better? If you feel better now than you did two weeks ago, or if you lost weight, you probably have some degree of CI, and you shouldn't eat as many carbohydrates as you did before the test. Some people who have a high degree of CI will feel dramatically better than they did before the test, especially if there was a large weight loss. Some people say they feel like a new person after taking this test. Others say after a few days of the test, they feel young again.

Check your weight. Any weight loss during the test is not due to reduced calories, as many people eat more calories than usual during this two-week period. It's due to the increased fat burning resulting from reduced insulin. While there may be some water loss, especially if you are sodium sensitive, there is real fat loss.

If your blood pressure has been high, and especially if you are on medication, ask your health-care professional to check it several times during the test, and especially right after the test. Sometimes blood pressure drops significantly and your medication may need to be adjusted, or eliminated, which should only be done by your health-care professional. For many people, as insulin levels are reduced to normal, blood pressure normalizes too.

### Finding Your Carbohydrate Tolerance

If nothing improved during the test—and it was done exactly as described above—then you may not be carbohydrate intolerant. In this case, the level of your carbohydrate intake may be balanced and my only recommendation is to avoid refined carbohydrates. But if the Two-Week Test improved your signs and symptoms, the next step is to determine how many carbohydrates you can tolerate, without a return of these problems. This is done by adding a single-serving size of natural unprocessed carbohydrates to every other meal or snack. This may be plain yogurt sweetened with a little honey for breakfast or an apple after lunch or dinner. For a snack, try tea with honey, or a healthy homemade energy bar (see the Phil's Bar recipe in chapter 18). Avoid all refined carbohydrates such as sugar and refined-flour products (like white bread, cereals, rolls, or pasta). In addition to fresh fruit, plain yogurt, and honey, other suggestions include brown rice, sweet potatoes, yams, lentils, and beans. If you can find real-food whole grain products, they can be used. These include sprouted breads, whole oats (they take thirty to forty-five minutes to cook), and other dense products made with just ground wheat, rye, or other grains. If in doubt, avoid them during this one- to two-week period.

The purpose behind gradually adding these carbohydrate foods is to determine if any of them cause the return of any of the original signs or symptoms, including weight gain, or even new problems. At this stage, having just completed the test, your body and brain will be more aware of even slight reactions to carbohydrate foods—basically, you'll be more intuitive to how your body responds to food. Yet I want to re-emphasize not to add a carbohydrate in back-to-back meals or snacks, because insulin production is partly influenced by your previous meal.

With the addition of each carbohydrate, be aware of any symptoms that you had previously eliminated with the test, especially for symptoms that develop immediately after eating, such as intestinal bloating, sleepiness, or feelings of depression.

Most importantly, if any signs or symptoms that disappeared during or following the Two-Week Test have now returned, you've probably exceeded your carbohydrate limit. For example, if your hunger or cravings were greatly improved at the end of the test, and now they've returned, you probably added too many carbohydrates. If you lost eight pounds during the test, and gained back five pounds after adding some carbohydrates for a week or two, you've probably eaten too many carbohydrates. Likewise, if blood pressure rises significantly after it was reduced, it may be due to excess carbohydrate intake. If any of these situations occur, reduce the carbohydrates by half, or experiment to see which particular foods cause symptoms and which don't. Some people return to the Two-Week Test and begin the process again.

In some cases, people can tolerate simple carbohydrates, such as fresh fruits, plain yogurt, and honey, but not complex carbohydrates such as sweet potato, whole grains, beans, or other starches. In other situations, some individuals don't tolerate any wheat products. During this post-test period, these factors are often easy to determine.

After this one- to two-week period of experimenting with natural carbohydrates, you'll have a very good idea about your body's level of carbohydrate tolerance. You'll better know which foods to avoid, which ones you can eat, and which must be limited. You'll become acutely aware of how your body feels when you eat too many carbohydrates. From time to time, you may feel the need to go through a Two-Week Test period again to check yourself, or to quickly get back on track after careless eating during the holidays, vacations, or at other times.

### Modified Two-Week Test

For those who want to take the Two-Week Test, but are performing anaerobic training or are in their competitive season, the Two-Week Test can be modified. The only change in this version is that fresh fruits are allowed, but fruit juice is not unless it is during training or racing. All fresh fruits are allowed with the exception of those that are high glycemic: large bananas, watermelon, pineapple, and all dried fruit should be avoided.

When performing the modified version, follow the same guidelines as above for the Two-Week Test, using the allowable fresh fruits as desired.

### Fiber

Many people find the loss of grains in the diet leaves the digestive tract sluggish and a little constipated. After years of eating lots of carbohydrates, your intestine gets used to that type of bulk. If you become constipated during the Two-Week Test, or afterward when you're maintaining a lower amount of carbohydrate in your diet, it could be due to a number of reasons. First, you may not be eating enough fiber. Bread, pasta, and cereals are significant sources of fiber for many people.

Psyllium is a high-fiber herb that is a very effective promoter of intestinal function. Adding plain unsweetened psyllium to a glass of water, tomato juice, or a healthy smoothie can keep your system running smoothly—start with a half-teaspoon a day for a few days to make sure it's tolerated, then use up to about one teaspoon a day or about six grams. Another way to add psyllium to your diet is to use it in place of flour for thickening sauces or in place of bread crumbs to coat meats and vegetables. If you require a fiber supplement, be sure to read the labels and use the ones that do not contain sugar. There are sugar-free psyllium products on the market, so you should not have trouble finding one.

Another reason for constipation at this time may be dehydration. If you don't drink enough water, you could be predisposed to constipation. During the Two-Week Test, you'll need more water—up to a total of two to three quarts or more per day. After the test, vegetables, legumes, such as lentils, and fruits are also great sources of both water and fiber. So if you become constipated, it may simply be that you need to eat more vegetables and fruits as tolerated. In addition, adequate intake of natural fats, discussed later in this book, can also be helpful.

Occasionally, some people get very tired during or after the Two-Week Test. This can be due to a number of factors. Most commonly it's from not eating enough food or not eating often enough. The most common problem is not eating breakfast. And many people should not go more than three to four hours without eating something healthy.

Once you successfully finish the Two-Week Test, and add back the right amount of tolerable carbohydrate foods, you should have a very good idea of your carbohydrate limits—the amount of carbohydrate you can eat without producing symptoms. This is best accomplished by asking yourself about your signs and symptoms on a regular basis: energy, sleepiness, and bloating after meals, and so forth. You may want to keep a diary so you can be more objective in your self-assessment. In time, you won't need to focus as much on this issue; your intuition will take over and you'll automatically know your limits.

### Ideal Carbohydrates

At the top of the list of unprocessed carbohydrates is fruit. In addition to containing vitamins and minerals, fruit includes important phytonutrients. Though fruit is a carbohydrate food, the glycemic index of most fruit is low to moderate because fruit has substantial amounts of fiber, and because fruit sugar, or fructose, possesses the lowest glycemic index of all sugars. Most fruits contain a combination of fructose and glucose, and those with the most fructose have a lower glycemic index. At the low end of the glycemic index are cherries, plums, grapefruits, apricots, melons, berries, and peaches. Apples, pears, and baby bananas have a more moderate glycemic index, with grapes, oranges, and large bananas scoring higher. Pineapple, watermelon, and dried fruits are among the highest-glycemic fruits and should be eaten sparingly, if at all. Most people who are CI can tolerate some amount of fresh fruits, although sometimes they can only eat from the low-glycemic group.

Legumes or beans can be tolerated by many people, but often only in small amounts. These foods are thought by many to be a protein food, but most contain much more carbohydrate than protein. For instance, a serving of red beans typically has six grams of protein and sixteen grams of carbohydrate, with five of these carbohydrate grams as fiber. Because of the presence of both protein and fiber, the glycemic index of red beans and other legumes remains relatively low for a carbohydrate food. In addition, other legumes may have even lower glycemic effects. Overall, because of their composition, most beans, including lentils, have a moderate glycemic effect, and are a good alternative to refined-carbohydrate foods.

Vegetables also contain carbohydrates, though most only small amounts. Vegetables are an extremely important item in the diet and are discussed in detail later in this section. Some vegetables, however, contain moderate to high amounts of carbohydrates and there-fore warrant discussion here. Among the higher-carbohydrate vegetables are corn and potatoes, which should be eaten sparingly, if at all. In fact, a baked potato has a whopping thirty-seven grams of carbohydrate—as much as a serving of cooked pasta—and a higher glycemic index than some cakes and candy. Potatoes and corn are such high-glycemic foods because they've been genetically changed to be sweeter than the same foods a generation or two ago. New potatoes have a much lower glycemic index than other varieties.

Many people consume the bulk of their carbohydrates as grains. Whole grains, and products made from them, are more healthful than their refined counterparts, containing more of the nutrients and fiber from the original grain. For instance, whole oat groats are better than the common processed oatmeal cereals, especially the "quick" oats. Long-grain brown rice is better than short-grain white rice. Wild rice, which isn't really rice but a seed from a reedy grass, is fairly low in carbohydrate and has a moderate glycemic index as well. There are a number of breads on the market made from whole sprouted grains, and most have a lower glycemic index. Processed wheat flour (white flour) can increase insulin levels two to three times more than true whole-grain products. But whether whole or processed, grains are starches and more difficult to digest than most foods, and many people, often unknowingly, are intolerant to wheat of any kind. Wheat is such a common problem for many people that I devoted the section below to it.

## Wheat: An Unhealthy Food Staple

Wheat may be the most unhealthy food staple of the Western diet next to sugar and contributes significantly to ill health and disease. We all know how bad sugar is for health due to its high-glycemic nature—but wheat and wheat products can actually be worse due to an even higher glycemic index. Eating that piece of bread is not unlike eating several spoonfuls of white table sugar, and your body turns much of this wheat into fat. Almost half of that so-called fat-free bagel can end up becoming stored fat.

Wheat is a lobbying success story, like the tobacco industry, as it's found in most people's media-driven diets. It's certainly not recommended for nutritional reasons as we can obtain whatever nutritional benefits wheat contains from many other healthy foods. And considering the health risks, wheat's place on any food pyramid can only be a scheme that serves those who are addicted and the companies that sell it.

Wheat is a common cause of intestinal problems, allergies and asthma, and skin problems; it can prevent absorption of various nutrients, contribute to weight gain, and occasionally causes death.

The reason for wheat's failure as a healthy item is twofold: the protein component of wheat, called gluten, causes allergies in many people, including infants who are unfor-tunately given this as their first food. And many people are adversely affected by gluten without realizing it, through a slow, silent buildup of chronic illness. Gluten is what makes bread rise, so most baked goods and packaged foods are full of it.

The second reason wheat is unhealthy is that almost all wheat products are high glycemic—from bread, bagels, and muffins to cereals and additives to many packaged foods to wheat flour itself, a staple in almost all kitchens and recipes. Gone are the days when people would buy real whole-wheat berries, grind them, and make flour or sprout them for use in food products. While the berries still contain gluten, they're not high glycemic. But almost all wheat used today is highly processed, making it high glycemic.

The list of specific conditions associated with consuming wheat keeps growing—from autoimmune diseases (such as arthritis, type 1 diabetes, lupus, MS) and chronic inflammation to infertility and skin disorders (such as eczema, acne, and psoriasis), and even cancer. Some people are more sensitive to the harmful effects of wheat than others. Wheat is among the most common cause of allergies in children and adults, along with milk, soy, peanuts, and corn. The most practical way to assess this is to note how you feel after ingesting wheat. The most common symptom is intestinal bloating, but signs and symptoms are associated with skin, breathing, and edema, and may be immediate or delayed. If you're sensitive to wheat, significantly reducing or eliminating it from your diet is the most effective remedy.

Here are some other points regarding wheat's harmful effects:

In the intestines, wheat can prevent the absorption of important minerals. These include calcium, magnesium, iron, zinc, and copper—all essential for good health.

Wheat can reduce digestive enzymes, especially those from the pancreas, rendering key foods less digestible—including protein and fats. Not digesting protein impairs amino acid absorption, and whole protein absorption can cause allergies. And if fat is not digested, essential fatty acids may not be absorbed, adversely affecting a whole spectrum of problems from skin quality to inflammation and hormonal balance.

Since refined wheat is higher glycemic, it can lead to the production of higher amounts of insulin by the pancreas. In addition to causing more fat storage, this can also increase your risk of various diseases including diabetes, cancer, and heart disease.

Combining exercise and wheat can trigger allergic reactions in some people, although it's not common. This occurs when a person eats some form of wheat and exercises within a given time period. This is followed by some allergic reaction, from mild problems (sometimes so mild people are used to it) like skin rash or hives to more severe problems including anaphylaxis and, in rare occasions, even death. This may also include breathing difficulty. It is sometimes difficult to diagnose because of the need for both triggers (wheat and exercise) around the same time period. It's conceivable that some of the deaths reported in athletes are due to this problem.

High-glycemic wheat products, which are often sweetened with more sugar, can result in a sweet tooth—or addiction—that not only perpetuates the desire for more sweets, but the dislike for health-promoting but bitter or less sweet-tasting foods, like vegetables.

Wheat can sometimes cause mental or emotional symptoms, including depression, mood swings, attention problems in children, and anxiety. One long-term illness associated with wheat allergy is dementia due to cerebral (brain) atrophy.

Osteoporosis may be strongly associated with wheat allergy.

Other quality of life issues can also be associated with wheat consumption. These include belching or gas, diarrhea, or other abdominal discomfort; reduced mental focus and poor concentration; and fatigue—some people actually fall asleep after a meal containing wheat, even just a sandwich.

A serious wheat-intolerance problem once thought of as rare is celiac disease, an autoimmune condition where patients must avoid any amount of wheat or risk serious, sometimes life-threatening reactions. Many professionals agree that even mild forms of wheat allergy are really the same thing—a subclinical celiac condition. In fact, this problem is more recognized today, with a recent article in the *Journal of Family Practice* showing that

for every person diagnosed with celiac disease, there are eight others who go undiagnosed. Millions of Americans—including
endurance athletes—and many more people
throughout the world have this condition.

If you're in doubt about what wheat may
be doing to your health, consider strictly
avoiding it for a couple of weeks or a month.
You just may become a new, healthier person,
and your training and racing can improve.

### What About Sweeteners?

Sweeteners are carbohydrates, or sugars,
in their purest form. They range from highly
processed and high-glycemic products such
as maltodextrin and table sugar, to the lower
glycemic sources such as honey and agave. As
with other carbohydrate foods, the least processed and more natural sugars are best for
use as a sweetener.

Most sweeteners are complex carbohydrates—high glycemic and more difficult to
digest. These include all maltose sugars (maltodextrin, malt sugar, maple sugar, and syrup),
corn sugars and syrups (such as high fructose
corn syrup), all cane sugars whether white or
brown, rice syrups, and molasses. Perhaps the
best sweeteners to use are simple carbohydrates that don't require digestion, are unprocessed and lowest in glycemic index. The best
is honey, but in moderation and not to exceed
your carbohydrate tolerance.

## HONEY!

Honey has been used for centuries as both a sweetener and a remedy for skin
problems. Even today, honey remains the most natural sweetener available. Honey
contains a variety of vitamins, minerals, and amino acids, including antioxidants. In
addition, honey has anti-inflammatory and antimicrobial effects. Recently a large
volume of scientific literature has substantiated honey's therapeutic value, as well as
its ability to improve endurance in athletes.

Honey is also perhaps the only carbohydrate food that does not promote tooth
decay through acidity. In general, proteins and fats raise salivary pH, making it more
alkaline, while carbohydrate foods lower pH, making it more acidic. Honey is the
sweet exception—a carbohydrate that may raise pH levels. In addition, honey has
an overall beneficial effect on oral health due to its antibacterial effect and ability to
reduce dextran, a sticky, sugary substance that helps bacteria adhere to the teeth.

Like fruit, honey is primarily a blend of fructose and glucose. Different types of
honey have different ratios of each type of sugar. Those that crystallize the fastest are

## Artificial Sweeteners

I recommend avoiding all artificial sweeteners in virtually all situations because I believe fake sugars can have an adverse effect on your health. These include the traditional ones such as aspartame and saccharine, to those considered natural such as stevia. Some say the research is still not clear on this issue, but I say why wait when there's enough information to suggest that they are harmful. Artificial sweeteners are used in many food items: diet soda, chewing gum, ice cream, iced tea mixes, and many other products. If you want to avoid them, you must read the labels.

While substances such as saccharin are not recommended for children or pregnant women, and aspartame has been related to an increased incidence of migraine headaches and allergic reactions, another fact has been ignored: The use of artificial sweeteners is most often accompanied by increased consumption of food. In other words, if you use artificial sweeteners, studies show you often end up eating more food, usually sweets. What's worse is that you may store more fat as well. Researchers are unclear why this happens, but certain factors seem to be implicated. It may be a learned process by the body. The tasting of sweet substances may cause the body to store, rather than burn, fat. Or, it may be related to the dehydration that accompanies consumption of artificial sweeteners. This

the ones with the highest glucose content, and thus the higher glycemic index. Since fructose has the lowest glycemic index of all sugars, honey with higher fructose content will have the lowest glycemic index. Sage and tupelo honey, for example, are known for their high fructose content, while clover honey has a medium fructose content, and alfalfa honey is higher in glucose.

When shopping for honey, look for a number of attributes. Dark honey may be the most therapeutic and have the most nutrients. Buckwheat honey is said to contain the highest amounts of antioxidants. Raw, unfiltered honey retains more beneficial qualities. Heat, light, and filtering remove some of the beneficial properties of honey.

Agave is often put in the same category as honey—it's a sweet natural syrup—but is very different. It's made from the cactus-like agave plant (similar to aloe vera), which is also used to make tequila. While it's very high in fructose with a very low glycemic index, it lacks the therapeutic benefits that honey contains. Due to its high fructose content, some individuals don't tolerate it. Intestinal distress is the most common symptom, and in those with high triglyceride levels, high fructose intake may worsen the condition.

**QA**

**Question:** I suffer from an eating disorder and yo-yo dieting. This, coupled with occasional training burnout—my maximum triathlon training is about fifteen hours per week—result in a weight gain/loss spread of thirty to forty pounds during the course of a year. I usually place in the top quarter of my age-group in races. I am forty-six years old. How can I hope to stabilize my diet and weight and maintain a constant training regimen?

**Answer:** First, understand that this is a truly serious health problem. Second, decide that you want to make the necessary changes in fitness and health a priority. Whether you do this on your own, with the help of a close friend, or with guidance from an appropriate health-care professional, one of the next steps is to build a great aerobic base. But in order to do this, you may have to make many significant changes in your life. One may be your diet. For example, if you're carbohydrate intolerant, fat burning may never improve significantly enough and brain chemistry may be unbalanced. Another change may be needed with training. You may have to come to the realization that training at the appropriate level—most likely a lot slower than you're used to—is an important part of the process. Learning about all the brain and body's physical, chemical, and mental aspects, focusing on areas most necessary to start, is a long process, but changes come quickly when you make the appropriate adjustments.

may trigger the brain to increase the appetite and food intake as a means of restoring water balance. In addition, eating low-calorie substances will lower the body's metabolism. This will not only cause the body to store more fat but will also activate the need to eat more food.

Some people argue that artificial sweeteners reduce calories. You may be fooled into believing that you are buying a more-healthful, low-calorie food when you choose a product made with fake sugar. But by using an artificial sweetener instead of a teaspoon of honey, for example, you're avoiding only fifteen calories or less. This is not a significant

caloric factor. Not only that, counting calories, as discussed elsewhere, is unhealthy.

Clearly if you want to be healthy and continually improve your aerobic system, fat burning, and endurance, it's important to understand how carbohydrates can affect overall health, especially in relation to your particular needs. In general, refined carbohydrates are best eliminated. The best choices are fruits, legumes, and unprocessed whole grains if tolerated, with small amounts of honey as a sweetener. As you begin to choose your carbohydrate foods more wisely, you will notice your endurance and overall health improve significantly.

# CHAPTER 15

# THE POWER OF PROTEIN—
## Going Way Beyond Building Muscles

We all need protein from our diet every day for optimal health and particularly for better endurance. This is true at all ages, for males and females, regardless of your sport . Larger body frames and those performing more extreme sports may need more protein. Growing children also need higher amounts of protein for development. But once optimal body size is attained and growth stabilizes, there is still a significant and continuous need for protein.

We tend to think of protein needs as being higher in weight lifters and bodybuilders, but endurance athletes have similar requirements, perhaps even greater.

In addition to helping build muscles, protein is necessary for many other activities:

Protein is necessary to make enzymes, important for balancing fats, digestion, and hundreds of other metabolic functions.

Protein is essential for maintaining neurotransmitters—the chemical messengers used for communication by the brain and nervous system, and especially the gut.

Protein is a key element for building new cells in bones, organs, glands, and elsewhere all throughout the body—and for the rest of your life.

Oxygen, fats, vitamins, hormones, and other compounds are regulated and transported throughout the body with the help of protein.

Protein is necessary to make natural antibodies for the immune system.

Protein contains key amino acids for health. For example, cysteine is necessary for the body to make its most powerful antioxidant, glutathione; glutamine is used as energy to fuel the intestine's *villi* for nutrient absorption.

Protein is important for the production of glucagon in relation to controlling insulin, blood sugar, and other key areas of metabolism.

### How Much Protein?

Studies continue to show that the protein recommendations by the World Health Organization, USDA, and other agencies are too low. These recommendations have resulted in reductions in protein intake by some people, with dire health consequences. Even the argument that protein can harm the kidneys, especially those with kidney problems, is losing ground as new studies show that restricting dietary protein in those with kidney disease can actually increase the risk of death.

How much protein do we need each day? The answer to this question depends on your lean body mass, your level of training, and other factors, including what makes you feel best. The range of healthy protein intake is wide. General estimates on protein needs can be made based on a percent of calories in your diet or with a more detailed approach using a range of normal based on the USDA's guidelines as the minimum needs. Both are very general and often inadequate for endurance athletes.

Based on research, we could estimate that endurance athletes could need up to 1.6 grams of protein per kilogram (2.2 pounds) of body weight each day.

Here are some examples you can use to help determine protein needs. If you have a training schedule of about ninety minutes a day, the following may represent typical protein needs:

For a 175-pound person, the daily protein intake may be 128 grams. The protein foods that would provide this include three eggs and cheese at breakfast, a salad for lunch with a hefty serving of turkey, and salmon for dinner.

For a 145-pound person, the requirement may be about 106 grams: two eggs for breakfast, a chef's salad for lunch, and a sirloin steak for dinner.

And for the person weighing 125 pounds, who would minimally require about 90 grams of protein: two eggs at breakfast, tuna salad for lunch, and lamb for dinner.

If your training is higher, your caloric needs will also be high and the need for protein increases proportionately. Or, if you weigh more or less, your protein needs may also be different. If you're 200 pounds or more, or appreciably less than 125 pounds, for example, just estimate the protein requirements based on the above numbers. For example 200 pounds is 25 percent heavier than 175 pounds, so 25 percent more than 128 grams of protein is 160 grams for the high end of the normal range, or 80 grams at the low end.

These are not meant to be perfect recommendations for at least two reasons. First, they're based on weight and not lean muscle. And second, we are all individuals with slightly different protein requirements. However, this provides a first step to guide you toward a good approximation of your protein needs. The next step is to determine what makes you feel best based on a little experimentation with your food intake. Once you've modified your carbohydrate needs according to the previous discussion, your protein needs will be relatively easier to determine.

Clearly, eating more protein than the body can utilize can be unhealthy—just like eating more carbohydrates or fat than the body needs is. But if you require more than 100 grams a day, that's not excessive; it's what your body needs. Eating the amount of protein your body requires is not a high-protein diet—it's getting your proper requirements! However, even moderate amounts of protein can be harmful for those who are not healthy. For example, as protein intake increases so does your need for water, which helps eliminate the normal by-products of protein metabolism through the kidneys. That's part of the old argument

that protein is a stress on the kidneys; it most certainly is if you are dehydrated. Or if you're under significant stress and your stomach does not make sufficient amounts of natural hydrochloric acid—the first chemical stage of protein digestion—undigested protein in the gut can cause significant intestinal distress. Addressing the cause of the problem—the stress and stomach, not the protein—is the best remedy.

### Amino Acids

Just as carbohydrates are made up of sugars, dietary protein is made up of building blocks called amino acids. In order to obtain these vital components, the intestine must do its job. First, protein must be efficiently digested in the intestine, breaking down into amino acids. Second, these amino acids must be absorbed into the body. Once absorbed, the amino acids are used either as individual products, or recombined as proteins. For example, the amino acid tryptophan is used to make certain neurotransmitters in the brain. Also, recombining many amino acids provides for the manufacture of new muscle cells.

There are at least twenty amino acids necessary for human nutrition, all of which are indispensable for optimal health and human performance. Some amino acids can be manufactured in the body by other raw materials from food, and others called "essential amino acids" must be taken in through the diet. While amino acids that are made in the body are sometimes referred to as "non-essential," this is misleading as all amino acids are essential.

### Best Protein Sources

In general, animal foods are the best sources of protein containing all the amino acids. Overall, the highest-rated protein food is eggs, followed by beef and fish. With the exception of soybeans, which are mostly carbohydrate, vegetable foods individually contain only some of the amino acids. Combining the right non-animal foods can provide a complete amino-acid meal. But eating all the amino acids at one meal is not necessary. For those who don't eat animal products, obtaining all your amino acids is accomplished by combining enough variety, since no one plant-based food (except soybeans, which have very low amounts of the amino acid methionine) contains all the amino acids. Certain combinations of plant foods, such as beans and rice, or whole grains and legumes, can provide a complete protein. However, combining meals high in carbohydrates (such as rice, beans, grains, etc.) with protein can reduce digestibility, with the result that some protein will not digest into amino acids, and some amino acids won't get absorbed.

Digestion of concentrated protein foods, such as eggs, meat, and fish, can be impaired by combining it with complex carbohydrates (or double sugars). That's because these two macronutrients digest at different rates. So eating foods such as a meat sandwich, pasta and fish, or eggs and toast, can result in less protein digestion. This can also cause indigestion. (Combining simple sugars with proteins should not cause these problems since these carbohydrates don't require digestion.)

For most people, getting enough protein should not be a problem as there are many healthy options. These include eggs, meats, fish, and dairy foods. Choosing the best animal proteins means finding the best sources: organic, grass-fed, free-range, kosher, and whatever other labels are used to differentiate the highest quality eggs, meats, fish, and dairy from those obtained from poorly treated animals. In some cases, visiting a small local farm will help you decide. Some of today's local farmers are not only health-conscious but actually care about their animals and how their operations impact the environment.

The human body, especially the intestine, is well adapted to digesting animal-source foods, having evolved on a high-meat/fish and low-carbohydrate diet with varying amounts of vegetables, fruits, and nuts. While the popular trend in recent decades has been toward the misconception that meat consumption is unhealthy, there are a variety of unique features of an animal-food diet that are vital for fitness and health. Here are some of them:

- Animal foods contain high levels of all essential amino acids.

- Vitamin B12 is an essential nutrient found almost exclusively in animal foods.

- EPA, a powerful essential fat important in controlling inflammation, is almost exclusively found in animal foods (conversion of omega-3 fats in plants to EPA is not always efficient in humans).

- Iron deficiency is a common worldwide problem and is prevented by eating animal foods containing this mineral in its most bio-available form.

- Vitamin A is found only in animal products (conversion of beta-carotene in plant foods to vitamin A is not always efficient in humans).

- Animal products are dense protein foods with little or no carbohydrate to interfere with digestion and absorption.

- People who consume fewer animal protein have a greater rate of bone loss than those who eat larger amounts of animal protein.

## The Incredible, Edible Egg

Eggs are a near perfect food all wrapped up in one single cell. Eggs contain the most complete and highest protein rating of any food. Two eggs contain more than twelve grams of protein, just over half in the white and the rest in the yolk. In addition, eggs also contain many essential nutrients, including significant amounts of vitamins A, D, E, B1, B2, B6, folic acid, and especially vitamin B12. Eggs also contain important minerals including calcium, magnesium, potassium, zinc, and iron. Choline and biotin, also important for energy and regulation of stress, are contained in large amounts in eggs. Most of these nutrients are found in the yolk.

The fat in egg yolks is also nearly a perfect balance, containing mostly monounsaturated fats and about 36 percent saturated fat. Additionally, egg yolks contain linoleic and linolenic acids—both essential fatty acids. Eggs have almost no carbohydrate (less than one gram), making them the perfect meal or snack for the millions who are carbohydrate intolerant. Ounce per ounce, eggs are also your best food buy with hardly any waste. And, with so many ways of cooking them, eggs are delicious and quick to prepare. For most people, eggs can be part of a healthy food plan; I eat several whole eggs a day.

While most people love the taste of eggs, many are still concerned about eating them because of cholesterol—it's one of the most misunderstood subjects related to heart disease. Abnormally high levels of cholesterol can be a risk factor for heart disease, although your total cholesterol is not the best—or only—measure for heart-disease risk. Many people who die of heart disease have normal total cholesterol numbers, and many with high cholesterol never develop heart disease.

Perhaps the greatest misconception about cholesterol is that eating foods containing it significantly raises levels in the blood. In truth, most studies have shown that eating cholesterol does not alone substantially increase blood-cholesterol levels. Moreover, some studies show that not eating cholesterol can prompt your body to make more—and that eating eggs can improve your cholesterol numbers!

While there is a correlation between higher total cholesterol in the blood and incidences of heart attacks, evaluating cardiac risk calls for a complete fasting blood-lipid profile that measures at least total, HDL (high-density lipoprotein), and LDL (low-density lipoprotein) cholesterol, and triglycerides.

The most important thing to know about cholesterol is that cholesterol itself isn't "bad," but rather something to be kept in balance. It's also important to understand that most of the cholesterol in the bloodstream is actually made by your liver. If you eat more cholesterol, your body prompts the liver to make less of it. But if you take in less, your liver makes more. That's why many people on a low-cholesterol diet still have high blood-cholesterol levels.

Actually, all cells in the body—including those of the heart—make cholesterol every day. That's because cholesterol is necessary for many essential processes that keep us healthy. For example, the outer surfaces of cells contain cholesterol that helps regulate which chemicals enter and exit. Cholesterol is also used to make many hormones, including sex hormones and those that control stress. Cholesterol is also a key component of the brain and nerve structure throughout the body, and a key compound in the skin, allowing us to make vitamin D from the sun.

HDL cholesterol is called "good" cholesterol because it protects against disease by removing accumulated deposits of cholesterol and transporting them back to the liver for disposal. So, higher HDL numbers are generally healthier. It's best if you can divide your total cholesterol figure by your HDL number and get a ratio below 4.0, which is about the average risk for heart disease. Aerobic exercise, monounsaturated fats, fish oil, and moderate alcohol can increase HDL. Excess stress and anaerobic exercise, hydrogenated fats, and excess consumption of saturated fats and refined carbohydrates lower it.

More importantly, the recommendation that people substitute polyunsaturated fats for saturated can be devastating for HDL levels. If the ratio of polyunsaturated fat to saturated fat exceeds 1.5, HDL levels usually diminish, raising your cardiac risk. If your fats are balanced, as discussed in the next chapter, you avoid raising your ratio above 1.5.

LDL cholesterol is known as the "bad" cholesterol. A recent trend in preventative medicine is to stress lowering LDL cholesterol with drugs. But it's really not the LDL itself that causes the potential harm or risk. It's only when the LDL oxidizes that it deposits in your arteries. Oxidation of LDL results from free radicals, in much the same way that iron rusts. While lowering LDL levels can make less of it available for oxidation, antioxidants from fruits and vegetables can help prevent oxidation. In addition, many of the factors just mentioned that raise HDL also lower LDL, which is best measured when blood is drawn after a twelve-hour fast for an accurate evaluation.

Excess dietary carbohydrates can especially adversely affect LDL levels. This is due to excess triglycerides from carbohydrates producing more, smaller, denser LDL particles, which are even more likely to clog arteries.

In addition, a lower intake of dietary cholesterol is linked to an increase of these more dangerous LDL particles. And to make matters worse, these types of LDL particles are also associated with the inability to tolerate moderate to high levels of dietary carbohydrates (i.e., insulin resistance) even in relatively healthy individuals.

One of the worst scenarios for your cholesterol is if the HDL is lowered while the LDL and total cholesterol are elevated. Hydrogenated and partially hydrogenated fats (trans fats) do this, and many experts now consider the intake of hydrogenated fat to be a risk factor for heart disease. So avoid margarine and products containing this dangerous substance.

Eating too much saturated fat can raise LDL and total cholesterol levels. The worst offenders may be dairy foods such as butter, cream, cheese, and milk. Red meat such as beef, while it does contain saturated fat, can actually improve cholesterol levels. This is partly because, just as in eggs, about half the fat in beef is monounsaturated. Grass-fed beef has the best balance of fats compared to most beef, which is corn-fed. In addition, much of the saturated fat in beef is stearic acid, a fatty acid that won't raise cholesterol and may actually help reduce it. (The fat in cocoa butter also contains high amounts of stearic acid.)

Fiber and fiber-like substances are also an important factor in decreasing total cholesterol and improving total cholesterol/HDL ratios. Most people don't eat enough fiber, especially from fresh vegetables and fruits. Eating at least one large raw salad daily in addition to cooked vegetables and one to three servings of fresh fruit or berries—totaling eight to ten servings—will provide significant amounts of fiber. These foods also provide natural phytosterols, which help reduce cholesterol and may be the reason early humans, who ate very large amounts of saturated fat, were well protected.

Back to eggs. Do you avoid eating eggs because you fear they will somehow raise your blood cholesterol to dangerously high levels? The fact is that eating eggs won't necessarily raise your total cholesterol. After decades of medical research, studies have never linked egg consumption to heart disease. Stephen Kritchevsky, PhD, director of the J. Paul Sticht Center on Aging at Wake Forest University, states, "People should feel secure with the knowledge that the [medical] literature shows regular egg consumption does not have a measurable impact on heart disease risk for healthy adults. In fact, many countries with high egg consumption are notable for low rates of heart disease."

Eggs are only as healthy as the hens that lay them, since the nutritional make-up of eggs, especially the fat, depends upon what the chickens eat. For this reason you should avoid run-of-the-mill grocery-store eggs that have been produced in chicken factories. Unfortunately this includes most eggs on the market. The healthiest eggs come from organic, free-range hens. Even better: buy eggs from a local farmer who lets chickens eat healthy, wild food and organic feed. Local free-range usually means that the hens are allowed to roam where they can eat bugs and vegetable matter, yielding more nutritious eggs. So-called omega-3 eggs come from chickens fed flax seeds. Often these hens are neither free-range nor certified organic and are still housed in very crowded hen factories.

### Beef

Beef has been one of the biggest casualties of the carbohydrate trend of the past few decades. The fact is, beef can be an important part of a healthy athletic diet. Consider that just three ounces of lean porterhouse contains twenty grams of protein, and just six grams of saturated fat, balanced by a healthy seven grams of heart-friendly monounsaturated fat. In addition to being an excellent source of high-quality protein, beef is also rich in B vitamins, glutamine, calcium, magnesium,

iron, zinc, and other vital nutrients. Organic and natural grass-fed beef are the very best choices as they have not been treated with antibiotics or given growth-stimulating hormones. And grass-fed beef not given corn to fatten the animals contains an excellent balance of fats.

You can buy naturally raised meats in some grocery and health food stores, and local sources may be even better. Look for nearby farms and ranches that sell meat from animals that have been raised on grass, not fed corn, and without the use of growth hormones, antibiotics, and other chemicals used by most stock-growers. Whether you live near a farm that sells natural or organic meat, or order from a ranch that can ship to you, you may wish to save money and buy a large quantity of beef so that you always have some on hand.

When cooking beef, keep it on the rare side. Studies show that beef cooked medium, medium well, or well done is associated with higher rates of stomach cancer. This is due to the production of carcinogens (certain nitrogen compounds) created during cooking. Heat-sensitive nutrients, such as the amino acid glutamine, are also significantly reduced in meat cooked beyond rare. The less cooked the better. Bacteria in beef are usually due to the food-handling process. While bacteria can reside on the surface of meat, it won't get inside unless the meat is ground. Almost all cases of food poisoning involving meat are from sources that have been ground ahead of

**Question:** I have been a vegetarian since my early twenties, I am a male, fifty years old now, and run about twenty miles a week. I want to take up triathlon but am worried that my increased protein needs won't be met by my current diet. I do eat eggs. What do you recommend?

**Answer:** Eggs are a great protein source, especially in whole forms—the white and yolk have about the same amounts of protein. It's easy to use whole eggs as a meal or in many different recipes. In addition, if you need more protein you can use egg-white powder to make a healthy shake for use as a meal or snack to supplement your nutritional needs. In addition, a whey protein concentrate is a great protein source, and can be used the same way as egg-white powder.

time. For this reason, ground meat should be thoroughly cooked unless it's freshly ground just before eating it.

## Poultry

I rate eggs and beef as the best sources of protein but give poultry a poor rating due to how most of these animals are raised and processed. However, if you find an excellent source of chicken and turkey, and you really enjoy eating it, these are great protein foods.

The poultry industry has done such a good job telling you on paper how healthy chicken is over other meats, but this is untrue. In fact, chickens are generally raised in more unhealthy environments than cattle and other animals because of lower standards. Most chickens are given many chemicals and drugs to counter common diseases and infections in crowded chicken farms.

The best birds for the table are organically raised—they've not been treated with or fed any chemicals or drugs; instead, they are given certified-organic feeds and filtered water. This may be the safest of all poultry. Many grocery stores and health food stores carry organic chickens and turkeys. In addition, you may be able to find birds such as these from a local farm. Turkey and duck are even better choices.

## Fish

While fish is a great source of protein, with some containing healthy omega-3 fats, some fish are healthier choices over others. The best sources are wild, cold-water fish; farm-raised fish should be strictly avoided.

In general, avoid seafood that includes the so-called bottom feeders, those fish and other sea species that eat from the ocean's floor, where the potential for consuming toxic material is highest. This is especially true for those species that feed close to shore. Flounder, sole, catfish, and crab are some examples of foods to avoid eating regularly. Oysters, clams, mussels, and scallops are also sources of potential pollutants. Clams are perhaps the worst seafood to eat, especially when raw, since they normally filter out and concentrate viruses and bacteria, heavy metals, and other chemical pollutants from the waters in which they live. If you enjoy eating seafood, here are some tips for doing so more safely and more nutritiously:

Choose fish caught in waters farther away from polluted, industrial areas. Some examples are Canadian salmon, sardines, and herring.

Look for cold-water fish like salmon, dark tuna, sardines, and other small fish that contain higher amounts of omega-3 fat.

Eat smaller fish and crustaceans: trout, bass, and shrimp, and avoid marlin, great white tuna, and swordfish. Smaller and younger fish have not accumulated the toxins found in larger and older species.

Limit your intake of shellfish, and choose smaller species such as the smallest shrimp.

Avoid precooked fish and prepared or processed seafood such as breaded fish or seafood, fish cakes, ground fish, and imitation crabmeat (common at sushi bars).

If you catch your own fish, ask local authorities about the limits of safety. Some regions recommend limiting how much of certain species you should eat in a year.

Unfortunately, the oceans, rivers, and lakes are becoming so contaminated that wild fish are containing levels of toxins that are dangerous. I recommend limiting fish to once or twice a month or less, and even less than that for children and pregnant women.

The picture is worse for farm-raised seafood—this should always be avoided. These foods often include antibiotics, pesticides, steroids, hormones, and artificial pigments. Unfortunately, they are becoming popular due to availability and cost. For example, farm-raised salmon makes up 95 percent of the American salmon on the market today. Since these fish are raised in confined, crowded, and unsanitary conditions, the threat of disease and parasites is great. To combat this, some fish farmers use antibiotics, pesticides, and even steroids to make the fish sterile and growth hormones to speed them to market size. In addition, since farm-raised salmon do not normally eat crustaceans that naturally make the flesh pink or orange, salmon growers often feed the fish color additives to pigment the flesh.

### Other Meats

In addition to beef, poultry, and fish, other meats are also potentially good sources of protein. Pork and lamb are popular meats, and recently meats such as buffalo and elk have appeared in some grocery stores. When choosing these meats, use the same guidelines as with beef and poultry—buy those that are organic or raised naturally at a local farm without corn feedings.

Wild game, including deer, rabbit, and game birds, is also another great source of protein. Wild-game meat is generally leaner but higher in essential fatty acids than domestic meats. While hunting your own meat is nearly ideal, there is a growing concern in some areas like the northeastern United States that the use of pesticides and other environmental chemicals has affected wild animals. But in general, wild game is much safer than store-bought meat.

Generally avoid ground meat of any kind unless it has been freshly ground right before deep freezing or eating it. Ground meat is a haven for bacteria. If you like ground meat or have a recipe that requires it, it's best to buy a large piece of meat and then grind it up just before cooking—most butchers, even those in large groceries, will do this for you. Also beware of other meats that have already been cut, such as sliced meat, chopped meat, and stew meat. Try to buy as large a piece of meat as possible and cut it yourself.

Processed meats can also be unhealthy. Most sausage, lunch meats, and other processed meats are not only ground but may also contain high amounts of sugar and chemicals that you want to avoid. However, it is possible to find organic bacon and hams that have been cured with honey and with no harmful chemicals.

The most nutritious parts of the animal to eat are the organs and glands. In our society, the liver is the most common organ food, with stomach, brains, kidneys, and others only rarely eaten. However, when a lion kills his prey, it's the organs and glands that are first devoured. The muscle, what we refer to as the "meat," is often left for the scavengers. Unfortunately, with our polluted environment, organ meats such as liver are becoming more dangerous since it's the liver's job to filter the blood and remove toxins from the body. If you enjoy liver and other organ and gland meats, be sure to find a reputable source.

### Cultured Dairy Products

Cheese and plain yogurt are dairy products that contain quality protein without many of the problems associated with milk. This is especially true if you can find products made from raw milk and that are also organic. Goat and sheep milk are much more compatible for humans than cow milk. These cheeses can be found in many stores and on the Internet.

Whichever type of milk they're made from, the culturing of these products makes them good sources of complete protein, with the lactose, or "milk sugar," reduced by friendly bacteria in the culture process. To be sure that an item is fully cultured, check the "Nutrition Facts" on the label; the carbohydrate count should be very low. (Of course you want to avoid the fruit-flavored and sweetened varieties of yogurt that are always full of sugar—sometimes a half-dozen teaspoons or more!)

It's important to remember that dairy is also high in certain types of saturated fats, more than any of the other protein sources listed here. As discussed later, this can contribute to chronic inflammation.

Avoid so-called American cheese, cheese spreads, and other processed cheeses. These highly processed products, which outsell natural cheese, are usually several types of unripe cheeses ground up with added chemical stabilizers, preservatives, and emulsifiers.

## Curds and Whey

Remember Little Miss Muffet, eating her curds and whey? These are the two proteins found in milk. Whey protein is the thin liquid part of milk remaining after the casein (the curds) and fat are removed. Whey is the part of the milk containing most of the vitamins and minerals, including calcium, and it's a complete protein. During the making of cheese, which mostly is produced from curds, whey is often fed back to the animals for nutritional reasons.

The whey component of milk contains a group of natural sulfur-containing substances called *biothiols* that help produce our most potent antioxidant, glutathione. Because it helps the immune system, whey has been used to help prevent and treat many chronic conditions, from asthma and allergies to cancer and heart disease. It can also help improve muscle function. Most people who are allergic to cow's milk can usually consume whey without problems because

the lactose content is very small. However, in those who are truly lactose-intolerant (probably less than 5 percent of the population), this amount of lactose could be a problem.

Some cheese is made from whey. Italian ricotta is the most common one; check the ingredient label on ricotta to make sure the main ingredient is whey. Whey is also made into powders for use in baked goods and smoothies as discussed below.

The curds from milk are used for most cheese making. Cottage cheese is the best example of what curds look like. However, the curd is the protein in milk most people are allergic to if they have a dairy allergy. Newborns and young children are especially vulnerable to curds because their intestines and immune system are too immature to tolerate this protein.

## The Soy Story

While soy is a vegetarian source of a complete protein, it often poses a problem because much of today's soy is highly processed and concentrated. Whole green soybeans, or edamame, are an example of a whole food and a good source of protein. With a relatively small amount of simple processing soy can be made into tofu, also a good food. This is how most soy has been consumed for centuries, and studies of these populations seem to show that soy has health benefits when consumed as a food.

But today, many soy powders used in food products and supplements are so concentrated

**Question:** I have been hearing and reading a lot about quinoa—and how this South American plant packs a lot of protein. What is your opinion here? Any recipe suggestions?

**Answer:** Quinoa is a grain-like food grown in South and North America, with commercial production highest in Peru and Bolivia. Closely related to the tumbleweed, quinoa has been heavily marketed in recent years with much hype. One drawback of quinoa is that it's high in starch, reducing digestibility. It is also processed to remove the outer coating, which contains bitter-tasting phytonutrients. While it's considered high in protein, it's a vegetable protein and not complete. It is gluten-free. So, one must weigh the positives and negatives of this food item. I don't eat it and have never prepared it, but there are many recipes online.

that a serving or two would be like eating a pound or two of real soybeans—something most people would never even consider. For this reason, it's best to avoid all processed soy products, especially soy-protein isolates and caseinates, and hydrolyzed soy. The more soy is processed, the worse it can be. Monosodium glutamate (MSG), a once commonly used powder that makes food seem to taste better (still used in Chinese and other restaurants), is made by processing soy. So products containing isolated or hydrolyzed soy also include some MSG (but it is not required to be listed in the ingredients).

Many athletes may be intolerant and even allergic to soy in all forms. In addition, concentrated soy isoflavones, used in dietary supplements, can pose serious dangers, including an increased risk of cancer, particularly for postmenopausal women—the very audience these products are marketed to by the big companies. They may also contribute to hormonal imbalance.

### Protein Powders

Soy, milk, whey, egg, and other foods are commonly sold to supplement the diet. These have value when used cautiously. Certainly avoid any of these powders if you're intolerant to those foods. In addition, avoid all powders that have been isolated, caseinated, or hydrolyzed. These products are touted as being highest in protein—which is true, but at the expense of being highly processed and containing MSG. Those marked "concentrated" are the least processed of the powders and are an acceptable part of a healthy diet. Egg-white powder is the least processed of all the powders. This and whey concentrate are the best and healthiest of all these products. (If you use egg-white powder in a blender, you must include a small amount of fat otherwise it will create a large volume of foam—great for meringue but not for smoothies and other recipes.)

All in all, protein foods are a key part of an athlete's diet. When choosing protein sources, look for real food, including fresh whole eggs, whole pieces of meat and fish, and raw-milk cheese as tolerated. Avoid the processed protein products—cold cuts, frozen foods, processed cheese, and so on. If you need to increase protein intake with a food supplement, use egg-white powder or whey concentrate. These foods also contain a variety of important vitamins, minerals, and phytonutrients.

# CHAPTER 16

# DIETARY FATS—
## Optimal Health and Recovery, and Avoiding Injuries

Yes, anyone can effectively learn to burn body fat for endurance energy—and that is a key to success for athletes. But there is another aspect of fat equally important for the endurance athlete. This is dietary fat—including oil—found in foods. These fats, when properly balanced, help one recover from a workout and racing, repair injuries by correcting inflammation, control pain, and perform many other critical tasks.

While most athletes take anti-inflammatory drugs, the fact is they don't work as well in controlling pain, inflammation, and speeding recovery. The body already possesses the natural ability to control pain and inflammation better than any drug—through the balancing of dietary fats. In addition, the balance of dietary fats can play a vital role in preventing chronic illness and help promote healthy aging.

The building blocks of dietary fats are called fatty acids, just like glucose and amino acids are the components of carbohydrates and protein, respectively. The relative balance of these fatty acids is a key for optimal health and endurance. Among the injuries common in endurance athletes are those associated with pain, bone loss, and muscle, joint, ligament, and tendon inflammation; many also have allergies and asthma.

These and many other problems are associated with an imbalance of specific fatty acids from dietary fat.

Do you have an imbalance of fats? This is the first question to ask yourself and it can be done with a simple checklist. Many athletes are unaware that their fats are not balanced until some injury or illness becomes obvious or chronic. These problems are typically accompanied by certain signs, symptoms, and lifestyle habits. The following checklist is a simple self-assessment survey that can help you determine the likelihood that you have an imbalance in fats. Check the items below that apply to you:

- ☐ Aspirin or non-steroidal anti-inflammatory drugs improve my symptoms.
- ☐ I have chronic inflammation or "itis" type conditions, such as arthritis, colitis, or tendinitis.
- ☐ I have a history or increased risk of heart disease, stroke, or high blood pressure.
- ☐ I often eat restaurant, take-out, or fast food.
- ☐ I follow a low-fat diet.
- ☐ I often feel depressed.
- ☐ I have a history of tumors or cancers.
- ☐ I sometimes suffer from reduced mental acuity.
- ☐ I have diabetes or family history of diabetes.
- ☐ I am over age fifty.
- ☐ My blood tests show increased triglycerides or cholesterol.
- ☐ I am carbohydrate intolerant.
- ☐ I have seasonal allergies.
- ☐ I suffer from intestinal problems such as diarrhea, constipation, or ulcers.

If you checked one or more of these items, there's a higher chance that you have a fat imbalance. The more items you check off, the more likely it is you have a problem.

### Acute versus Chronic Inflammation

Acute inflammation is the body's way of responding to and repairing itself from the daily wear and tear of physical stress. All this activity requires recovery. An easy bike ride or even just a walk produces chemicals that cause mild inflammation throughout the body as part of a complex recovery process. An acute injury produces inflammation too—a cut hand, a damaged joint, or an irritated stomach. The reddish, swollen, hot area of a cut finger is an example of this normal inflammatory process. Once the initial inflammation has got the healing under way, the body produces anti-inflammatory chemicals to stop the inflammation process and allow the healing to be completed.

Problems arise when the body is unable to produce sufficient anti-inflammatory chemicals because of an imbalance of fats (excess physical stress or even a lack of recovery may also contribute). When this happens, chronic inflammation can develop. Without proper balance of fats and adequate anti-inflammatory actions, even an easy workout can contribute to an ongoing chronic inflammation.

### The Big Fat Lie

For decades, fat has been widely criticized as the "bad" component of our daily diet. Low- and no-fat foods have become synonymous with losing "weight" and being healthy. These notions, of course, are untrue when we look at the macro picture. The fact is, fat is one of the most beneficial substances in our diet, and is often the missing ingredient for endurance athletes in developing and maintaining optimal health and human performance. But the food industry's ongoing, well-financed misinformation campaign against fat has misled the public. No wonder there's an epidemic of fat phobia. Just think of the billions of dollars spent each year on low-fat and fat-free foods and you'll understand why you might not have been told the whole truth about fat. In addition, this anti-fat campaign has contributed to actual deficiencies in fat that have contributed to inflammatory conditions such as heart disease, osteoporosis, and others. The bottom line on dietary fat: Too much or too little is dangerous. It's simply a question of balancing the good fats and avoiding the bad.

The good fats are those that nature has provided, including olive oil, coconut oil, and the fats from fish and other animals.

The bad fats are the artificial and highly processed ones, such as trans fats and overheated fats in fried foods, all of which can cause serious health problems. Foods such as potato chips, french fries, and fried chicken, to name just a few, are examples of those containing bad fat. Many of these bad fats are found in packaged foods and restaurant meals. Consume these and you can disturb the balance of fat and promote chronic inflammation.

### Some Benefits of Fat

Scientists have known of the importance of fat in the diet since discoveries made in 1929 by researchers who demonstrated that certain fats were essential for human health. Let's highlight some of the many healthy functions of fat in a healthy diet.

*Disease prevention and treatment.* Certain dietary fats consumed in balanced proportions can help prevent many diseases. For instance, we now know that dietary fats are central to controlling inflammation, which is the first stage of most chronic illness. Increasing certain dietary fats has been shown to reduce the growth or spreading of cancer and improve recovery in heart disease. Many brain problems, including cognitive dysfunction such as Alzheimer's disease, can also be prevented with fats. A healthy brain is made up of over 60 percent fat.

*Energy.* Fat not only produces long-term energy but prevents excessive dependency upon short-term energy needs from sugar. Fat provides more than twice as much potential energy as carbohydrates do: nine calories per gram as opposed to only four calories.

Your body is capable of obtaining much of its energy from fat, if your fat-burning mechanism is working efficiently. Even the heart muscle uses fat for energy.

*Hormones.* The hormonal system is responsible for controlling many healthy functions in our brain, muscles, metabolism, and elsewhere. The hormones produced in various glands are dependent on fat—in the adrenal glands, the thymus, thyroid, kidneys, and other glands. Cholesterol is one of the fats used for the production of hormones such as progesterone and cortisone. The thymus gland regulates immunity and the body's defense systems, especially earlier in life. The thyroid regulates temperature, weight, and other metabolic functions. The kidney's hormones help regulate blood pressure, circulation, and filtering of blood.

*Eicosanoids.* Hormone-like substances called *eicosanoids* are necessary for such normal cellular function as regulating inflammation, hydration, circulation, and free radicals. These substances are produced directly from fat in the diet. In addition to chronic inflammation, eicosanoids are also important for regulating blood pressure and body-wide hydration. An imbalance can trigger constipation or diarrhea, especially during long endurance events. Eicosanoid imbalance may also be associated with menstrual cramps, blood clotting, tumor growth, and other problems, and may increase pain.

*Insulation.* The body's ability to store fat permits humans to live in most climates, especially in areas of extreme heat or cold. It also enables athletes to compete in these environments. In warmer areas of the world, stored fat provides protection from the heat, preventing too much water from leaving the body, which can result in dehydration. Some evaporation is normal, of course, especially for temperature regulation, but fats under the skin regulate evaporation and can prevent as much as ten to twenty times more water from leaving the body. In colder lands, increased fat stored beneath the skin prevents too much heat from leaving the body. An example of fat's effectiveness as an insulator is in the Eskimo's ability to withstand great cold and survive in good health. Eskimos eat a high-fat diet (and despite this have a very low incidence of heart disease and other ailments).

*Healthy skin and hair.* Fat has protective qualities that also give skin the soft, smooth, and unwrinkled appearance which many people try to achieve through expensive skin conditioners. The healthy look of skin comes from the fat inside. The same is true for your hair. Fats, including cholesterol, also serve as an insulating barrier within the skin. Without this protection, water and water-soluble substances such as chemical pollutants would enter the body through the skin. With the proper balance and amount of fats in your diet, your skin and hair develop a healthy appearance.

*Digestion.* Bile from the gall bladder is triggered by fat in the diet, which helps aid in the digestion and absorption of important fats and fat-soluble vitamins. Most of the fats in the diet are digested in the small intestine—a process that involves breaking the fat into smaller particles. The pancreas, liver, gall bladder, and large intestine are also involved in the digestive process. Any of these organs not working properly could have an adverse impact on fat metabolism in general, but the two most important organs are the liver, which makes bile, and the pancreas, which make the enzyme lipase. Without sufficient fat in the diet, the gall bladder will not secrete enough bile for proper digestion.

Fat also helps regulate the rate of stomach emptying. Fat in a meal slows stomach emptying, allowing for better digestion, especially of proteins. If you are always hungry it may be because your meal is too low in fat and your stomach is emptying too rapidly. Fats also slow the absorption of sugar from the small intestine, which keeps insulin from rising too high and too quickly—essentially, fat in a meal lowers its glycemic index. Additionally, fats protect the inner lining of the stomach and intestines from irritating substances in the diet, such as alcohol and spicy foods.

*Support and protection.* Stored fat offers physical support and protection to vital body parts, including the organs and glands. This is particularly important for runners who have higher levels of gravity stress. Fat acts as a natural, built-in shock absorber, cushioning the body and its various parts from the wear and tear of training, and helps prevent organs from sinking due to the downward pull of gravity.

Fats also can protect the body against the harmful effects of X-rays. This occurs through physical protection of the cell, and by controlling free-radical production, generated as a result of X-ray exposure. In addition to medical X-rays, we are constantly exposed to X-rays from the atmosphere in the form of cosmic radiation. This is important as most endurance athletes train and compete outdoors. Cosmic radiation also penetrates most objects, including airplanes. The average person gets more cosmic radiation exposure during an airline flight from New York to Los Angeles than from a lifetime of medical X-rays.

*Vitamin and mineral regulation.* Most people know that vitamin D is produced by exposure of the skin to the sun. However, it is actually cholesterol in the skin that allows this reaction to occur. Sunlight chemically changes cholesterol in the skin through the process of irradiation to vitamin D3. This newly formed vitamin D is then absorbed into the blood, allowing calcium and phosphorous to be properly absorbed from the intestinal tract. Without the vitamin D, calcium and phosphorous would not be well absorbed and deficiencies of both could occur. But without cholesterol, the entire process would not occur.

Besides vitamin D, other vitamins, including A, E, and K, rely on fat for proper absorption and utilization. These important "fat soluble" vitamins are present primarily in fatty foods, and the body cannot make an adequate amount of these vitamins on its own to ensure continued good health. In addition these vitamins require fat in the intestines in order to be absorbed. A low-fat diet could be deficient in these vitamins to begin with and also could further restrict their absorption.

Certain eicosanoids from dietary fat help carry calcium into the bones and muscles. Without this action, calcium levels in bones and muscles can be reduced, resulting in the risk for stress fractures, muscle cramps, and other problems. Unused calcium may be stored, sometimes in the kidneys, increasing the risk of stones, or in the muscles, tendons, or joint spaces as calcium deposits.

*Taste.* A favorite function of fat is that it makes food delightfully palatable. Low- and no-fat products are usually quite bland, and often manufacturers add sugar to these products to improve taste. Fat also satisfies your physical hunger by increasing satiety (the signal given to the brain that the meal is satisfying and you can stop eating). With a low-fat meal, the brain just keeps sending the same message over and over: Eat more! Because you never really feel satisfied, the temptation to overeat is irresistible. In fact, there's a good chance you can actually gain weight on a low-fat diet by overeating to try to get that "I'm not hungry anymore" feeling.

## The Balance of Fats

Now that we've discussed the importance of natural dietary fats and the necessity of healthy body fat, it's just as important to outline how to balance your consumption of certain fats in the diet. It's accomplished in three simple steps:

When using fats and oils, use only olive oil, butter, coconut oil, or lard for cooking, and primarily olive oil for salads and other dishes.

Avoid all vegetable oils and trans fats (hydrogenated or partially hydrogenated).

Balance consumption of foods high in omega-6 and omega-3 fats.

The issue of balancing fat consumption is quite complex; volumes of studies have been written on the subject and many scientists have devoted their entire careers to this topic. But I have simplified the explanations to help you achieve this important task. First, let's look at three common types of dietary fats: monounsaturated, polyunsaturated, and saturated.

### Monounsaturated Fat

This type of fat should make up the bulk of dietary fat. Monounsaturated fat, also referred to as "oleic" or "omega-9," has been shown to have many health benefits, including helping to prevent cancer, heart disease, obesity, and other chronic illnesses. The Mediterranean diet, with its lower incidence of obesity and diseases, is relatively high in monounsaturated fat, which may be the key reason for its health benefits. In some cases, we know how monounsaturated fat can prevent disease. This fat is known to raise "good" HDL cholesterol and lower "bad" LDL cholesterol, which can greatly improve cardiovascular health.

Monounsaturated fat is also very stable. As discussed later, polyunsaturated fat is easily oxidized and can form dangerous oxygen free radicals from exposure to air, light, and heat. These free radicals can lead to bodily dysfunction, contributing to injuries and even disease. Due to its chemical structure, monounsaturated fat is virtually immune to oxidation through cooking or exposure to air and light.

Monounsaturated fat is found in many foods, and some oils are predominantly this type of fat. Foods highest in monounsaturated fats include avocados, almonds, and macadamia nuts, with other nuts and seeds containing moderate amounts. Olive oil is very high in monounsaturated fat and is one of the best oils for both cooking and use on salads or other foods.

The best olive oil to use is the least processed and most nutritious—extra virgin olive oil. This is obtained from the whole fruit by using a cold-press technique, which does not alter the natural antioxidants, phytonutrients, or quality of the oil. The most potent phytonutrients are phenols, which give the oil its slightly bitter taste. Very high amounts of phenols are found in extra virgin olive oil. Phytonutrients, including phenols, are virtually absent in almost all other oils.

By using extra virgin olive oil for most of your oil needs, as well as eating foods that are high in health-promoting monounsaturated fat, such as avocados and almonds, you'll be taking an important step to balancing your dietary fats.

### Polyunsaturated Fat

Many foods naturally contain polyunsaturated fat. They include omega-6 and omega-3 essential fatty acids that play a vital role in regulating inflammation and other key functions. Concentrated and potentially dangerous amounts of omega-6 fat are in vegetable and other omega-6 oils, with the highest levels contained in safflower, peanut, corn, canola, and soy oil. Many processed foods contain high amounts of these oils. Too much omega-6 polyunsaturated fat, whether from vegetable oil, processed food, or dietary supplements, can adversely affect health in two significant ways. First, an excess of omega-6 oil can contribute significantly to chronic inflammation, increase pain, and adversely affect muscle function, important factors in most physical injuries.

Second, polyunsaturated fat is easily oxidized to substances called free radicals, making it a potentially dangerous food. Oxidation occurs when this type of fat is heated or exposed to light and air. When we consume oxidized fat, this free radical stress can damage cells anywhere in the body, speed the aging process, turn LDL cholesterol "bad," and significantly increase the need for antioxidant nutrients.

Many fats contained in dairy foods—such as butter and cheese—are also an omega-6

# TWO TYPES OF BODY FAT

The human body possesses two distinct types of body fat, referred to as "brown" and "white." Both forms of body fat are active, living parts of us, heavily influencing our metabolism. Most of this is in the form of white fat, which totals from about 5 percent of total weight in very lean male athletes to more than 50 percent of total body weight in obese individuals. Brown fat makes up only about 1 percent of the total body fat in healthy adults, although it's much more abundant in healthy babies.

Brown fat, also called brown adipose tissue or BAT, helps us burn white fat; this is important for endurance. Without adequate brown fat activity, we can gain body fat; it's most noticeable in cold weather when we can become sluggish like a hibernating animal. There are a number of ways to increase brown fat activity.

Certain foods can stimulate brown fat and increase overall fat burning. Eating several times a day, five to six smaller, healthy meals instead of one, two, or three larger ones, for example, can trigger a process called thermogenesis—an important post-meal metabolic stimulation for fat burning. However, if our caloric intake is too low, brown fat can slow the burning of white fat. This can happen on a low-calorie diet and when we skip meals.

Brown fat is also stimulated by certain dietary fats. The best ones are omega-3 fat from fish oil and extra virgin olive oil. While supplements of fish oil may be the only way to obtain adequate amounts of EPA, some supplements can be harmful; a popular supplement, CLA (conjugated linoleic acid), can actually reduce brown fat activity.

Capsaicin, the substance responsible for the pungent flavor of chili peppers, can stimulate brown fat. Use this in cooking and even on salads.

Other foods that increase brown fat activity include those with caffeine, but only if it's tolerated. Tea, coffee, and chocolate contain small to high amounts of caffeine. However, if under stress, the adrenal glands become overworked, which can promote fat storage and reduce fat burning; caffeine may worsen adrenal stress in many athletes. Also, avoid coffee, tea, and chocolate products if they contain sugar, which can reduce fat burning.

Brown fat is greatly controlled by skin temperature. If we get too hot during training, brown-fat activity can lead to less burning of white fat. Dress light for training, or remove clothing as you warm up. Even sitting in a hot tub, sauna, or steam room regularly after an aerobic workout may offset some of the fat-burning benefits. Hot tubs and saunas do come with health benefits, but to avoid the reductions in fat burning take a minute or two to cool the body in a cold shower or tub afterward. In contrast, brown fat is stimulated by cold. Cooling the body's brown-fat areas can help stimulate fat burning.

Brown fat is found around the shoulders and underarms, between the ribs, and at the nape of the neck. These are important areas to keep cool and from overheating after training. (Low body temperature is associated with reduced fat burning; this is often related to low thyroid function.)

fat. The fat content of most people's diet is very high in concentrated omega-6 fats from vegetable and other oils and dairy products; this poses a serious imbalance. To accomplish a better balance of fat, begin by avoiding all vegetable and omega-6 oils and processed food; instead, use extra virgin olive or other recommended fats.

### Saturated Fat

Of all the dietary fats, saturated fat is always considered the worst. But saturated fat is important for energy and hormone production, cellular functioning, and other healthy actions much like other fats.

Similar to other fat, saturated forms are made up of many different fatty acids, some of which have been linked to ill health when in excess. The worst may be palmitic acid, high in dairy fat. This fatty acid can raise cholesterol, and some of the dietary carbohydrate that converts to fat becomes palmitic

acid. High blood levels of palmitic acid may be associated with type 2 diabetes, heart disease, stroke, and carbohydrate intolerance. However, when fats are balanced, palmitic acid does not seem to be such a health problem.

Arachidonic acid (AA) is another component of saturated fat that gives it a bad name. While small amounts are essential for health (it's considered an essential fat), high AA levels are very unhealthy. AA is found in dairy, egg yolks, meats, and shellfish. However, the amounts in these foods are relatively small compared to the amount of AA produced by the conversion of omega-6 fats from vegetable oils in the average diet. Like many other situations regarding fat, balance is the key. In the case of AA, it's an essential fat, especially for the brain, the fetus, newborns, growing children, and athletes. But in larger amounts it can cause problems. Too much AA, either from saturated fat or vegetable oil, can contribute to chronic inflammation, bone loss, and increased pain.

The good side of saturated fat is important too. Stearic acid, for example, has various health benefits on the immune system. This saturated fatty acid is found in cocoa butter and grass-fed beef. And stearic acid can be converted to monounsaturated fat. Another healthy saturated fatty acid is lauric (called a medium chain fatty acid or MTC), which plays an important role in energy production and has antiviral and antibacterial actions, especially in the intestine (and the stomach in particular, against H. pylori). Coconut oil, high in saturated fat, is also high in healthy lauric acid (and contains very little polyunsaturated fat, making it an ideal fat for cooking).

In animal foods, which contain relatively high amounts of saturated fat, the most important factor that determines the fatty acid profile is the food consumed by the animal. Grass-fed beef, for example, contains a much healthier content of fatty acids compared to corn-fed beef. For the same reason, wild animals usually contain healthier fatty-acid profiles than animals that are fed grain in confinement. In plants, the soil plays a certain role in determining fatty acid content.

Before discussing a key feature in balancing dietary fats, it's worth looking at the fat content of various foods to demonstrate the mixture of mono, poly, and saturated fat in each. A few foods contain predominantly one type of fat or another, but most foods, even oils, contain a combination of all three. Many people are surprised to learn, for instance, that the fat in an average beefsteak is about half monounsaturated and half saturated, with a small amount of polyunsaturated.

The table below shows approximately how much of each type of fat is contained in some foods.

## The ABCs of Fats: Optimal Balance

Together, the two forms of polyunsaturated (omega-6 and -3) and saturated fats contain three important fatty acids I'll call A, B, and C fats. In the body, each of these fats is converted to three different groups of hormone-like substances called *eicosanoids* (pronounced i-cos-an-oids). I'll call these groups 1, 2, and 3. Basically, A fats make group 1 eisosanoids, B fats group 2, and C fats group 3. This is a very simplified explanation, but fairly accurate.

Group 1, 2, and 3 eicosanoids regulate inflammation: group 1 and 3 produce anti-inflammatory chemicals, and group 2 produces inflammatory chemicals.

An imbalance of eicosanoids resulting in too much of group 2 not only promotes inflammation but also pain, bone loss, muscle problems, allergy, asthma, and, potentially, can lead to cancer, Alzheimer's, diabetes, stroke, heart disease, and other chronic illness. The right balance of eicosanoids can prevent, postpone, and even treat these conditions. Eicosanoid balance is so powerful—so influential to overall health—that billions of dollars are spent by pharmaceutical companies to research and develop new drugs that attempt to balance the body's eicosanoids. But you can do it for pennies by eating the right foods! And while drugs that attempt to balance fats have some short-term success, they come with significant unhealthy and sometimes deadly side effects. Balancing fats by eating right only has healthy—nearly miraculous—benefits.

The term eicosanoid is a general one that encompasses a variety of very different compounds with names such as prostaglandins, leukotrienes, and thromboxanes. They're involved in complex reactions from moment to moment in all cells throughout the body. An understanding of how to balance the A, B, and C fats, and the 1, 2, and 3 groups of eicosanoids is most important. First, let's discuss A, B, and C fats in more detail.

## "A" Fat

The highest amounts of A fats are found in many vegetable oils: safflower, soy, corn, peanut, and canola. These omega-6 fats contain an essential fatty acid called linoleic acid—LA. They are "essential" because we require a certain amount and the body can't make them, so we must eat them for optimal health. When we do, LA is converted to other fats, including GLA (gamma-linolenic acid), with the end result being the group 1 eicosanoids. These have powerful anti-inflammation effects, reduce pain and the risk of many problems, and prevent chronic illness throughout the body. Common

dietary supplements of omega-6 products that contain high amounts of GLA include black-currant seed, borage, and primrose oils.

A serious potential problem, as noted above, is that A fats can convert to B fats and group 2 eicosanoids, causing chronic inflammation, pain, and other problems associated with this imbalance.

## "B" Fat

The B fats are sometimes considered bad fats because of the effects they can have on the body. But these effects are only bad when in excess and not balanced. B fats contain the essential fat AA (arachidonic acid), as noted above, and produce group 2 eicosanoids. These eicosanoids promote inflammation and pain, among other problems. But these so-called problems can actually be important for health at the right time. For example, inflammation is a vital first stage of the healing process. Following this acute inflammatory process, as healing proceeds, anti-inflammatory eisocanoids in groups 1 and 3 are produced to reduce inflammation. Another example is pain; the body uses pain to help us be aware of problems so we can remedy them. Chronic pain is not normal, or healthy, and is usually associated with an unresolved problem associated with an imbalance of eicosanoids.

Another important function of AA (which is also considered an omega-6 fat) is that it's very important for the repair and growth of the brain. This is especially vital in the fetus, newborns, and developing children; but as adults, we should continually be repairing and growing the brain as well.

B fats are highest in dairy products such as butter, cream, and cheese, and in lesser amounts in the fat of meats, egg yolks, and shellfish. However, for most people, the largest source of AA is from A fats, usually from vegetable and other omega-6 oils, creating the potential of significant problems. By eliminating these oils and using only olive or coconut oil, the overall balance of fats is usually greatly improved. In addition to the common use at home, vegetable and other omega-6 oils are often used in packaged foods, and in restaurants.

### "C" Fat

The C fats are termed omega-3 and are found mostly in cold-water ocean fish, with lesser amounts in beans, flaxseed, and walnuts. Smaller amounts are found in vegetables and in wild and grass-fed animals. These fats contain ALA (alpha-linolenic acid), an essential fatty acid that is converted in the body to EPA (eicosapentaenoic acid), with the final production of group 3 eicosanoids.

| Approximate Percentage of Mono, Poly, and Saturated Fats/Oils in Some Foods | | | |
|---|---|---|---|
| Oil | Mono | Poly | Saturated |
| Olive oil | 77 | 9 | 14 |
| Canola oil | 62 | 32 | 6 |
| Peanut oil | 49 | 33 | 18 |
| Corn oil | 25 | 62 | 13 |
| Soybean oil | 24 | 61 | 15 |
| Safflower oil | 13 | 77 | 10 |
| Coconut | 6 | 2 | 92 |
| Egg yolks | 48 | 16 | 36 |
| Steak | 49 | 4 | 47 |
| Cheese | 30 | 3 | 67 |
| Butter | 30 | 4 | 66 |
| Almonds | 68 | 22 | 10 |
| Cashews | 62 | 18 | 21 |
| Peanuts | 50 | 32 | 18 |
| Sesame | 40 | 42 | 14 |

| The ABCs of Fats | | |
|:---:|:---:|:---:|
| A Fats | B Fats | C Fats |
| ↓ | ↓ | ↓ |
| Group 1 eicosanoids | Group 2 eicosanoids | Group 3 eicosanoids |

Fish oils derived from cold-water ocean fish already contain EPA. This is a very useful supplement for those needing to balance fats, as C fats are usually the most difficult to obtain through the diet. (EPA also exists in conjunction with another fatty acid, DHA, which is especially important for the fetus through childhood.)

Flaxseed oil is a popular omega-3 fat but does not contain EPA. While some of the omega-3 fat in flax can convert to EPA, this process requires various nutrients and, in humans, conversion to EPA is very inefficient, so the amount converted to EPA may be small. Flaxseed oil is also very unstable and can turn unhealthy if not fresh.

### Balancing the ABCs

It's relatively easy to balance A, B, and C fats to promote a balance of the 1, 2, and 3 groups of eicosanoids. There are three main ways to do this:

1. First, eat approximately equal amounts of A, B, and C fats in your diet. It does not necessarily have to be at each meal, but in the course of a day or week, balance is of prime importance. And by eating a balance of A, B, and C fats, you'll consume polyunsaturated (A and C) and saturated (B) fats in the optimal ratio of 2:1. In the typical Western diet, many people consume ratios of 5:1, 10:1, or even 20:1! It's no wonder there's an epidemic of chronic inflammation, pain, injury, and disease. (If you don't eat meat or dairy, consume approximately an equal ratio of A and C fats; in this case, some of the A fats will convert to B fats.) Fat imbalances typically occur from some combination of eating too much A or B fats or too little C fats.

2. Limit or avoid the two most common foods that cause an imbalance in fats: vegetable and omega-6 oils and refined carbohydrates, including sugar. Recall that insulin can be produced in higher amounts when these carbohydrates are consumed. This causes more A fats to convert to B fats and the group 2 eicosanoids. Two foods that can help prevent too much A fat from converting to B fat are EPA in fish oil and raw sesame oil, which contains the phytonutrient sesamin.

3. Maintain a healthy diet and lifestyle. Certain factors can impair the conversion of A and C fats to their respective group 1 and 3 eicosanoids (but unfortunately, these factors won't impair the conversion of B fats to group 2). These include reduced consumption of specific vitamins and minerals (such as vitamins B6, C, E, niacin, and the minerals magnesium,

calcium, and zinc), trans fat contained in hydrogenated or partially hydrogenated oil, low protein intake, excess stress, and aging (although this can be compensated for by maintaining an optimal balance of fats).

Eat the best diet possible to ensure you obtain all necessary nutrients, avoid bad fats, and moderate stress. As noted earlier in this chapter, when using fats and oils:

- For cooking, use only olive oil, butter, coconut oil, or lard, and primarily olive oil for salads and other items.
- Avoid all vegetable and omega-6 oils such as soy, safflower, corn, and peanut, and avoid trans fats.
- Balance consumption of omega-6 and omega-3 fats.

## Anti-inflammatory Drugs—How They Work and Cause Harm

Many endurance athletes take various types of painkillers and other drugs, especially non-steroidal anti-inflammatory drugs—NSAIDs—in hopes of improving their competitiveness, while alleviating chronic aches and pains. Unfortunately, these drugs most often cause more stress on the whole body. Controlling pain and inflammation is instead best accomplished by eating adequate amounts of healthy fats and maintaining their proper balance.

Anti-inflammatory drugs work as follows: In the conversion of A, B, and C fats to eicosanoids, an important enzyme called cyclooxygenase, or COX, is required. There are actually two COX enzymes, and many people are familiar with the term "COX-2 inhibitors." These are drugs that attempt to inhibit these enzymes. Aspirin and all other NSAIDs, including ibuprofen and Naprosyn, temporarily block the COX enzyme, so much less of the inflammatory series 2 eicosanoids are formed. While this reduces the inflammatory group 2 eicosanoids, these drugs can also eliminate groups 1 and 3, along with their beneficial properties. This may result in an improvement of symptoms, but it also turns off the important anti-inflammatory mechanism. In addition, the cause of the problem—fat imbalance—goes untreated. *Most importantly, if aspirin or other NSAIDs makes you feel better, it usually indicates that your fats are not balanced.*

Here's how these non-steroidal drugs cause the body harm:

- They slow the process of recovery and repair.
- They cause gut problems, including bleeding, in almost everyone taking them (even if it's not noticeable).
- They can cause muscle dysfunction and don't necessarily reduce muscle pain associated with training and competition.
- They can reduce the body's ability to repair joint and bone stress.
- They can cause kidney damage, especially when you're dehydrated.
- They can disturb sleep.

| The ABCs of Fat: A Summary | | | |
|---|---|---|---|
| Type of Fat: | A | B | C |
| Food Source: | vegetable oils | animal fats | fish, flax |
| Contains: | LA | AA | ALA |
| Converts to: | GLA | | EPA |
| Eicosanoids: | Group 1 | Group 2 | Group 3 |
| Response: | anti-inflammatory | inflammatory | anti-inflammatory |

- They may not necessarily reduce inflammation.
- They cause immune system stress.
- They can actually contribute to injuries.

Other issues regarding pain are discussed later in the book, but controlling pain is one of the common reasons why athletes take NSAIDs and other drugs—but as noted, NSAIDs don't always control the pain of training and competition very well. Controlling pain and inflammation is best accomplished by eating adequate amounts of healthy fats and maintaining their proper balance.

### So How Much Fat Should You Eat?

Once you are equipped with the knowledge of how important balanced fats are for the body, the next question is this: How much fat should you have in a healthy diet? The amount of fat in a healthy diet depends on the individual. We now know that natural dietary fat is very important for all athletes. A diet that gets 10 or 20 percent of its calories from fat is probably inadequate for most people. In fact, a low-fat diet can be very unhealthy because you risk reducing essential fats, and most people on low fat diets have a significant imbalance of A, B, and C fats. There are many populations in which fat intake exceeds 40 percent of calories, like the Eskimos and people living in the Mediterranean region, who on average are healthier than people who eat a lower-fat diet. In addition, many health-care professionals and health organizations have recommended a diet that's 30 percent fat, not one that's 20 percent or even 10 percent.

Over the years, I have found that most people are healthier with at least 30 percent fat in their diet. Some may need more—35 or even 40 percent—but everyone is individual in their particular needs. Rather than strictly follow these percentages, I recommend that you experiment and find what works best for you. Your diet should be personalized, just like your training and racing.

# CHAPTER 17

# WATER AND ELECTROLYTES—
## Critical Ingredients for Endurance

**W**ater is among the most important nutrients for athletes. Unfortunately, it's also the most common nutritional deficiency. Proper intake of water is vital to overall fitness and health, with normal fluctuations in water loss of less than 1 percent of body weight. A loss of as little as just over 1 percent of water may begin the process of dehydration and start signs and symptoms of dysfunction. A loss of water that is 2 percent of body weight or more can result in significant performance loss. For a 150-pound athlete, this is only 3 pounds. Assessing yourself for proper hydration can be as simple as weighing yourself on an accurate scale, without clothes, immediately before and after a long training session, for example, to gain a better idea of how much water you've lost. Any level of dehydration can affect the brain, muscles, and metabolism.

Certain minerals, called electrolytes, are also very important in relation to water regulation. The key to maintaining proper hydration is to drink plenty of water throughout the day and consume adequate amounts of electrolytes, especially sodium, in the diet. As previously discussed, adrenal function, important for water and electrolyte regulation, is also key to maintain proper hydration and mineral balance.

## H₂0

A key ingredient in maintaining optimal function and balance throughout the body is water. It helps transport other nutrients to the cells, maintain the function of blood, and eliminate wastes from the lungs, skin, and colon. Water also plays a major role in hormone regulation and balancing acid-alkaline levels in the body. More importantly, water is like your car's radiator, cooling the metabolic reactions that create heat in your body. For example, muscle contraction produces large amounts of heat, which must be cooled by water. If this regulation did not occur effectively, your temperature would rise to a level that would destroy your enzymes and other protein-based substances and you would function very poorly or, worse, could die. The water literally absorbs the excess heat and carries it to the skin, where it is dissipated through evaporation and sweating.

About 60 percent of the body is made up of water, with different areas accounting for various percentages. For example, about 80 percent of your blood, heart, lungs, and kidneys are water; your muscles, intestines, and spleen are about 75 percent water. Even areas like your bones, which are 22 percent water, and fat stores, 10 percent water, require a specific level which, if not maintained, results in poor function.

Very slight reductions in water can have adverse effects on training and competition. That's because dehydration can lower blood volume. This reduces blood flow to the brain, muscles, organs, glands, and other areas. Lower blood volume causes other problems too, including:

- Reduced oxygen and red blood cells going to the muscles
- Reduced transport of nutrients, including glucose, fats, and amino acids
- Reduced removal of carbon dioxide and other byproducts of metabolism
- Reduced transport of hormones that help regulate muscular activity
- Reduced regulation of lactic acid and lactate
- Reduced cardiovascular function
- Reduced effectiveness of muscle contractions
- Reduced effectiveness of the sweating mechanism

In addition, lowered blood volume raises the heart rate, which negatively affects athletic performance, as indicated by poor MAF Test results. Muscle cramps are also associated with dehydration, along with sodium loss.

For the same reasons, dehydration can affect your brain, creating moodiness and reducing memory. It can also influence perceived exertion, making an average workout feel more difficult. And those athletes relying on eye-hand coordination (tennis, ball sports, etc.) can also be adversely affected by dehydration. Other symptoms of dehydration include headache, dizziness, high heart rate, and dry mouth. But these indicators are also felt after you're dehydrated.

## Evaluating Dehydration

Thirst is how most people remember to drink water. But this is not the best way to stay hydrated, since the brain's thirst center does not send a message until you are almost 2 percent dehydrated. By then, you already have lost function associated with dehydration. The kidneys, however, respond to dehydration much sooner than the brain tells you you're thirsty. If your urine output is diminished, it may be one of the first indications that you're beginning to dehydrate. What is meant by diminished? This, of course, varies with the individual. If you're not urinating at least six to eight times each day, for example, or if each time you urinate the volume is noticeably reduced, you may be dehydrated.

While the best measurement of dehydration involves blood tests such as isotope techniques and plasma osmolality, most healthcare professionals and athletes can rely on other practical evaluations. These include urine-specific gravity and urine osmolality.

Even more practical, and quite accurate, is the color of urine.

All athletes can learn to evaluate the color of their urine regularly. It may be the best and earliest indicator that you need more water. Pale or light yellow color or clear urine usually indicates good hydration status. But if urine color is brighter yellow or a darker brown/tan color, this it may indicate dehydration. The exception is for the first urine in the morning, which is darker because you're mildly dehydrated due to no (or reduced) water intake during the night. (This is the reason drinking water should be one of the first things you do upon awakening.)

Synthetic vitamin B2 (riboflavin) typically produces a very bright yellow color of the urine within hours of taking it. This chemical typically comes from a vitamin supplement.

## Water Loss—Sweat

Evaporation from the skin, important for controlling body temperature, is also a major source of water loss. Even under cool, resting conditions, about 30 percent of water loss occurs here. Water in exhaled air is also significant, as the air going in and out of your lungs is humidified. A small but significant water loss (about 5 percent) occurs through the intestine.

During training and racing, water loss increases dramatically. The body attempts to conserve water, and loss through the kidneys becomes limited. In this case, sweating increases significantly, and water lost from

**Question:** What happens when you get an IV after a race? I did the Hawaii Ironman one hot year, and I was amazed to see so many triathletes in the medical tent getting intravenous treatments. How does an IV speed up rehydration? Are there any side effects?

**Answer:** If you are in need of medical assistance during or after a race (as determined by someone on the medical staff), you may be given an intravenous (IV) solution. Depending on your particular needs, this may provide your body with much needed water, sodium and other electrolytes, and glucose. This procedure can quickly restore these nutrients to your bloodstream to help your body speed recovery. There are no real side effects, other than the rare risk of improper insertion of the needle into your vein or secondary infection. An important point to emphasize is to prevent finishing a race in such poor health.

the skin through sweating is about three hundred times the amount lost during rest. This water loss can be as high as a liter an hour in longer activity. In a typical four-hour event, for example, an athlete can lose about four liters (about a gallon) of water (and a significant amount of sodium). But in a very hot, dry climate, the same event could result in twice the amount of water loss through sweat. *It's very important for athletes to replace this much water throughout the race to avoid stress on the body and reductions in performance.*

The amount of water loss during activity is determined in part by a number of factors that include:

- Air temperature (The higher the temperature is, the more water loss.)

- Humidity (Drier climates result in more water loss.)
- Body size (Larger athletes lose more.)
- Level of fitness (Those more fit may regulate water better.)
- Level of health (Those with good adrenal function regulate water better.)
- Heat acclimation (If you're used to the race climate, you'll regulate water better.)
- Clothing (Too much or too little during a sunny race, for example, can cause poor regulation.)

Along with water, sweat causes significant losses in sodium. For each liter of water lost in sweat, there is a loss of between one and five grams (1,000 to 5,000 mg) of sodium—as sodium chloride—lost *per hour* of hard training or competition.

Photo credit: Timothy Carlson

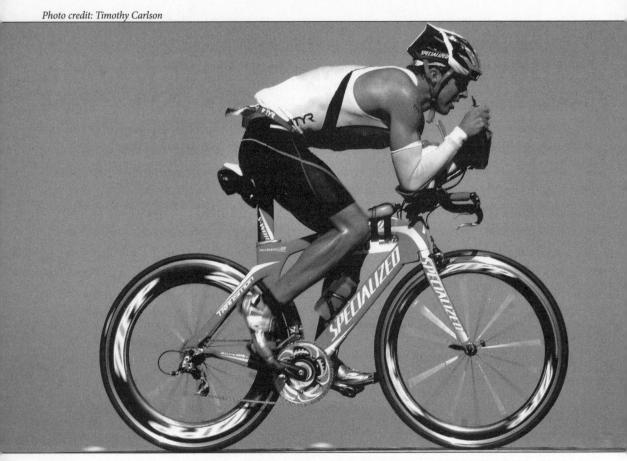

**Always stay properly hydrated, especially when racing.**

### Rehydrating

If you're dehydrated, just drinking a glass of water may not immediately solve the problem, although it certainly starts the rehydration process. Complete water replacement throughout the body—rehydration—may take twenty-four to forty-eight hours no matter how much you drink at one time. Unfortunately, the human body does not function like that of many other animals. By drinking a large volume of water, dehydrated animals can consume 10 percent of their total

body weight in a few minutes and rehydrate quickly.

Humans, however, need to drink water in smaller amounts much more frequently to correct dehydration and maintain proper water balance. For example, after a long or hard workout, drinking sixteen ounces (500 mL) of water every thirty minutes is more effective for rehydration than drinking a very large amount at one time. A large dose of water at one time can impair the thirst mechanism and promote a diuretic response—so you can actually lose more water than normal through urine. (In addition, when drinking a large amount of water at one time, many athletes inadvertently swallow too much air, which can cause bloating.)

Here are some general guidelines to prevent dehydration and maintain proper water balance:

- Drink water every day, throughout the day—don't wait until you're thirsty.
- Drink smaller amounts every couple hours rather than larger volumes at one time.
- Have water available at all times, and get into the habit of drinking small amounts all day.
- Avoid carbonated water as your main source; the carbonation may cause intestinal distress.
- Learn to drink water without swallowing air—drink slowly and without tilting your head up and back. Air in the stomach is a common cause of distress, especially during competition.
- Avoid chlorinated and fluoridated water; chlorine can be toxic, and fluoride impairs energy production.
- An average-sized athlete may need about three to four quarts of water each day, depending on the individual, the types of training, and the environment.
- Get used to drinking water before and immediately after workouts. When training for more than about an hour, drink small to moderate amounts of water during the workout.
- About three hours before long, hard, or competitive events, drink at least sixteen ounces of water, and about half that much water about fifteen minutes before the start of activity.
- During activity lasting more than an hour drink about ten ounces of water every twenty minutes.

Over-hydrating—drinking high volumes of water right before training or competition—does not help reduce the effects of dehydration. Also avoid glycerol-based products, which may not help hydration and can cause intestinal distress. Instead, maintain adequate water intake every day up to and during physical activity as needed.

In addition to the above recommendations, get used to drinking water as your main source of liquid in the course of the day between meals. While it's true you obtain some of your water needs through food and other beverages, most should come from plain water, consumed between meals. Certain drinks such as coffee, tea, and alcohol can increase your need for water because of their diuretic effect (causing the body to lose water). So don't rely on these beverages as part of your water intake. (Even decaf coffee and tea can contain small amounts of caffeine.) Higher levels of protein consumption also increase the need for water.

Retaining the water you drink following workouts and competition can also be accomplished with the addition of sodium, from food or drink. Tomato or vegetable juices, soups, and other salty foods can be very helpful to rehydrate. Sodium tablets can also be effective if the dose is carefully calculated. The addition of sodium also will also stimulate your desire for more water intake.

Athletes are quickly affected by dehydration. Runners can reduce their pace by 2 percent for each percentage of body weight lost by dehydration. Water losses of 6 percent to 10 percent may occur in a triathlon or marathon. Even shorter events are affected by dehydration; a 10K race run in thirty-five minutes under normal hydration can slow to almost thirty-eight minutes when the runner is 4 percent dehydrated. In addition, since dehydration causes an elevated heart rate, it's not unusual to find a plateau or worsening in the MAF Test when an athlete is dehydrated.

In addition, temperature regulation can be significantly affected during dehydration. The ability to expel heat, especially during long or hard events or in hot weather, is reduced. This can raise body temperature, reducing the function of the brain, muscles, and metabolism. Cooling the skin with water, especially dumping water over your head, can be helpful.

The aerobic system can help water regulation, in part due to the significant amount of blood vessels that make up the aerobic fibers. In athletes with a good aerobic base, water regulation is more efficient and body temperature and sweating function more effectively.

Athletes completing long or hard training, and especially competition, who have nausea, vomiting, or diarrhea, or those who are unable to consume water because of the same problems, may require intravenous fluid replacement. This often occurs in triathlons, marathons, and ultramarathons, especially in hot weather. It's not uncommon for those in team competition to have intravenous fluid replacement, including those in football, soccer, and other sports.

### Excess Water and Low Sodium

In some athletes, the body does not properly regulate water and sodium. The result is that the body holds too much water. In some athletes, this abnormal fluid retention results in diluting the blood's sodium levels, potentially causing abnormally low sodium, a condition called hyponatremia.

Various theories exist as to why this happens. Some think it is due to abnormal hormone actions or the over consumption of water (often caused by the abnormal thirst that accompanies this problem). My contention is that athletes who are optimally fit and healthy will effectively regulate water and sodium; those who are not can have an overload of water sometimes seen only following endurance events, although a similar condition, albeit less extreme, may occur after long a training session. Abnormal hormone function, including those in the adrenal

# DRINK CLEAN, SAFE WATER

Make sure your water is safe. Only 1 percent of the world's water is safe to drink. Today, more people are questioning not only the quality of their drinking water but the container it comes in. If you are concerned about your health, you should not just assume your water is safe to drink—you need to take active steps to find out for sure. And if there is a problem, you need to correct it. Most contaminants in water fall into four categories:

- Environmental chemicals, including pesticides, herbicides, and trihalomethanes, a by-product of chlorination, and chemicals that can leach out of plastic bottles
- Heavy metals, including lead, copper, and nitrates
- Bacteria, including the most common coliform bacteria
- Radiological pollution, including radon, radium, and uranium

If you're concerned about your water, the first step is to analyze it to find out what, if any, contamination exists. Once any questions about the quality of the water are answered, necessary steps to improve it, including filtration and finding safe sources, can be taken more logically.

## Problems with Plastic

Water (and other foods) stored in plastic containers may not be as safe to drink as once thought. For many years, plastic has been suspect regarding the possibility that harmful chemicals contained in many plastic materials can leach into water. Research continues to show this as a real hazard. Here are some recommendations:

- Avoid using plastic as long-term storage containers for water or other foods. Instead, save all your glass containers to use for food storage.
- Certain foods react strongly with plastic. Avoid buying vinegar, tomato, alcohol, and similar products housed in plastic containers.
- Remove the plastic parts to bottles containing these foods. For example, some bottles of vinegar contain plastic pouring spouts that can be removed.
- Use glass bottles for water when away from home.

For everyday water bottles, it's best to avoid water from the store as these products are months or years old and thus have a higher risk of plastic chemicals in the water. Instead, add fresh water to your bottles each day. Water in your bottle for a day poses little if any risk compared to water that's been there for months. Having a healthy source of water at home, such as well water or filtered water from your tap, is key to having safe drinking water during training. When bottles are empty at the end of the day, rinse them with water and let dry overnight (this will also help prevent mold or bacteria from growing).

glands and the brain, which regulate water and sodium, may be a common cause of these problems.

A healthy endurance athlete should be able to properly regulate significant amounts of water consumed during a race—even up to a gallon an hour in extreme conditions (although there is usually no need for this amount of water intake). This is because the body has effective mechanisms to regulate water. In addition to brain and adrenal hormones, both the kidneys (which remove excess water from the blood) and an effective sweating mechanism prevent water from accumulating in the body. Even water loss through the intestines and lungs contributes slightly to this regulation.

The fact is, however, that athletes can weigh more after a race due to abnormal holding of water. This can result in abnormally (sometimes seriously) low sodium as previously discussed. The problem of low sodium associated with excess water has been called *exertional hyponatremia*. In my experience, many, if not most, of these athletes are in Stage 1 or 2 of the overtraining syndrome.

Generally, athletes who gain weight during endurance events—typically about 10 percent of all those in a race—may be those individuals with some type of health problem, often one of a functional nature. Of these, about 30 percent develop hyponatremia.

This issue is complex and very individual. Rather than suggesting that athletes restrict water consumption (which may only be treating the symptoms) and risk further dehydration, addressing potential health problems that could affect how the body regulates water and sodium should be a priority. Many of these potential health problems, including adrenal dysfunction, can be evaluated at rest in athletes, while others may be very subtle and appear only following long training. The right health-care professional can be a valuable asset in helping to resolve these cases.

### Electrolytes

Two commonly discussed electrolytes are sodium and potassium (chloride is also an important electrolyte). These nutrients are vital in maintaining optimal function throughout the body at all times. These minerals are regulated by water, by certain adrenal hormones, and by the brain. Sodium plays the most important role because it can easily be influenced by common problems, such as dehydration and adrenal function.

Sodium from the diet helps regulate our appetite for thirst and salt. This regulation occurs through the brain, with the help of the kidney and adrenal glands. Sodium can also help maintain rehydration after water ingestion, even when consumed before and during competition.

The excess loss of sodium is often associated with overtraining syndrome and poor adrenal function. As discussed previously, the adrenal glands produce the hormone aldosterone, which regulates sodium and potassium. Reduction in levels of aldosterone, however, may occur in association with excess cortisol production and any type of excess stress, especially overtraining. This can result in excess sodium and water loss and increased potassium levels in the body. In this situation, taking potassium in dietary supplements or as a salt substitute should be avoided.

Chronic adrenal dysfunction, causing excess sodium loss, may also be associated with so-called athlete's diarrhea. This condition may produce more signs and symptoms with the stress of competition.

### Sodium Replacement

The use of sodium during competition, added to water, carbohydrate drinks, or by tablet, can help many athletes, especially in long endurance events, as sodium loss can still occur in a healthy athlete due to high stress. Consuming sodium helps replace these loses,

**Question:** Is table salt more effective than sea salt for sodium replacement? Do you also recommend eating a bag of potato chips if you feel in need of salt, say, on a long bike ride?

**Answer:** I use sea salt for all cooking and table use. It has a similar amount of sodium as plain sodium chloride, although often slightly less because it also contains many other minerals such as calcium, magnesium, and others in small amounts. You can also use sea salt in your water bottle. I always suggest carrying salt tablets (sodium chloride) during your long ride as this is a better way than potato chips to get sodium. Or, add sodium to your water bottle before starting your ride. Potato chips often contain other chemicals besides salt, and potatoes are a starch that requires digestion—something your gut may not do well, causing bloating.

# WATER, SODIUM, AND MUSCLE CRAMPS

Also called heat cramps, muscle cramps can occur at any time but are more common in longer events during hot weather. They are usually associated with dehydration and sodium loss, more often in athletes with reduced fitness and health. For example, those with adrenal dysfunction will often have low sodium levels and be less likely to regulate water efficiently, causing muscle cramps. Muscle imbalance and muscle fatigue can also be associated with muscle cramps during training and competition, with or without dehydration and sodium loss.

Regularly consuming sufficient amounts of water, along with sodium, can be very helpful to treat and prevent this type of cramping. However, potassium—traditionally suggested for muscle cramps—may be less helpful and can even be harmful in athletes whose sodium levels are very low. That's because potassium levels in most of these athletes are already normal or too high.

## Serious Heat Illness

Heat exhaustion and heat stroke are two examples of severe illness in athletes. The problem more commonly occurs during competition in hot environments, where athletes are unable to regulate their body temperature, resulting in very high temperatures and dehydration (of over 3 percent body weight). Athletes typically complain of fatigue, lightheadedness, feeling hot (sometimes cold), stomach and muscle cramps, nausea, headache, and sometimes heart palpitations. In more severe cases, vomiting, diarrhea, hyperventilation, altered mental states, rapid heartbeat, and the inability to perform, or even to walk, can occur. The symptoms of heat stroke may also include confusion, amnesia, disorientation, visual disturbance, seizure, and even coma. Most of these signs and symptoms are due to the effects of dehydration on the brain and body.

Remaining hydrated, rehydrating quickly following hard training and competition, and maintaining proper overall fitness and health is the best remedy to avoid heat illness. Treatment requires medical attention, and often includes immediate submersion of the athlete's trunk, legs, and arms into cool or iced water to reduce body temperature. If not available, the use of ice packs or ice water towels around the trunk, legs, and arms can also be helpful.

Regulating the consumption of water and electrolytes, especially sodium, should be a primary focus for all athletes. This goes beyond drinking enough water when working out or racing and includes maintaining high levels of aerobic function and overall health.

helps maintain hydration, and promotes the desire to drink water. Significant losses can occur in athletes with adrenal dysfunction—these individuals should not be competing if they have adrenal dysfunction affecting sodium regulation.

Small amounts of sodium, in the form of sodium chloride (salt), can be added to water throughout the event. In addition to replenishing sodium, this can increase stomach emptying to get more fluid and sodium (and carbohydrate when used) absorbed into the blood. This can include about 500 mg per hour, although this procedure, like all experimentation, should be tried during training to assure no intestinal distress is created.

The addition of sodium can especially be helpful in longer events of more than about four hours, or if you've just traveled to an event and have not had one to two weeks to acclimate to hot weather.

While water and sodium regulation may be more difficult in athletes who are physically larger (due to increased water loss), athletes who are older or very young may have similar problems. By their mid-sixties, for example, many athletes have less tolerance to heat stress. In addition, their heart rates are higher with less blood flow (cardiac output); and both their sweat mechanism and thirst regulation are less effective. These factors may be less significant in those who are healthier and fitter.

On rare occasions, it is possible for adrenal dysfunction to produce excess aldosterone, typically during the early stages of overtraining. This could potentially contribute to increased potassium loss, although this situation occurs infrequently.

# CHAPTER 18

# EATING AND DRINKING YOUR WAY TO BETTER ENDURANCE—
## The Role of Ergogenics

**E**rgogenics is not an easy word to say, or rather, people often have different ways of pronouncing it (the first g is hard, the second one soft). It is a term, however, that should be part of every endurance athlete's vocabulary. Properly defined, ergogenics refers to the enhancement of physical performance by consuming nutrients in liquid or solid form to help your body perform better.

Foods that can do this include carbohydrates in liquid and solid forms, protein and fat, and other drinks and solid food consumed before, during, and after very long training sessions and competitions. However, using a carbohydrate beverage, for example, when the rest of the body is not functioning well will not make up for a lack of endurance. In addition, it's important to individualize your intake of nourishment, whether it's water, sodium, carbohydrate drink, the addition of fat and protein, or other combinations.

I can provide some general guidelines, but all athletes have different sweat rates, fat-burning capabilities, and nutritional needs. With some trial and error during training, a better understanding of your particular needs can be easily accomplished.

Research on ergogenic nutrition has traditionally looked at the use of carbohydrates to help maintain glycogen stores and blood glucose during endurance events. While this is important for endurance athletes, most of these studies, and the strategies that are used, focus on increasing the use of glucose—not fat—for energy during competition. Recently, more studies have considered additional protein as part of pre- or post-competition meals. However, most of these studies have not considered the condition of the athletes tested with regards to their aerobic function and increased fat burning.

With a high level of fat burning, the need for additional nutrients during long training and competition is reduced, since your energy reserves from fat are extensive. Many properly trained athletes find that two- or three-hour training sessions or even longer, depending on the individual, do not require any additional nutrients except water. During competition, these athletes are able to race for two hours and often more, relying only on the addition of water. Whether you can perform your best at various distances depends on your level of fitness and health.

## Liquid Carbohydrates

Drinking a carbohydrate beverage that provides thirty to sixty grams of carbohydrate per hour during long competition can help improve endurance. In addition to helping maintain fat burning for muscle energy, it can also help maintain brain function, including coordination and prevent negative perceived exertion (a subjective feeling, for example, that your effort is more difficult and painful). While these liquid drinks are high in water content, they should be consumed in addition to, rather than in place of, water and sodium.

There are two important factors to consider in relation to carbohydrate beverages: The strength of the carbohydrate solution you choose is important, and so is the type of sugar contained in the beverage.

### Strength of the Carbohydrate Solution

The concentration or strength of the carbohydrate solution refers to the amount of sugar and water in the drink. Whether homemade or one of the many retail products available, this is a very important factor that can influence how your intestines handle the drink, which then affects your metabolism. Homemade liquid carbohydrate drinks are best because they are simple to make, are made from basic natural foods, don't contain unwanted or unhealthy ingredients (some are not listed on the label), and you can adjust the amount of water, carbohydrate, sodium, and other components to your particular needs.

A 6 to 8 percent carbohydrate solution is ideal for most athletes during competition or very long training. This can be made by adding six to eight grams of carbohydrate (approximately one heaping teaspoon), such as honey, to 180 ml (six ounces) of water. For store-bought juices and other beverages, read the label for the carbohydrate content.

This concentration will not remain in your stomach for too long but will empty into the small intestines at a similar rate as water. Liquids that are concentrated with more than 8 percent carbohydrate can remain in the stomach longer, not allowing the stomach to empty as fast and delaying the absorption of sugar.

My suggestion is to always start by using liquids made of simple sugars such as fruit juice, with apple working well and citrus being too acidic for most athletes. The sugar content of most commercial juices is 6 to 8 percent (not the concentrated versions, which are much higher). Honey is another option. Both honey and fruit juice also contain fructose, which is a sugar that eventually converts to glucose. But some athletes don't tolerate as much fructose because in high amounts it causes lower intestinal discomfort.

In addition, some sugars, such as the various forms of sucrose, malt sugars, and others, require digestion and can cause intestinal distress.

### Types of Sugars: Digestibility and Potential Gut Problems

A second factor to consider when choosing the form of carbohydrate drink is the type of sugar. Not all carbohydrates are the same when it comes to digestion. Some can cause excess stress to the gut. Intestinal distress is a common complaint from athletes. It can occur before, during, and after training and competition. And it often affects performance. While swallowing air during eating and drinking is one cause, most gut problems are due to the ingestion of certain types of carbohydrates. Simple sugars that don't require digestion include fruit juice and honey; their glucose and fructose is readily available without digestion. Other sugars, such as sucrose, maltose, and corn and rice syrups, must be digested in the gut before their glucose is available for absorption.

Other potential digestive problems can occur when double sugars and complex carbohydrates are combined with protein. This is due to the fact that both foods digest at very different rates. When combining protein liquids or foods with carbohydrate liquids or foods, use simple sugar sources, such as fruit juice, honey, or ripe fruits. In addition, the use of amino acids, which don't require digestion, can help avoid the potential of digestive stress.

Experiment to find out which liquid and solid carbohydrates work for you—meaning which don't cause intestinal distress, which make you feel the best, especially in your gut after consuming, and which seem to give you more energy and better recovery. The use of a heart-rate monitor can be helpful in your efforts to find the best combination of liquid

**QA** **Question:** It seems that come race day—I primarily run 10Ks and half-marathons—my stomach gets upset in the early hours. I have to get up quite early for these dawn starts to make sure my stomach settles down. Are there any food or drink supplements that you can recommend that will calm my pre-race jittery stomach?

**Answer:** This is often not food-related but rather your sympathetic system keeping you overactive. In this situation, food will not digest well and could give you a jittery stomach. I would be careful with caffeine as it can further upset your stomach. One way of calming down your overactive nervous system is to use some deep breathing relaxation techniques (see chapter 28). Regarding diet, make sure all you eat is healthy food. Then, experiment to see which food and drink helps relax you more, or which items don't trigger stomach symptoms.

and solid during a long training session. For example, you'll be able to run or bike slightly faster with more comfort at the same heart rate after consuming certain liquids or foods, compared to others.

This trial and error period should be done during training, not competition—especially training that mimics your competitions in relation to time of day, total time, similar course and weather, and other factors as best can be matched.

## Pre-Race Meals

Your meals leading up to competition should not be any different from your regular meals, assuming they are healthy. Many athletes change their meal plan for various reasons; for example, they attempt to improve glycogen stores by eating high amounts of refined carbohydrates. The problem is that this is often done at the expense of health, as the food and liquid consumed is often junk food or other unhealthy items. This can cause additional stress and often trigger high amount of insulin, reducing fat burning, lowering blood sugar, and potentially, depending on timing, even reducing glycogen stores. My recommendation has always been this: Once you find the best daily eating plan for your body's needs, maintain those eating habits in the days leading up to competition. This will keep your blood sugar stable, optimize glycogen stores, and moderate insulin levels. Why change your body chemistry and risk additional metabolic stress by eating very differently before an event? As an endurance athlete, your goal is to maintain a high level of fat burning and utilize this during your event.

## CAFFEINE?

Many athletes consume caffeine before or during training and competition. By now, you know that experimentation is key. If you don't normally drink coffee or tea, avoid it before or during competition. If you normally drink coffee or tea, sometimes avoiding it can be more of a stress because you may be addicted to it and could cause a number of symptoms before your race, including headaches, disorientation, and sluggishness from the lack of caffeine your body is used to.

If you consume and tolerate caffeine regularly, consider the amount you ingest. A single six- to eight-ounce cup of coffee, for example, may be sufficient no matter how much you're used to. This can especially help with your morning bathroom ritual. Caffeine can also stimulate fat burning. But it can disturb blood sugar, speed stomach emptying, and increase your anxiety if you're not used to it or take too much. It can also increase the stress hormone cortisol. For most athletes who drink coffee or tea, consuming it with food is best.

The use of carbohydrates can greatly help in this endeavor during competition, but a pre-competitive meal should include a healthy balance of low to moderate carbohydrates, complete proteins, and healthy fats, which will fill glycogen stores while satisfying other nutritional requirements.

I remember my first pre-race, carb-loading dinner: it was in Boston around 1981, the night before the marathon. While I usually avoid these activities, I was a speaker on a panel. I ate dinner elsewhere before the event expecting little healthy food. And that was the case: white pasta, white bread, white rolls, and some kind of sugar-laden carbohydrate drink. And for dessert, white cake with white icing. The pre-race feast was a sacred event, a ceremony of sorts that millions of endurance athletes have participated in ever since. However, I decided then to not only avoid these pre-race events but make sure the athletes I worked with didn't participate either.

For most athletes, it's important to consume some type of breakfast on the day of competition. After an all-night fast of not eating, liver glycogen stores are typically very low and your body needs fuel. This is another important experiment to perform during training. Many athletes find a blended shake made from real food is very effective in accomplishing this task. Your normal healthy breakfast—what your body is most used to—if containing adequate fruit and protein, is your best bet.

Here is an example of the caffeine content of some single-serving drinks. The amounts are in milligrams of caffeine, and the dose varies with how you make it, the specific product, and the exact size:

- Regular coffee: 85–300
- Double espresso: 120
- Decaf: 3–5
- Black tea: 50–140
- Green tea: 20–50
- Real cocoa: 25–50

**Note:** Most herbal teas don't contain caffeine, but some over-the-counter drugs do, in a range of 15–300 mg (read labels).

In addition to consuming small amounts of water before your event begins, some athletes feel the need to consume more carbohydrates. This can easily be taken as part of breakfast, as a healthy energy bar or shake, or as a 3 to 4 percent carbohydrate solution consumed between breakfast and your event. This drink is made by diluting the 6 to 8 percent solution with equal amounts of water; or, by combining a heaping teaspoon of a simple sugar (such as honey) in twelve ounces (360 ml) of water. This will not produce a high amount of insulin, which could impair fat burning, but will still provide carbohydrates. A small amount of salt can be added as well—just enough so the salty taste is hardly noticeable.

Here are some other hydration considerations:
- Cool fluids, between about 60 and 72°F (15–22°C), empty from the stomach a bit more quickly than body-temperature fluids. But this does not mean iced drinks are best—these may stimulate stronger stomach contractions and gut discomfort.
- The amino acid L-glutamine improves water and electrolyte absorption, and may be useful before activity. However, glutamine is broken down quickly in water, so don't add it to your water bottle the night before. You can add it to your morning meal and pre-event drink the same morning, or use a tablet or capsule—about 500–1,000 grams should be sufficient.

## PHIL'S SHAKE—THE ULTIMATE HEALTHY BEVERAGE

My favorite pre-training morning meal is a healthy smoothie (or shake). I also have one midafternoon. I soft-boil a dozen eggs at a time and keep them refrigerated, so preparation for this shake is about five or six minutes. Here's my large one-serving recipe:

**Ingredients:**
2 soft-cooked eggs
1 large or 2 small apples, pears, peaches, or the best in-season fruits
1 raw whole carrot
Spinach, kale, and/or cilantro to taste
About ½ cup blueberries
1 teaspoon plain psyllium
1 tablespoon raw whole sesame or flax seeds
8–10 ounces water

**Directions:**
Add all ingredients to a good blender and blend well.

The best blenders will do a great job on the whole fruits, including the core and all the seeds, and the raw whole carrot, raw spinach, kale, cilantro, or other vegetables. With enough fruit for sweetness, none of the bitter taste from the vegetables is noticeable—you'd never know there were so many healthy ingredients!

## Fuel During Competition

Many endurance events result in dehydration despite fluid intake, since it's almost impossible to balance water loss and intake. However, the more water you can drink in smaller amounts throughout your event, the less dehydrated you will become by the finish. In long events, this water should be consumed in addition to carbohydrate drinks.

As discussed above, a 6 to 8 percent carbohydrate solution is best for most athletes during long competition. This should also contain about 500 mg of sodium. Consume eight to sixteen ounces of this solution about every fifteen minutes. (Over the period of about an hour, this should provide about thirty to sixty grams of carbohydrate in addition to water and sodium.)

Many athletes find that the addition of protein during exercise is also very helpful in long events. Whey protein concentrate powder is an effective source of protein. Mix about ten to fifteen grams of protein from whey powder into your carbohydrate drink. Avoid all hydrolyzed, isolated, and caseinated protein powders.

Many athletes prefer solid food to obtain some of their carbohydrate and protein needs, especially in very long events such as an Ironman or ultramarathon. In this case, a homemade energy bar recipe is provided at the end of this chapter and provides a good mixture of calories from carbohydrates, protein, and fat in an easy-to-digest form, and is easy to carry and chew.

A small amount of fat can also be helpful during competition and help in recovery after competition. A small amount of coconut oil, for example, cannot only make some solutions or foods more palatable but provides MCTs (medium chain triglycerides), which can contribute to energy needs.

## After Competition

Recovery from a long event is important, not just for glycogen replacement but for the entire repair process that must occur throughout the body. Some key factors that greatly help; cooling the body in water, drinking smaller amounts of water often, and avoiding alcohol until food intake and hydration are near normal are all very important. And, of course, a healthy athlete will generally recover much better than one less healthy.

Consuming food can be helpful too. Immediately following your event—within fifteen to thirty minutes of finishing—consuming certain foods can significantly help in the recovery process. In addition to water, carbohydrate, protein, and fat are also important—much like the foods used during activity. Use the same carbohydrate-protein-sodium solution or homemade energy bar for this food and water replacement. Try to include 50 to 100 grams of carbohydrate, depending on your weight, within the fifteen to thirty minute period. Protein and fat also contribute significantly to replacement of glycogen stores.

After the post-event window of fifteen to thirty minutes, continue eating regular food (such as your energy bar) and drinking smaller amounts of water every two hours for a few hours, or until you feel hydrated and less fatigued. Do not drink alcohol or caffeine during this period as it can contribute to dehydration.

### Healthy Snacking

A snack is really just a small meal. Depending on what it is made from, snacks can be useful before, during, and after long workout sessions and competitions to satisfy all the needs I discussed above. In addition, snacking can be very healthy and useful during travel to your events, as restaurant food is often limited to unhealthy choices. On

## PHIL'S BAR—THE ULTIMATE HEALTHY SNACK

A favorite snack food is my homemade Phil's Bar. Use it as a pre- and post-competition food, and even during competition. It's also a great in-between meal snack, main meal when traveling, and even a healthy dessert. It's a complete meal—low glycemic carbohydrates—that includes protein and good fats. And it tastes great. Here's the recipe:

### Ingredients:
3 cups whole almonds
⅔ cup powdered egg white
4 tablespoons pure powdered cocoa
½ cup unsweetened shredded coconut
Pinch of sea salt
⅓ cup honey
⅓ cup hot water
1 to 2 teaspoons vanilla

### Directions:
Grind dry ingredients. Mix honey, hot water, and vanilla and blend into dry ingredients. (At this point, you may have to mix it all by hand if your mixer isn't very efficient). Shape into bars, cookies, or lightly press into a buttered muffin tin. You can also press the batter into a dish (about one-inch deep) and cut into squares. Allow to dry. Adjust the water/honey ratio for less or more sweetness. Keep refrigerated (they'll still last a week or more out of the refrigerator). For other flavor options, use fresh lemon instead of cocoa, or use more coconut. Makes ten to twelve bars.

race day, snacking can be your way to obtain a healthy pre-race meal as well as the necessary solid food during and after your event. In fact, perhaps no other single dietary habit can make a more positive difference than healthy snacking.

The key to healthful snacking during your normal week is to reduce the amount of food eaten at regular meals and to distribute this nutritional wealth throughout the day. Eat five or six smaller meals that add up to the same amount of food that you would normally consume in a typical two- or three-meal-a-day routine. After a good breakfast, eat every two to four hours, based on how good it makes you feel. Those under more stress or with blood sugar problems usually need to eat more frequently. An example of a daily meal schedule starts with breakfast, a midmorning snack, lunch, a midafternoon snack, a light dinner, and if necessary a small snack (which can be a healthy dessert) in the early evening.

Healthy snacks can be almost anything you like, just as long as they are made from real, healthy food. For many people, snacks, like regular meals, should contain protein. Experiment to discover how much food you need and which types work best. Some people may need to eat much larger snacks but others can get by on minimal amounts. Snacks should be just like any other healthy meal, just smaller, and still supply adequate nutrition. This might include:

- Vegetables and fruits, such as an apple or pieces of carrot and celery
- Raw almonds or cashews, or almond butter with apple slices
- Leftovers
- Plain yogurt and fresh fruit

- Cheese and fruit
- A boiled egg
- Homemade energy bar or healthy smoothie

Healthy snacking will quickly suppress cravings, especially for junk foods, improve physical and mental energy, and can even stimulate fat burning. Since snacking stabilizes blood sugar and prompts your body to produce normal levels of insulin, your body will store less fat and use more of it to fuel all your training and competition. Snacking can also help your body counteract the harmful effects of daily stress. In this way you reduce the overproduction of the stress hormone cortisol and insulin (both can prompt your body to store more fat). Snacking also helps to reduce cholesterol. Studies show that eating more frequently can lower blood cholesterol, specifically LDL, the "bad" cholesterol. In addition, studies show a staggering 30 percent increase in heart disease in those eating three meals or less per day.

# PHYTONUTRIENTS AND GOING ORGANIC—
## Eat Your Vegetables and Fruits!

What are phytonutrients? Where are they found? And why should endurance athletes include an abundance of them in their diet?

The term "phyto" originally comes from the Greek word meaning plant. Phytonutrients refer to those organic components of plants that are known to promote health and immune function—and there are literally thousands of them. Unlike the traditional nutrients—carbohydrates, protein, fat, vitamins, and minerals—phytonutrients are composed of chemical compounds such as carotenoids, which are the red, orange, and yellow pigments in fruits and vegetables.

Basically, all vegetables and fruits should be considered plant foods. Generally, fruits are foods that contain a seed or seeds inside, whereas vegetables have separate seeds usually not contained inside but found on a stalk or other part of the plant. Both vegetables and fruits contain some carbohydrates, some high enough for those who are carbohydrate intolerant to avoid. These include most potatoes, corn, watermelon, and pineapple (these are less natural as they've been genetically modified through the years to produce much higher levels of starch and sugar). All types of dried fruits, including raisins, are also very concentrated carbohydrates that may be problematic for those sensitive to carbohydrates.

Some foods that are technically fruits are usually thought of as vegetables: avocados, tomatoes, eggplant, peppers, squash, and other fruits that are not sweet, although healthy. What's important to know is that vegetables and fruits should make up the bulk of your diet. Most people don't eat enough vegetables and fruits, and there are very, very few who eat too much of this good thing. I often recommend as a general guideline that adults try to eat at least ten servings of vegetables and fruits per day. Many of these should be raw and most, if not all, should be fresh.

What is a serving? Traditionally, many have considered a serving to be a half-cup. More recently, however, many dietary guidelines have recommended different approaches for measuring servings. For instance, a serving of lettuce might be a cup and a half; a serving of carrots might be one medium carrot; a serving of broccoli is one medium stalk; and a serving of asparagus is five spears. Using guidelines like these will help you to eat more vegetables than using the traditional half-cup serving.

## Eat Your Vegetables

Consider vegetables as an important part of each meal. Including a spinach and tomato omelet at breakfast; a large salad of lettuces, carrots, cucumbers, and onions at lunch; and some lightly cooked mixed vegetables with dinner can easily provide you with adequate intake. Even a favorite like meat loaf can be made so that up to half of it is vegetable content; add chopped onions, red or yellow bell peppers, zucchini, fresh parsley, and garlic.

Vegetables, such as lightly steamed greens, are quick and easy to prepare and are tasty. Depending on the season and markets you shop, produce such as kale, mustard greens, rapini, Swiss chard, collards, and common spinach are also some of the most nutritious. These bitter leafy vegetables are full of valuable phytonutrients, as well as a host of vitamins and minerals. Greens can be served as a delicious bed for just about any protein food from beef to fish, or steamed and served with a little butter or extra virgin olive oil and sea salt as a side dish. Also add these and others to homemade soups, with leeks, white or yellow onions, mushrooms, or red and yellow peppers.

It is also important to eat a variety of vegetables because they contain varying amounts of specific nutrients. For instance, a serving of leaf lettuce supplies a high amount of beta-carotene but only a small amount of vitamin C, while a serving of brussels sprouts contains high levels of vitamin C with a small amount of beta-carotene.

One of the easiest ways to ensure that you eat enough vegetable variety is to choose them in a rainbow of colors. Carrots and winter squash, which are orange, are high in beta-carotene, which is converted by the body to vitamin A. Many green vegetables are high in vitamin C—a serving of broccoli, for example. In addition to orange and green vegetables, consider purple eggplant and cabbage; red peppers; white, green, and red onions; white cauliflower; yellow summer squash; brown mushrooms; and many others. Each of these colorful vegetables contains its own unique set of vitamins, minerals, and phytonutrients.

### Have at Least One Salad Each Day

In reaching your goal of ten servings of vegetables and fruits per day, it's important to make sure much of this is raw. Salads, large and small, can easily provide this full amount. Your salad can be a snack, a side dish, or, with some added protein, it can be a meal in itself. Fresh lettuce, spinach, young kale, Swiss chard, and other greens are the foundation of a great salad. Add a variety of raw vegetables such as carrots, chopped red and yellow peppers, purple cabbage, tomatoes, and avocados. Separately, these can be used for meals that don't contain a salad. In addition, steamed and chilled green beans and asparagus liven up a salad. Chopped walnuts or almonds, gourmet olives, capers, and artichoke hearts make a salad even more interesting and tasty. You can even include fruit in your salad, such as an arugala and pear salad with olive oil and goat cheese. These and many other recipes are found at the end of chapter 22.

To make your salad into a main meal, add some protein. Lightly grilled tuna, wild shrimp, sliced beefsteak, hard-boiled eggs, or crumbled goat cheese are some options.

Of course, a great salad requires a delicious dressing. My healthy salad dressing is great, but simple extra virgin olive oil or vinegar is fine too. Always use your own homemade dressing and avoid the additives that come out of a bottle.

The best way to add fruits to your diet, including berries, is to use them as they are—as a snack, a healthy dessert, or made into recipes such as smoothies. Some of these were discussed in the last chapter under "snacks." Fruits are also a delicious part of a salad, as mentioned above; another example is an apple walnut salad with greens.

## Phytonutrients

The thousands of nutritional components in natural foods can help protect you from chronic inflammation. This will help you avoid certain injuries and speed recovery from workouts and races. In addition, reducing chronic inflammation helps prevent cancer, heart disease, and other degenerative conditions.

Phytonutrients—also called phytochemicals—are chemical compounds made by plants from sunlight (via photosynthesis) when grown in good-quality soil. These substances have been researched in the labs for decades and used therapeutically for centuries by many cultures. Scientists now know there are thousands of these natural chemicals that have potent healthy actions.

Phytonutrients comprise three main groups of plant compounds that include phenols, terpenes, and nitrogen-containing alkaloids. Some of the names may be familiar to you while others may not. And many have been appearing on store shelves as dietary supplements for years. Some common phytonutrients include a group of carotenes (including alpha and beta, and lycopene), a group of bioflavanoids (including hesperetin and lutein), and isothiocyanates (including sulforaphan). There are also seven phytonutrients contained in what I call the vitamin E complex. These include four tocotrienols and three tocopherols (the component most people are familiar with is alpha tocopherol, which is technically not a phytonutrient but vitamin E).

Don't be concerned about remembering all the names, but do remember to consume a variety of foods. In addition to vegetables and fruits, raw nuts and seeds contain the best sources of many phytonutrients. They're even found in other foods, including green and black tea, and grass-fed beef.

Some plant compounds in this category that are commonly synthesized as drugs include caffeine, nicotine, morphine, and cocaine. These compounds are not considered nutrients, so the term "phytochemical" would best apply.

The presence of phytonutrients is one reason studies continue to show that eating vegetables and fruits prevents cancer and most other chronic diseases, while the common dietary supplements containing vitamins don't. More than fifteen years ago, epidemi-ologist John Potter, of the University of Minnesota, was quoted in *Newsweek*, providing us with a snapshot of the bigger scientific picture: "At almost every one of the steps along the pathway leading to cancer, there are one or more compounds in vegetables or fruit that will slow up or reverse the process." Unfortunately, most people don't eat enough of the foods that contain these powerful nutrients.

### Bitter Is Better

Scientists now understand that naturally occurring phytonutrients found in vegetables and fruits may be even more important to good nutrition than the vitamins in these foods and can help prevent chronic inflammation and halt the production of cancer-causing agents in the body, blocking activation of these chemicals or suppressing the spread of cancer cells that already exist. The vegetables and fruits researchers think are most capable of preventing cancer and other diseases, including heart disease, are green leafy vegetables, broccoli, brussels sprouts, cabbage, onions, citrus fruit (not the juice), grapes, red wine, green tea, and others. One common theme in many of these types of foods is their taste: the more bitter or pungent, the better.

For plants, these bitter-tasting phytonutrients serve as natural insect repellents and pesticides. Some are even toxic to small animals like birds, mice, and rats, including some compounds in cabbage and brussels sprouts. Generally, higher amounts of bitter-tasting phytonutrients are found in sprouts and seed-lings than in mature plants. This provides young plants with natural protection from being eaten at an early stage of life, before the chance of reproduction. But you would have to consume pounds and pounds of vegetables daily to ingest toxic amounts of phytonutri-ents.

Despite the therapeutic and nutritional value of phytonutrients, the food industry is solving the so-called problem of bitterness in vegetables and fruits by removing these healthful chemicals through genetic engi-neering and selective breeding. Unfortu-nately, our culture has associated bitterness with bad taste instead of health promotion. Now many agricultural scientists, who want foods sweeter, are artificially changing our natural food supply for us—they are literally removing the healthy components from cer-tain foods in order to sell more food prod-ucts. And they are succeeding. Canola oil, for example, has had its phytonutrients signifi-cantly reduced through selective breeding. And transgenic citrus is now common as both fruit and juice—it's sweeter but it's also free of limonene, the bitter substance that can help prevent and treat skin cancer. With the consumption of more sugar, and with packaged and processed foods being sweeter than ever before, many humans have not only lost their taste for vegetables because of bitterness, but find the natural taste of such foods as leaf lettuce, parsley, and zucchini offensive.

Cancer researchers propose that a height-ened sense of bitterness might be a healthy trait, allowing people to select foods with the highest phytonutrient content. This view contrasts with the food industry's practice of measuring the content of these bitter phyto-nutrients merely as a way of developing new non-bitter, phytonutrient-deficient strains. So while some nutrition scientists propose enhancing phytonutrients in foods for better health, the standard industry practice has been to remove them for better taste. Indeed, the lower amount of bitter compounds in the modern diet reflects the "achievement" of the food industry. The irony is that as agricultural scientists remove more phytonutrients from plants, farmers have to use even more chem-ical pesticides to protect their crops; thus, consumers are left with the double whammy of vegetables and fruits with less nutrition and more harmful pesticides.

In addition to bitterness, an astringent taste is also associated with healthy phyto-nutrients. These tastes can actually be quite attractive. Consider a fine-aged Bordeaux wine or a high-quality green tea. Unfortu-nately, these are exceptions, and sweetness is a dominant taste preference, or perhaps "addiction" is a better word.

You can get more phytonutrients into your diet by eating foods that have a natural bitter or astringent taste. In addition to zucchini and other squashes, pumpkins, cucumbers, melon, citrus, and many other vegetables and fruits, along with almonds and many types of beans, contain natural phytonutrients, as do red wine, green tea, and cocoa.

## Going Organic

Many master athletes are quite familiar with the organic food movement that became popular in the 1960s. Today's athletes seeking the healthiest foods can find a large variety of certified-organic produce, meats, and other foods in traditional "health food" stores, and now even in conventional grocery stores. Two common questions are whether it's worth the extra price to buy organic food versus conventional, and whether we can trust the sign that says "certified organic."

With great hesitation my answer to both questions is yes, but with an asterisk. The USDA's organic program is now part of an international movement. The regulations are better than the previous unregulated organic movement, where anyone could say a product was organic. Many of the guidelines are potentially good for consumers—organic animals must be raised with organic feed, filtered water, and certified organic pastures, and many commonly used drugs can't be used. Organic produce must be grown without commonly used pesticides, herbicides, and other chemicals. Many food product ingredients—additives, chemicals, preservatives, and others are not allowed in organic foods. And the program is relatively strict, helping to rid the market of dishonest vendors. So if a product has the USDA organic label, it's as good as the USDA's ability to police the program, just like the rest of what the agency does for all foods sold to consumers. But like the rest of our food supply, you have to be a careful consumer, reading labels and being aware of and avoiding organic junk food, which makes up most of today's organic products.

True to Jerome Irving Rodale's ideas of the mid-1900s, organic food is better, whether certified by today's standards or not. For example, organic vegetables and fruits usually taste better. They've not been genetically altered and contain much smaller amounts of chemical fertilizers or none at all. Moreover, many studies indicate that organic produce is more nutritious, containing more vitamins, minerals, and phytonutrients. Some of the organic produce studied had twice the nutrients of conventional equivalents. Many vegetables have been studied, including carrots, cabbage, lettuce, kale, tomatoes, and spinach, as well as a variety of fruits. The increase in nutrients found in certified-organic vegetables and fruits is most likely due to better care of the soil through organic farming methods, including composting, crop rotation, and cover crops.

I've also conducted my own research and found with independent laboratory analysis that some organically grown vegetables had significantly higher levels—ten times or more—of certain important nutrients such as folic acid compared to the same vegetables tested and listed in the USDA database.

For years, nutritionists insisted that today's conventionally grown foods were as high in vitamins and minerals as the meals of our grandparents. There is now sufficient evidence indicating this is not necessarily the case. Reductions in food quality have taken place since the mid-1940s, when the use of chemical fertilizers and pesticides rapidly became the norm in U.S. farming. A study in the *British Food Journal* compared the 1930s nutrient content of twenty vegetables and fruits with foods grown in the 1980s. Significant reductions were found in the levels of calcium, copper, and magnesium in vegetables; and magnesium, iron, copper, and potassium in fruit. Similar trends can be found in foods produced in the United States, with reductions in some nutrients of as much as 30 percent.

Most foods are farmed with chemical fertilizers and pesticides, with the exception of certified organic foods, which contain significantly less nitrates and heavy metals—both of which can be very harmful, especially to the brain and in particular for children. Heavy metals enter the plants through certain chemical fertilizers—some of these fertilizers are even derived from industrial waste. As discussed previously, through genetic engineering, phytonutrients have been removed from some common foods to make them less bitter. Organically grown foods don't contain genetically engineered ingredients or genetically modified organisms, making them a better choice.

However, the organic movement has created a whole new line of products for unsuspecting consumers—organic junk food. These include many of the same packaged foods much of the population has gotten sick and obese on, but which have been certified organic by the USDA. When in a health food or other store that carries organic products, avoid those containing organic sugar, white flour, bad fats, and other unhealthy ingredients that happen to also be organic. At one time, the term organic referred to being healthy—but that's certainly not the case today.

## Other Health Foods

With the problems in the organic industry, including the dilution of a strict standard in growing and producing the cleanest and highest quality foods, and the added costs due to a highly bureaucratic certification process that can cost a company or farm tens of thousands of dollars a year in fees, many truly health-conscious consumers once again are looking for healthy options. They're seeing the potential of the traditional farmers' markets, community organic cooperatives, roadside farm stands, and "pick-your-own" programs. Internet shopping for organic food is growing, especially in bulk quantity. These modern markets feature products grown in a "green" way—produced in line with the original organic movement, which had its name taken away by the USDA and other agencies worldwide. And they often include a "buy local" slogan.

The problem is that there is no regulation regarding whether these products are "green," organic, or beyond organic. One result is that, in some cases, authorities have stopped farmers from selling their products. Another problem is the notion that products that are better than organic—the "beyond organic" movement—should be more expensive. But just because products are grown with care, without chemicals, doesn't mean they should be more expensive. Without the "middlemen"—typically two, three, or more of them taking a share before products get to the retail stores—most of these products should be less expensive than the same or similar products in retail stores.

Despite these issues, if you're a careful consumer and talk to the farmers and producers, and even visit their farms, you can usually find high-quality, healthy products that are often better than the organic version in retail stores, and often for less cost. Supply and demand will help weed out the overpriced products.

Virtually all the food I buy is organic, although more and more is not USDA-certified organic. And I buy the basics—vegetables, fruits, meat, eggs, cheese, nuts, and seeds (although most of the vegetables are grown in my garden).

The most impressive operation I've seen is the Double Check Ranch in central Arizona, where I buy all my beef. While they don't participate in the national organic program, I have inspected their ranch and would certify them as "beyond organic." This ranch is clean, efficient, inspected by local government, and has a philosophy of not just producing healthy food but also incorporating an approach to farming that's good for the land as well. (Its Web site provides many informative articles at www.DoubleCheckRanch.com.)

I also buy food from local farmer's markets if I know the food is from a good source. And I have bulk items shipped. Most of these foods are cheaper than the organic versions in the retail stores. Additionally, my large garden provides a significant amount of food that is also "beyond organic."

If you really want the highest-quality produce, the best option is to grow your own. If you have any yard space at all, a small vegetable plot—even ten feet by ten feet or smaller—properly tended, can yield significant amounts of vegetables in season for your entire family. Many areas have community gardens, where many individuals share a larger plot of land. By growing your own vegetables, you can ensure their quality, reduce the price of your produce, and revel in the enjoyment of growing your own food.

Eat as much of as many types of organic vegetables and fruits as you can, both cooked and raw. Try to eat about ten servings per day. In addition to variety, the highest quality vegetables and fruits may be those that are organically grown—or those that are truly "beyond organic." Making all these healthy vegetable and fruit choices is just another journey on the road to optimal endurance performance and better health.

# HISTORY OF THE ORGANIC MOVEMENT

We're not exactly sure just when the organic movement started, since that would depend, in part, on how you define it. Certainly, in the early stages, the word *organic* was not part of this movement. The word *organic* would not be introduced until around 1941 by a British chemist, Sir Albert Howard. But by then, the movement was decades old and had more than one front. There were those who promoted the scientific reasons for natural farming; those who had more spiritual reasons to care for the land; small farmers who were being left out of big business; those with strong social attitudes who wanted to help the "little guys" get a fair share of the profits; and consumers, who eventually had the greatest numbers and created the real change. But even before the movement was noticed, there were those few who made the observations that growing food in the most natural soils produced better food and healthier people.

In the 1830s, German chemist Justus von Liebig was formulating his agricultural biochemistry theories, which he published in the 1840s, discussing how plants utilize nitrogen in the soil along with various minerals. Natural fertilizers, he theorized—including manure from healthy animals—would provide these vital nutrients. This was the beginning of modern farming, and the movement soon branched into two: one that became big business farming, with newly developing chemical fertilizers and pesticides, and the other that became the organic movement.

Sir Albert Howard may be one of the earliest "organic" farmers—he was from a British farming family but learned about natural soil production and organic gardening in India in 1905. The influence of Howard's writings—he called the introduction of chemical fertilizers and pesticides a great threat to the future of human health—created a clear separation of the organic movement and conventional farming. His writing spread throughout Europe and eventually to America.

By the early 1900s, American food manufacturers, as an integral part of the "modern farming" movement, began mass-producing the first packaged foods. This coincided with a major change from the farmers' market with its many single-food stands to one store that would sell all types of food—a "super market"—complete with the latest technology of packaged foods. Small groups of concerned citizens immediately and openly protested against the mass packaging of food. Some, including Dr. Royal Lee, began growing high-quality food with natural composting, and in 1929, Dr. Lee began manufacturing the first dietary supplements in America using these foods.

By the 1930s, with the influence of Howard's writings and others in America, the organic movement was organized, albeit small. One person who jumped on board was an engineer named Jerome Irving Rodale. He not only bought a farm and began gardening organically, but started publishing a magazine on organic methods in the 1940s—and none other than Sir Albert Howard contributed articles. Rodale also started a printing business that went on to publish books—a business that thrives today as a multi-million-dollar corporation.

I was introduced to Rodale's books on organic gardening in the 1960s and soon after planted my first organic garden. As a student working part-time in a health-food store, and having studied basic chemistry, I realized almost all the vitamins on the shelves were synthetic, not natural as they claimed. Seeing a growing market in the young organic industry, the pharmaceutical companies had quietly jumped on board by producing virtually all the synthetic vitamins for the health food industry, a problem that continues today.

After studying organic gardening and natural health, and many different health-care philosophies, I decided to go back to college, become a doctor, and focus on helping people get healthy.

Into the 1970s and '80s, the organic movement continued to hold its social, fair trade, and health-oriented subgroups. Even up to the time when the USDA decided to take charge of the movement by creating a National Organic Program (NOP) in 1990 that would define organic and certify growers, manufacturers and others involved in the organic movement, there continued to be different philosophies associated with organics.

The NOP would spend the next decade gathering information from the organic movement to create standards, rules, regulations, and a system to certify all those it would allow into the organic movement—often for a hefty price—under the guise that the USDA needed to control the process. The result was the "certified organic" regulations, released in 2002, complete with a seal of authenticity. They established three levels of organic: 100 percent, 95 percent, which allowed 5 percent non-organic material, and 70 percent organic.

There was one big problem with the process: During this decade big business lobbied heavily for regulations that would make it easier and cheaper to jump on the "certified organic" bandwagon. Not only that, the large manufacturers of processed foods, the sugar industry, large food chains, and a variety of other lobbyists made sure they were part of the process too. The result was a massive growth of organic junk food that coincided with the NOP's "organic" launch in 2002.

Just before the NOP became law, I created, in 1999, the first line of certified organic dietary supplements made from real food. I followed the developments of the USDA's certified organic program and prepared my formulas based on what I thought would be the requirements for organic certification. While these products were launched, it did not take long for the major players in the industry to keep them from taking hold in a marketplace run by a few large conglomerates.

The Organic Trade Association (OTA) evolved from part of the movement that was the political tail. Its goal was to help large companies involved in certified organic activities work with other large companies and the NOP. Unfortunately, they were a political organization not oriented to health. I attended their first national trade show, and was shocked at the number of organic junk food companies represented—the first day I watched overweight people sample organic cookies made from organic white flour and organic white sugar, eat processed organic corn chips, drink organic beer, and even smoke organic cigarettes. This was the modern health-food industry! The next day was even worse.

There were a number of speakers discussing the value of organic certification during the next day's events. A keynote speaker was J. I. Rodale's granddaughter, who was a main player in the Rodale publishing empire. She was so excited to see the organic movement get this far and be so "successful." After her talk, she took questions. I asked, "Are you concerned that the organic industry is made up of so much junk food that it adversely affects people's health?" Her answer was an emphatic "No." She said that people can make their own choices about what to eat.

Marie Rodale's grandfather, J. I., promoted the relationship between organic farming and optimal health and helped launch the organic movement. But now, companies making organic junk food have become the biggest advertising revenue for the modern Rodale publishing empire. In joining with big business and the USDA, the small farmers and start-up companies making healthy foods were left out.

Meanwhile, consumers jumped in too. They were the ones eating all the organic junk food. This was evident just by looking—at the owners, employees, and others working in the "health food" industry, including those in the stores. Go into Whole

Foods, for example, and you'll see the shelves full of organic junk. And a large part of the store is the bakery section—complete with white flour and sugar cakes, cookies, and pies.

My level of disappointment in the organic movement has reached a high, while my enthusiasm had bottomed. My first article after returning home from the OTA show, "Organic Junk," brought praise by a few but anger from industry people. Making money, it seemed, was the goal of certified organics, even if it contributed to the explosion of obesity not only in adults but now also in young children. Along the way, the large companies, including manufacturers and grocery stores, and the "new" health food chains, successfully pushed for the NOP regulations to be diluted—many unhealthy foods, food additives, and other ingredients would now be allowed in organic foods. I began writing and lecturing more on the dangers of organic junk food and "beyond organic"—those small farmers, companies, and consumers left out of the original organic movement who were still there hoping for healthy changes. The organic movement had left them behind. And many legitimate farmers, manufacturers, and food companies that were too small to pay the thousands of dollars to be part of the USDA's organic movement were actually creating healthier food.

Now, in 2010, I'm very disillusioned with the government-sponsored organic programs. And because the USDA took the word "organic" for itself, products or companies would not be allowed to use the word "organic" unless it was certified by the USDA. In addition, small farms, legitimate companies producing healthy foods, and others involved in the organic movement are even being harassed by federal and local authorities because they have not embraced the movement. The result is that a small but growing movement continues, made up of consumers and health-care professionals like myself, seeking the best food from good and honest people all working together for a healthier planet.

# CHAPTER 20

# DIETARY SUPPLEMENTS—
## Beware of What You Put in Your Body!

I have always recommended that athletes try to obtain all their nutrients from a healthy, real-food diet. This provides micronutrients (vitamins and minerals), macronutrients (carbohydrates, proteins, and fats), and phytonutrients (thousands of other plant compounds). This is not always possible. If you have increased nutritional needs or an inability to obtain certain nutrients in adequate amounts from a healthy diet, you may need to supplement your diet. Supplementing with products made from real foods is the most effective approach but is not always an easy task.

Many of the popular dietary supplements available can be dangerous, especially for endurance athletes. For example, a recent study published in the *American Journal of Clinical Nutrition* showed that common doses of vitamin C—1,000 mg a day—can actually reduce oxygen uptake and significantly diminish endurance. Another recent study published in *Medicine & Science in Sports & Exercise* demonstrated that an antioxidant supplement, comprised of vitamins E and C, beta-carotene, zinc, and others in common use, did not prevent exercise-induced abnormalities, including inflammation, and may actually delay muscle recovery.

It's important to note that the same nutrients in a healthy diet will not cause these problems. The fault is in the dietary supplement—and this includes the source (natural versus synthetic) and types of nutrients as well as the dosage. While the two studies cited here are recent ones, there are many more; it's been known for a long time that popular dietary supplements can be dangerous.

## Do You Need to Take a Supplement?

Knowing whether you need to take a dietary supplement is obviously the first question to answer. The notion that it "can't hurt," that a supplement is "like an insurance policy" or "your body can eliminate what it doesn't need," is a myth perpetuated by companies making supplements, and is simply untrue. In addition, some athletes take supplements because their training partner takes them, or because they saw ads for them.

A more individual determination of your nutritional needs is the first step in determining that you might need a dietary supplement. This can be accomplished in a variety of ways. One way is with the help of a health-care professional who may determine this through a variety of methods, including a good history, blood and urine tests, and other evaluations. However, with some exceptions, blood and urine tests are generally not the best ways to determine nutritional needs. While they can uncover the more obvious

and serious deficiencies, they won't show many other needs that may be more subtle or indicate that your diet is deficient.

Other ways to determine your potential needs for supplementation include experimentation, diet analysis, and symptom surveys. Let's consider each of these.

### Experimentation

Some people may effectively determine the need for a dietary supplement through careful experimentation. A health-care professional might conclude, after evaluating you, that you have a need for a particular nutrient. But the best indication that you need a particular nutrient is if taking it improves some aspect of body function. An improvement of body chemistry most likely will also improve some aspect of your endurance. This may include the successful treatment of a particular problem, such as fatigue or asthma, or the elimination of an abnormal finding in a blood test or other evaluation, such as an abnormal C-reactive protein test (a measure of chronic inflammation). In some cases, a particular supplement can help improve your MAF Test. For example, an iron or vitamin B2 deficiency can significantly reduce aerobic function. In this case, taking an iron supplement can help get more oxygen to the aerobic muscles to burn more fat. In a short period, your MAF Test could noticeably improve. However, taking iron when your body does not need it can be harmful.

In almost all cases, seeing some improvement from a particular supplement may occur within a relatively short time. If you have exercise-induced asthma and want to see if the nutrient choline can help improve your symptoms, taking this supplement for a month or two will almost always either help or do nothing. If it helps, you may want to continue taking it while you also consume more foods high in this nutrient (in this case the best food source is egg yolks).

## Diet Analysis

An excellent way to determine the need for a dietary supplement is to analyze your diet. This is a common tool used by some health-care professionals, researchers, and even individuals to evaluate nutrient intakes. It makes use of a computerized program and provides information about your levels of nutrients compared to the recommended daily allowance (RDA) or another standard reference (such as the USDA's Dietary Reference Intakes, or DRIs). Studies using this approach and other methods continue to show seriously low intakes of many nutrients by large numbers of people, including athletes. For example, a USDA survey estimated that 80 percent of American women did not achieve RDA levels of folic acid, iron, zinc, vitamin B6, magnesium, and calcium. This problem, of course, is due to poor dietary habits.

I performed a diet analysis, usually two or more, on almost all the athletes I've worked with throughout my career. Just as other surveys have shown, many people had serious nutritional imbalances in their diets. Even when I factored in dietary supplements some athletes took, they were frequently below RDA levels of various nutrients. Today there are many computerized diet analysis programs available and the USDA Web site (www.usda.gov) provides a simple one online that is free.

If a diet analysis shows that specific nutrients are below a minimum level, there are two important steps to take:

- First, improve your diet to include or increase foods containing these nutrients.
- Second, you may need additional nutrients from a dietary supplement—at least temporarily until your nutrient levels return to normal and you can maintain these levels with your diet.

## Symptom Surveys

Another approach that can help determine the potential need for a dietary supplement, and one used throughout *The Big Book of Endurance Training and Racing*, is the use of a survey. In this instance, it's a group of questions based not on nutrient levels in the body or in the food you eat but on certain signs and symptoms associated with a low level of a particular nutrient. For example, fatigue, excess blood loss, and the habit of chewing on ice may be associated with the need for iron, a micronutrient. Sleepiness after meals, intestinal bloating, and frequent hunger and craving for sweets may be associated with excess intake of carbohydrates, a macronutrient. Symptom surveys are based on commonly defined changes in the body when particular nutrients levels are low.

Here is an example of an actual survey I've used in private practice. Use it and see which items apply to you:

1. History or risk of heart disease
2. History or risk of Alzheimer's disease or other reduced mental capacity
3. Female (childbearing age)
4. Outdoors often in sun or use tanning salons
5. Live in Southern climate (below San Francisco or Washington, D.C.)
6. Over age fifty
7. History of anemia or other red blood cell problem
8. Feelings of depression
9. History of taking doses of vitamin C above 500 mg
10. Reduced intake of meat, fish, and eggs
11. Increased caffeine intake (coffee, tea, soda—more than three per day)
12. Increased alcohol intake (more than two drinks per day)

If you check even one or two questions, it could indicate a need for more vitamin B12 and/or folic acid, with the likelihood increasing significantly as you get past two checked items. The necessary dose can not be determined from a survey as other follow-up tests as noted above may be necessary; dosing is very individual. While most vitamin B12 and folic acid in dietary supplements are synthetic, natural forms are available (and are discussed later).

## Hidden Dangers of Dietary Supplements

Unfortunately, many athletes believe they need dietary supplements through unreliable means. The usual persuasive culprits are advertising, anecdotal evidence from a training partner, and bloggers. At one time the notion was that a dietary supplement could only help and not hurt. We now know clinically this is not the case, and many studies are showing the potential dangers of many types of dietary supplements. In addition, these extra nutrients will not improve body function if the body's need for these nutrients does not exist. In other words, taking more B vitamins won't help you if your levels of these nutrients are already normal.

If you take supplements because you feel it offers some safeguard against deficiencies, that could be a problem too. First, it may mean that you're not focusing on eating the best diet possible; dietary supplements usually won't provide all the nutrients you can obtain from a healthy diet. Second, you risk causing other imbalances. For example, taking too much omega-6 oil can cause an imbalance of fats.

The fact that a dietary supplement contains nutrients does not mean it's natural, or even safe. The vitamins in most dietary supplements are synthetic. Most are made from artificial chemicals in some manufacturing plant and not obtained from a nutritious, natural plant grown on a farm or in nature.

Most dietary supplements on the market do not provide vitamins and other nutrients as they naturally occur in real food. Although these supplements may be labeled "natural," their vitamins are usually synthetic and often provide doses much higher than foods in nature. Other supplements contain natural nutrients but are separated from the foods where they originated, leaving behind many important associated phytonutrients. I call these supplements HSAIDS, which stands for "High-Dose Synthetic and Isolated Dietary Supplements." When consumed, HSAIDS act more like drugs in the body than like real food.

HSAIDS are not necessarily bad, although some can be deadly, but they're not what most people think they are—equivalent to the same nutrient counterpart in food. The most important nutrients are those contained in foods, and if you supplement, products made from food are the best and safest choice.

In some instances, such as with the careful direction of a health-care practitioner trained in nutrition, HSAIDS may be useful. In the case of anemia, they may be beneficial for a relatively short period of time to correct a specific condition. Others may have long-term needs or require a high dose of a particular nutrient, such as an active form of folic acid, to address a common genetic problem.

The primary difference between HSAIDS and products made from real food, which contain truly natural nutrients in food doses, is how the body responds to them when consumed.

## Biological versus Pharmacological Responses to Supplements

When one takes a dietary supplement, just like when one eats food or takes a drug, the body has particular physiological responses. In general, nutrients in their natural state and natural dose have a biological effect, just like eating a healthy meal of real food. HSAIDS, however, have a pharmacological effect in the body, like a drug.

Examples of dietary supplements that clearly act in more of a biological fashion include products made from foods, including vegetable and fruit concentrates, fish oil, and protein powders made from whey or egg whites. These supplements provide nutrients in a concentrated form, acting essentially the same as when you consume the real food. They provide natural doses of vitamins, minerals, macronutrients, or phytonutrients helping to generate energy, regulate immunity, control aging, and perform countless other functions that improve health and human performance—just like real food.

Nutrients with pharmacological effects generally include HSAIDS and have actions like those of drugs rather than foods. These include synthetic vitamin C (ascorbic acid being one of many common forms), isolated high-dose vitamin E (alpha-tocopherol), and popular B complex supplements. These are almost always in doses much higher than a person could possibly consume during a meal or even a day's worth of food intake—even when consuming foods naturally high in these nutrients. Many contain doses that would take weeks of eating foods rich in these nutrients to get to the same levels—in other words, five, ten, even a hundred times normal amounts. By looking at the labels of supplements, you will see that most, even those labeled "natural," contain doses much higher than you would get from real food and much higher than the RDA. These unnaturally high doses are one reason they can be harmful.

Dietary supplements that promote pharmacological activity, like most drugs, are capable of modifying brain and body function, often in powerful ways. This is one reason they are accompanied by the risk of adverse side effects—we just don't have control over how they will act. These pharmacological effects of dietary supplements can vary with individuals, and many are not clearly known. HSAIDS with pharmacological actions can also interfere with other nutrients, whether from the diet or other supplements, or with over-the-counter and prescription drugs.

## The Contrasting Examples of Vitamins C and E

As an example of the difference between HSAIDS and truly natural nutrients, consider vitamins C and E. Food sources of naturally occurring vitamin C have biological effects, acting as antioxidants and protecting DNA from oxygen damage—something that occurs in endurance athletes often during training and especially when anaerobic. The dose of vitamin C contained in a high-quality meal of vegetables and fruits may be 100 mg or less. However, the synthetic counterpart (ascorbic acid and the various similar forms), found in almost all dietary supplements, may function differently. High doses of synthetic vitamin C, typically 500 to 1,000 mg tablets, can perform as an antioxidant but can also transform to a deadly pro-oxidant—which can cause excess free-radical activity and inflammation.

Another illustration of the difference between HSAIDS and truly natural nutrients is found in vitamin E. A natural dose of vitamin E is really quite small. For example, the amount of naturally occurring alpha-tocopherol in a loaf of whole-wheat bread made fresh from wheat berries—a relatively high source of natural vitamin E—may be only 2 to 4 IU. In contrast, vitamin E supplements typically come in extremely high doses of 400 to 800 IU. You'd have to eat 200 loaves to reach these supplement doses. This unnatural dose of vitamin E can interfere with other more effective antioxidants in the diet. And worse, these doses of vitamin E have been shown to significantly increase your risk of death!

Vitamins C and E are often sold under the "natural" label—as are most others, including all the synthetic vitamins. In nature these vitamins occur with other chemical components including a wide variety of phytonutrients. In addition, synthetic supplements have lower bioavailability. Synthetic vitamin C, for example, is not as biologically available and the body gets rid of it more quickly, in comparison to vitamin C in real foods. Studies have shown that vitamin C from food is 35 percent better absorbed, and excreted more slowly, than synthetic vitamin C.

There are also other potential side effects associated with HSAIDS, including the following:

- Popular doses of vitamin C supplements can be toxic when they react with the iron in the body or iron in dietary supplements. This is because of the powerful free radicals produced by iron.
- Consuming popular doses of iron can result in excess ferritin (the body's storage form of iron), which has been associated with an increased risk of heart disease and liver stress. High iron intake can also produce damaging excess free radicals and intestinal distress.
- Common preparations of copper, zinc, or selenium supplements can be toxic and can even cause disease.
- Popular doses of vitamin K and B6 can be toxic.
- Consuming popular high doses of vitamin A can result in bone loss and increase the risk of hip fractures in the elderly.

- Consuming popular doses of beta-carotene has been shown to increase lung cancer risk.

Other important considerations:

- None of the nutrients that can cause harm in the body from dietary supplements are harmful when consumed in real food.
- Taking a dietary supplement can promote a false sense of security that you're getting all the nutrients needed for optimal endurance and health.
- While researchers have found for decades that consumption of vegetables and fruits significantly decrease the risk of many diseases, most studies have concluded that dietary supplements containing the same vitamins and minerals do not.
- The International Olympic Committee states that up to one in four dietary supplements can produce a positive test for banned substances.

### HSAIDS Are Not Whole Foods

Another problem with most dietary supplements, even those made from natural nutrients, is that they have been isolated from foods, causing many valuable nutrients to be left behind. Some of these are more important than the one that is isolated. A common example is alpha-tocopherol, also referred to as vitamin E. Alpha-tocopherol does not normally exist alone in nature but occurs with three other tocopherols—beta, delta, and gamma—and four tocotrienols—alpha, beta, delta, and gamma. Together these seven other components of the vitamin E "complex" can be more important than alpha-tocopherol alone. For example, gamma-tocopherol is commonly found in natural foods and is more effective than alpha-tocopherol as an antioxidant. The common use of alpha-tocopherol supplements can be a problem since popular doses of alpha-tocopherol can displace gamma-tocopherol in the body, lowering the overall oxidative protection of the vitamin E complex. This is especially important for endurance athletes.

In addition, the tocotrienols are powerful substances that have potent anti-inflammatory and anti-cancer actions, reduce cholesterol, and perform other vital tasks. Too much alpha-tocopherol can interfere with some of these functions. Even moderate amounts, such as 100 IU of alpha-tocopherol, can block the ability of tocotrienols to control cholesterol.

Unbalanced, isolated high doses of alpha-tocopherol can interfere with body chemistry in other ways, too. They can have a negative effect on anti-inflammatory chemical production, cause generalized muscle weakness, lower thyroid hormone levels, and slightly increase fasting triglyceride levels. Like high-dose vitamin C, alpha-tocopherol may also become a pro-oxidant—which would be counterproductive to its antioxidant function.

## Supplement Hype

Within the dietary supplement industry, the biggest players—those that manufacture the synthetic vitamins and raw materials used to make HSAIDS—are the pharmaceutical companies themselves. The natural foods companies that make real food dietary supplements are generally small and not as welcomed into the natural foods market yet. However, the image that "natural" dietary supplements are prevalent, and the marketing of supplements as "real food" is widespread. But most of these claims are untrue when you read the fine print or know how products are actually made.

Because of the wholesome image of "natural foods," some supplements may contain food concentrates such as blueberry, broccoli, or spinach. However, these plant materials are not only added in minuscule amounts, they also are often made from foods cooked at very high temperatures. The reason for their inclusion, as market researchers tell us, is that it looks good on the label; an ad can even say the product contains real food, or some other claim about being made from fruits and vegetables. But a careful look at the label shows that the vitamins in these products are usually synthetic, were added separately, and are not from those "real" foods. Discerning and uncovering these hidden tricks is often not easy for the average consumer.

Another gimmick commonly used in the supplement industry is the use of yeast that's been fed synthetic vitamins. The technique is simple: feed a nutrient to living yeast, then dry the yeast and add it to a dietary supplement as a source of nutrients. In the case of minerals it may be a useful technique, and claims of "natural" can be made honestly since all minerals—from calcium and magnesium to manganese and zinc—exist on earth in a natural form (most carried to this planet from the sun during the earth's creation). But feeding a synthetic vitamin made by a drug company to yeast, adding the yeast to a supplement and then calling it "natural" and "real-food" is grossly misleading and deceptive.

## Real-Food Supplements

Most companies don't produce supplements made from whole foods. It's difficult and costly to find foods dried with a low-heat process that preserves heat-sensitive nutrients, including the phytonutrients. It's even more difficult to find supplements made from certified-organic materials. In addition to these issues, many dietary supplements contain unwanted added ingredients. These fillers, binders, and other chemicals are quite common. Avoid products containing casein, gluten, soy, wheat, artificial colorings, artificial flavorings, and especially sugar (even if it's organic!).

## The Antioxidant System

Endurance athletes often require additional nutrients because of high levels of training and competition. But the most important fact is that you can obtain most of the nutrients your body needs for optimal endurance from a healthy diet. So where does that leave the role of supplements? Should

they ever be used? And, if so, in what special circumstances? To answer these questions, we need to turn our attention to the athlete's body—and how it functions under the stress of training and racing.

One of the most important aspects of nutrition for endurance athletes is associated with the antioxidant system. This part of our body is related to immune function, and when it's not working well, training and competition can lead to illness and poor muscle function. This is a common problem and an important aspect of the overtraining syndrome.

Physiological stress triggers the release of a variety of chemicals that can influence muscle function and recovery. Some of these chemicals promote acute inflammation to help in the recovery of muscles and other areas following training. Aerobic training offers improved immune function because it produces these chemicals in sufficient amounts, but does not overproduce them.

Anaerobic training, competition, and probably long aerobic training sessions can overproduce these same chemicals, and the body cannot control them as easily. That's why a longer period of recovery is necessary. The problem is that sometimes these chemicals impair performance because the body doesn't have all the nutrients to recover properly. For example, these same chemicals produced in high levels can disturb muscle function, increase muscle fatigue, promote chronic inflammation, hinder protein and fat metabolism, and slow muscle recover. They can also reduce immune function, leading to more illness, such as infections. They can even to be the start of a long process leading to chronic disease including cancer and heart disease.

Many of the chemicals triggered by training and competition are associated with oxygen. These are called oxygen free radicals. Fortunately, the human body is equipped with a system to control these free radicals—the antioxidant system. This system, an important component of aerobic muscle fibers, uses a variety of nutrients called antioxidants to break down oxygen free radicals into safe chemicals. However, in high amounts these free radicals are not well controlled by our antioxidant system and they turn harmful. The antioxidant system works throughout the body, and developing the aerobic system enhances the body's antioxidant system significantly and offers protection during the racing season. However, if the aerobic system is not well developed or the anaerobic system is overworked, our antioxidant mechanism can be less effective, leading to the problems noted above.

Likewise, if you don't provide the antioxidant system with the raw materials it needs to function well, problems can occur. One of the most important groups of nutrients is the antioxidant group. These include vitamins C and E, beta-carotene, selenium, zinc, and others that are easily obtained by eating a variety of fresh vegetables and fruits, nuts and seeds, and other foods. Athletes who don't consume sufficient antioxidants can run into health problems because the body is making more oxygen free radicals than it can control with its antioxidants. This problem can be even worse with the addition of anaerobic training and or racing.

Even athletes consuming the recommended daily amounts of antioxidants from their diets can become deficient during longer periods of anaerobic training and competition. This scenario has led many athletes to consume dietary supplements composed of antioxidants. Unfortunately, antioxidant supplements don't provide the same nutrients that are obtained from the diet, even though the names of these nutrients are often the same. And these dietary supplements don't accomplish the task that the dietary nutrients provide. In fact, recent studies show that dietary supplements of antioxidants not only don't help our antioxidant mechanism, but can also impair its function and even have side effects.

## Immune System

In addition to antioxidants, other nutrients related to the immune system are often low in athletes. As noted above, this is because of a relatively high oxygen uptake from training and racing. Many athletes often get sick following competition, or they get a cold that lasts more than the few days it should take the body to recover from that illness. This problem is, in part, associated with poor functioning of the immune system.

Nutrients that help support the immune system are many—the most important and most powerful is a substance called glutathione. You can't take this in supplement form because it's digested in the intestines before you can absorb it; those products that claim to be glutathione are really the raw materials the body needs to make glutathione, the inclusion of which should be an important focus of your diet. These include:

- Natural forms of vitamin C and E and lipoic acid. Vegetables and fruits, along with raw almonds, cashews, and sesame seeds, will provide sufficient levels of these nutrients.
- The amino acid cysteine is even more important and is a component of whey—in powder form it's a common dietary supplement.
- Sulforaphan, a sulfur compound in cruciferous vegetables such as broccoli, kale, brussels sprouts, and cabbage, is very potent in helping the body produce glutathione. Two- to three-day-old broccoli sprouts (before their leaves turn green) have the highest levels of sulforaphan (these are easy to sprout at home for use in salads, smoothies, etc.).

Common herbs that contain phytonutrients include turmeric and ginger. These can be obtained in their fresh state—ginger, especially, is available as a root in most stores that carry fresh vegetables. These can be used regularly in many different recipes. Ginger tea made with honey is a great refreshing drink that can significantly help immune function and provide carbohydrates following a hard workout or competition.

## Omega-3 Fats

Because endurance athletes create high levels of wear and tear on their bodies, which promotes acute inflammation as part of the normal repair process, an imbalance of fats is not unusual. And with a fat imbalance comes the risk of chronic inflammation and pain. The most common problem that causes this imbalance is low levels of omega-3 fat, the best source being from fish oil. In my practice, I found through dietary analysis that significant numbers of patients had diets very low in omega-3 fats. It has been estimated that more than fifty million people in the United States alone have this problem. The addition of cold-water fish, especially salmon and sardines, can supply more EPA to help balance fats. (Farm-raised fish contain little if any EPA.)

Unfortunately, fresh-water and ocean fish are increasingly being polluted, and eating fish regularly may pose toxin risks. Most fish oil supplements containing EPA are carefully produced without oxidized oils and to remove any heavy metals and other toxins. When buying oil-based dietary supplements, read the labels and make sure the oil has been tested for oxidation and for heavy metals and other potential toxins found in the oceans. A good guide is to use fish oil labeled as containing "0" cholesterol. Many have levels of only 2 or 4 mg of cholesterol, but this may imply that they have not been cleaned of potential toxins.

Some people like taking flaxseed oil as an omega-3 supplement. But since flaxseed oil is extremely susceptible to oxidation when exposed to air or heat, it is best to purchase it in capsules, or refrigerate its liquid form. However, flax oil does not contain EPA, and its conversion to EPA in the body is not very effective, requiring additional vitamins C, B6, niacin, and the minerals magnesium and zinc.

Also note: Avoid refrigerating capsules of dietary supplements containing oils as the cold environment may cause air to leak into the oil inside.

## Omega-6 Fats

Black-currant seed, borage, primrose, and other omega-6 oils are popular dietary supplements. They contain high amounts of GLA (gamma linolenic acid), which is converted to the group 1 anti-inflammatory eicosanoids. People with allergies, especially in the spring when these natural eicosanoid levels are low, often need this supplement. GLA is also essential for carrying calcium to muscle and bone cells. Without it, the calcium in your diet won't be as useful and some may be stored as calcium deposits. It's important when taking any product containing GLA to make sure your fats remain balanced; make sure to also take an EPA (fish oil) or raw sesame seed oil to help prevent GLA from ultimately converting to arachidonic acid, which promotes inflammation. Both sesame and all the GLA-containing oils are also very sensitive to oxygen and should be purchased in capsule form or, if liquid, kept refrigerated.

## Vitamin B Complex

Along with vitamin C, the B vitamins are the most common synthetic nutrients in the marketplace. Almost all B vitamins available in supplement form, whether the whole B complex or single vitamin products, are synthetic—even those labeled as "natural."

In the case of the B vitamins, those that are synthetic are also referred to as *inactive*—in order for the body to utilize these vitamins they must be converted to an *active* form. This requires other nutrients and energy, and conversion is not always effective.

As in the case with natural versus synthetic vitamin C, the body may not utilize the synthetic B vitamins as well. For example, up to 30 percent of the population may be unable to utilize synthetic folic acid. The only way for these individuals to obtain folic acid is from the diet (vegetables and fruits, especially green leafy foods) or by taking an active (natural) form of folic acid.

You can usually determine the type of individual B vitamins a bottle contains by reading the labels. Below is a list of some active (natural) forms of B vitamins:

- Thiamin (B1): thiamine pyrophosphate and thiamine triphosphate
- Riboflavin (B2): riboflavin-5-phosphate
- Niacin (B3): nicotinamide adenine dinucleotide (NADH)
- Pantothenic acid (B5): pantethine
- Pyridoxine (B6): pyridoxal-5-phosphate
- Folic acid: 5-methyl tetrahydrofolate and folinic acid
- Cobalamin (B12): methylcobalamin

The B vitamins are important for so many functions throughout the body. If levels become low, virtually any body area can break down. Those who don't get enough vitamins B1 and B2 typically are low in other B vitamins, too.

High doses of the B vitamins are not well absorbed or utilized. So if a supplement is needed, it's best to take lower doses two or three times daily than one larger dose. For B1 and B2, doses above 5 mg are considered high.

Foods high in B vitamins vary considerably and are not difficult to obtain in a healthy diet. Good sources include eggs and meats, nuts and seeds, legumes, whole grains, and some vegetables such as broccoli, spinach, and mushrooms, which have moderate amounts. Significant losses occur

## B1 AND B2

Here are two important surveys associated with the need for more B vitamins. The first one specifically relates to B1 and the second to B2.

*Survey 1: Check the items below that apply to you.*

☐ Carbohydrate intolerance, including diabetes
☐ Body temperature below normal
☐ Diuretic use (typically used for patients with high blood pressure and heart problems)
☐ Regular alcohol use
☐ Regular caffeine use (coffee, tea, cola)
☐ Moderate to high levels of training and competition
☐ Fatigue
☐ Regular headaches
☐ Reduced mental productivity
☐ Heart problems
☐ Poor appetite

☐ Tendency toward anxiety, phobia, panic disorder
☐ Sleep problems

*Survey 2: Check the items below that apply to you.*

☐ Skin problems
☐ Gingivitis (gum problems)
☐ Discomfort or pain on lips, tongue, or in mouth (non-dental)
☐ Cataracts
☐ Hair loss
☐ Anxiety, tension, or personality changes
☐ Sleep less than six to seven hours per night
☐ Use of antacids
☐ Reduce immune function (cold, flu, or other illness more than twice yearly)
☐ Over age fifty
☐ Increased need for antioxidants
☐ Frequently low hemoglobin or short of breath

The more items that apply to you, the more your levels of B1 or B2 may be too low.

in cooking and freezing, so fresh, raw vegetables are important sources. However, avoid the following foods in their raw state: red chicory, brussels sprouts, red cabbage, clams, oysters, squid, and other mollusks—these all contain the chemical thiaminase which destroys vitamin B1. Some antibiotics can also destroy thiamine. Light (especially the sun) can destroy B2, and sunlight on the skin can reduce some of the body's folic acid, a reason many athletes have a higher need for this B vitamin.

# Calcium

True calcium deficiencies are uncommon in the Western world, regardless of what the dairy industry tells us. The bigger problem is that many athletes are unable to use the calcium they already have in their bodies. Poor calcium metabolism, rather than a deficiency, is almost at epidemic proportions. The end result is that not enough calcium gets into the muscles, bones, and other tissues, with the remaining excess calcium potentially depositing in the joints, tendons, ligaments, or even the kidneys as stones. (Plaque that clogs the arteries can also contain this calcium.)

In order for your body to properly metabolize calcium, and more effectively absorb it from food, you must have sufficient vitamin D. This nutrient is free and plentiful, yet many are surprised to find that some athletes don't have enough. (The important issue of vitamin D and the sun is discussed in chapter 32. Just remember that without sufficient vitamin D, calcium cannot be properly absorbed and regulated, and that most problems of insufficient calcium are really due to low levels of vitamin D.)

Another important issue regarding calcium is to consume enough calcium-rich foods; this is easily done without supplementation through good dietary practices. And it does not necessarily mean eating a lot of dairy foods. (Recall that dairy fats are highest in B fat and can contribute to inflammation.)

Consider the moderate amounts of calcium in the following single servings of non-dairy foods:

- Salmon: 225 mg
- Sardines: 115 mg
- Almonds: 100 mg
- Seaweed: 140 mg
- Rainbow trout: 100 mg
- Spinach: 135 mg
- Green beans: 100 mg
- Collards: 125 mg

Two other important issues regarding calcium are absorption from the intestine (which is significantly influenced by vitamin D) and, after absorption, getting the calcium into the bones and muscles. Absorption is the first step to using calcium in the body.

In general, smaller amounts of calcium are better absorbed than larger amounts, whether from food or supplements. If a small amount of calcium is present in the intestine, 70 percent may be absorbed, for example, while a larger amount of calcium may have only a 30 percent absorption rate. If you're taking calcium supplements, it may be best to take a lower dose several times a day rather than a large dose once daily. Even though vegetables contain smaller amounts of calcium, larger percentages are absorbed compared to milk. So in some situations, a serving of broccoli may result in more calcium getting into the body than a serving of milk.

The stomach's natural hydrochloric acid is also very important in making calcium more absorbable. Neutralizing stomach acid has a negative effect on calcium absorption and a serious impact on digestion and absorption of all nutrients.

Excess phosphorus intake can be very detrimental for calcium use, pulling it out of muscles and bones. Most soft drinks contain large amounts of phosphorus—and the people who drink them risk significant calcium loss from bones, muscles, and other areas of the body.

The type of calcium supplement may be associated with absorbability. For example, calcium carbonate is more poorly absorbed than calcium lactate or calcium citrate. This is due to the alkaline nature of carbonate and the acidic nature of lactate and citrate.

Taking too much calcium in supplement form can disturb the body's complex chemical makeup. For example, too much calcium can reduce magnesium. Most athletes may be in need of more magnesium than calcium—it's necessary for most enzymes to work, including the ones important for fat metabolism. And the best sources of magnesium are vegetables.

## Iron

Most people think of anemia when the mineral iron is discussed. But iron is an important nutrient for all areas of the body, especially the brain and the aerobic muscles; it aids in the production of neurotransmitters and other brain chemicals, is in the protective covering of nerves, and helps carry oxygen in the blood to all parts of the body. Most people can obtain sufficient iron from a healthy diet, especially from beef and other meats. Vegetable sources of iron, such as spinach, are not as well absorbed. If supplements are necessary because of a clear indication of need, such as a blood test that shows low levels, a relatively low daily dose such as 10 mg for a month or two may be enough. Higher doses of iron can be irritating to the intestine and very unhealthy for the whole body. If you have a continuous need for iron, something more important may be missing (sometimes riboflavin—vitamin B2).

Iron is efficiently recycled in the body, with some loss occurring through sweating, or for women, through menstruation. The combination of excess iron loss and decreased intake may produce a serious deficiency.

## Choline

Like all essential nutrients, choline is required for most of the body's basic functions, but many athletes don't get enough. Choline is critical for proper fat metabolism, is associated with the adrenal glands' regulation of stress, and has anti-inflammatory effects. It also prevents the deposit of fat in the liver, helps transport other nutrients throughout the body, and is important for the brain's production of acetylcholine (a neurotransmitter used throughout the brain, especially for memory). Egg yolks may be the best source of choline in the diet, along with fish.

Asthma is a common condition associated with low levels of choline. Wheezing, coughing from bronchial spasm, and excessive mucous production during exercise has been termed "exercise-induced asthma," although it also occurs in those who don't exercise. During training, the body normally dilates the airways to allow for better air passage into and out of the lungs. In those with asthma, the dilation of the airway is followed by excessive narrowing, causing breathing difficulties.

Choline can help the nervous system control proper bronchial action. In this situation, a moderate dose of choline may be needed initially: for example, 500 mg several times daily until breathing improves and dietary choline is increased. (In addition, the excess intake of refined carbohydrate can maintain inflammation, which could also contribute to chronic asthma.)

To illustrate the importance of choline, I am reminded of one patient named Roy. He was a slim, forty-four-year-old construction worker who wanted to "run with the guys" after work; but after fifteen minutes he had trouble breathing due to severe asthma that had plagued him since childhood. Roy's asthmatic reaction was due in part to several factors: the stress of running at too high a heart rate without proper training; a diet high in refined carbohydrates; and, in particular, a significant need for choline. After two weeks of taking a choline supplement (600 mg, five times throughout the day), his breathing symptoms during running were mostly gone. Roy was so elated that he wanted to learn all he could about proper diet and exercise. I spent a significant amount of time helping him in his endeavors.

Roy focused on improving his aerobic system and eating well, including several eggs daily to keep his choline intake adequate. After about three months, he was able to eliminate the choline supplement without any recurring breathing problems. While he ultimately enjoyed road racing in 5K and 10K events, his passion was most evident on the track. As a masters' sprinter, Roy started performing extremely well in 100- and 200-meter races, and anchoring an impressive team relay, all in the New York area. He also expanded his events to include triple jump and long jump. About eighteen months after first visiting my clinic, Roy qualified for and competed in the world masters' track and field meet in Australia, where he won a number of medals in sprint and field events.

## Skin and Hair Care

The best way to maintain healthy and good-looking skin and hair is proper nutrition. This starts with a great diet, especially balanced fats, adequate protein, good intestinal function, and proper hydration. If your skin or hair is very dry and unhealthy, or you have other skin problems, this is usually a sign of reduced health, including the need to improve the diet.

Below are some specific issues pertaining to skin and hair:

- For sun protection, and because you're probably in the sun often when training and competing, which uses up a lot of nutrients, a number of nutritional substances from foods can be helpful. These include folic acid, beta-carotene, and lycopene, which are provided by a variety of vegetables and fruit. Tocotrienols, from raw nuts and seeds, and a part of the vitamin E complex, can help protect

# NATURAL FOLATES

Two of the many naturally occurring forms of folic acid include folinic acid and 5-methyl tetrahydrofolate (5-MTHF), the most common forms found in the foods we eat. Unfortunately, the most common form of folic acid in our food supply is synthetic and not well utilized by the body. Because it is much cheaper, it is used in food fortification and virtually all dietary supplements on store shelves. This synthetic form of folic acid is inactive and must first be converted to an active form to be useful in the body.

A significant number of people are unable to absorb or otherwise utilize synthetic folic acid. The numbers are difficult to determine, but scientists have estimated that perhaps up to 30 percent of the population has this inability (which is genetically determined). These individuals must rely on natural folic acid from food, or the 5-methyl or folinic acid versions in supplements.

Consumption of natural folic acid is not just important for prevention of neural tube defects, one of many types of birth defects. It's a necessary nutrient with body-wide benefits for all adults and children. These include the following:

- Brain function—the natural forms of folic acid are the only ones that can get into the brain. It is especially important for those who don't sleep well or are depressed.
- Intestinal function—it can help food digestion and absorption, heal the intestines, and, as studies have shown, prevent colon cancer.
- Liver detoxification of substances like estrogens in both men and women—it removes their harmful metabolites and prevents breast cancer.
- Protein metabolism and for regulation of certain amino acids
- The production of new blood cells
- Cardiovascular health (by reducing homocysteine)

In addition, unlike synthetic inactive folic acid, natural folic acid does not mask anemia if not taken with adequate vitamin B12.

the skin directly, and limonene, found in citrus peel, can protect against skin cancer. All the antioxidants, from all those vegetables and fruits, can also help with sun exposure since increased free radicals are one harmful effect of too much sun. In addition, fish oil, by mouth, helps protect the skin during sun exposure.

- Many skin problems are associated with low or deficient levels of vitamin B2 (riboflavin).
- Pure shea butter is a unique skin-care product made from an African nut extract (similar to a coconut) and has been used for centuries as a beauty product. European studies have shown that shea butter is remarkably active against skin blemishes and irritation. It's also useful as a daily hand, face, or body ointment. As a moisturizer, it is helpful against the damaging effects of the sun and also helps maintain the skin's elasticity. Pure coconut oil is also great for the skin, as is extra virgin olive oil.
- The omega-6 fat GLA is perhaps the best remedy for localized skin problems. Breaking open a gel cap of black-currant seed oil and rubbing it into the skin is a great remedy for dry skin, wrinkles, or even the most stubborn skin problems, and is as good if not better than all the expensive skin remedies on the market. It's also good for burns, including sunburn, but only after the skin has been thoroughly cooled. If you've been training or competing in

the sun and get burned, cool your skin in a cold tub, pool, or shower sufficiently until it stops feeling burned (this could take time depending on the severity of the burn).

Finally, don't put anything on your skin you're not willing to eat! That's because you absorb most ointments, creams, lotions, soaps, and other items commonly used on the skin and scalp. Most especially avoid fragrance, which is listed on the label as such. Use only plain, pure liquid and solid soaps without chemicals—not easy to find when shopping but these products are available. Some are scented with lemon, peppermint, or other natural oils, which are healthy components.

## Conclusion

The most important factor associated with whether you need to take dietary supplements is that you should first focus on obtaining all your nutrients from a healthy diet. Only after you've done the best job with your food intake should a dietary supplement be carefully considered. This may best be accomplished by evaluating your diet, so as to provide a more objective view of your nutrient intake and to determine if any nutrients are low. A health-care professional may also be of assistance in performing certain tests that may help determine the need for a dietary supplement. Just be wary of all those heavily marketed supplements promising great, unsubstantiated results.

# TAKING GOOD CARE OF YOUR LIVER AND KIDNEYS—
## Detox and pH Balance

The liver and kidneys are two of your body's best friends, performing all types of necessary metabolic housekeeping to help training and racing. But overwork or otherwise abuse them through a bad diet, and they can easily turn into your worst enemy, leading to all kinds of health issues. While scientists and clinicians have long known about the importance of liver detoxification and kidney function to balance body pH, and how diet plays a vital role in keeping them working well, manufacturers have created so-called nutritional products to take the place of a good diet. Unfortunately, consumers are never told that these expensive supplements are full of synthetic vitamins and other unwanted ingredients, and that diet is a better and much less expensive way to accomplish the task. For this reason, I have decided to devote this entire chapter to the liver and kidneys in order to emphasize these organs' importance for the well-being of all endurance athletes, and to show how diet plays a crucial role in their proper functioning.

A healthy, fully functioning liver can make your training go much more smoothly. It's an important organ (technically, more of a gland) to help detox unwanted chemicals created in your body during the course of training and racing and those taken in through food, air, and water. An unhealthy liver can derail your best training plans and, worse, lead to reduced fitness and health. Instead of expensive store-bought liver detox shortcuts, which may not do you or your body any good, rely on your diet.

As for the kidneys, one of their important functions is to help maintain the correct body pH, or biochemical acid-alkaline, balance to help your metabolism function better, something heavily influenced by the diet. For example, training and racing produce lactic acid and other chemicals and can lower body pH; this must be countered by raising the pH, best accomplished with well-functioning kidneys and certain healthy foods.

## The Liver

The largest of your internal organs, the gland-like liver is located under the front ribs on your right side. It weighs about three pounds, more in larger and less in smaller people. It performs thousands of important jobs for the body's metabolism. It maintains blood sugar during the night (by storing glycogen that converts to glucose), makes bile for digestion of fats, and even produces the hormone somatomedin for building muscle and cartilage. All these actions significantly affect

your training, racing, and overall health. One of the liver's most important tasks is removing toxins.

The liver filters the blood, and by doing so it breaks down and eliminates an untold number of chemical compounds. Some of these are normally produced within the body during metabolism, while others are consumed even in a healthy diet (with many more toxins in bad foods). In doing its job, the liver regulates hormones, cholesterol, fats, proteins, caffeine, sulfur (from cruciferous vegetables like broccoli and cabbage), various phytonutrients, iron, and many other compounds. Even healthy substances, such as hormones and nutrients, when completing their tasks in the body, are disposed of by the liver. But if this does not happen, the continuous actions of hormones causes an imbalance—just as if there was too much of that hormone. The brain also plays an important role in this regulation process by helping the liver decide how to regulate the breakdown of various substances.

Just as important, toxins that enter the body through food and our environment are filtered out and eliminated in the liver. These include pesticides and other toxic chemicals that find their way into our food and water, chemicals from air pollution (auto exhaust, cleaning products, perfumes, and toiletries), medications, and others. The liver accomplishes this through a complex process called detoxification. Once filtered, the liver disposes of all these substances, via the gall bladder, into the gut for removal from the body. Thus, optimal gut function also plays an important role in this process.

## Liver Detox

To be successful with detoxification, the liver requires a variety of nutrients. Unfortunately, among the advocates of liver detox, many scams lure the public into buying their products by promising miracle detox potions. Most won't be as effective as eating real food because they contain synthetic vitamins and other chemicals—all of which must be broken down and eliminated by the liver. The very best way to promote healthy liver function comes from eating real food and avoiding environmental toxins as much as possible.

To obtain the many nutrients required for liver detox, focus on a regular diet full of a variety of organic, unprocessed foods—fresh vegetables and fruits, whole raw nuts and seeds, and high quality protein (including whole eggs). Organic foods have more of these important nutrients and fewer toxins such as pesticides.

The signs and symptoms of poor liver detox may be subtle. So how do you know if your liver function needs more support? Ask yourself the following questions:

- Are you sensitive to caffeine (you can consume only small amounts or none at all)?
- Are you sensitive to perfumes, paints, and other chemical smells?

- Are you sensitive to certain drugs: benzodiazepines (Valium, Ativan, Xanax), antihistimines (Benadryl, Claritin), certain antibiotics (Bactrim, Erythromycin) and antifungals (Lotrimin)?
- Are you sensitive to certain foods: grapefruit, turmeric, curry, chili (capsaicin), or cloves?
- Do you eat less than two servings a day of animal protein (meat, fish, whole eggs)?
- Are you taking non-steroidal anti-inflammatory drugs (Advil, Aleve)?
- Are you taking more than one dose of Tylenol or aspirin per week?
- Are you sensitive (even to the smell) to high-sulfur-containing foods such as egg yolks, onions, garlic, broccoli, or cabbage?
- Do you consume more than two alcoholic drinks per day?
- Do you eat less than about eight servings of vegetables and fruits per day?

If you answered "yes" to even one or two of these questions, it could indicate that your liver detoxification pathways are not as efficient as they should be. Liver function also slows down with age if we don't keep it going with adequate healthy food.

For ease of study, researchers and clinicians discuss liver detox as two different chemical pathways, called Phase I and Phase II. Each is associated with specific toxins and nutrients. Through a careful evaluation of an athlete, I could often determine which pathway needed more support, something difficult to do here. For simplicity, I discuss Phase I and II together as one general category of liver detox. It is important to understand that too much of one nutrient may help one phase while hurting the other. This is another reason why many detox supplements can be harmful—they're too general and may not be specific for your needs. But a healthy diet will provide a natural balance of nutrients for the liver to use.

The most important compound for liver detox is a substance called glutathione. Fortunately, the body makes glutathione when we eat a variety of foods rich in specific nutrients. It's important to consume these foods regularly. Some of the key nutrients the body needs, and some foods containing them, to make glutathione include:

- Lipoic acid found in spinach, broccoli, peas, brussels sprouts, and many other bitter-tasting vegetables
- Sulforaphan from broccoli and kale (highest in broccoli sprouts)
- Gamma tocopherol and alpha tocotrienol from fresh vegetables and raw nuts and seeds
- The amino acid cysteine, highest in certain animal proteins, especially whey

In addition, the process of detoxification normally produces large amounts of unstable chemicals called oxygen free radicals. A diet rich in antioxidants helps sweep up this radical "fallout" from liver detox. Potent antioxidants found in brightly colored vegetables and fruits—tomatoes, yellow summer and winter squash, cilantro, kale, carrots, melons, blueberries—include the carotenoids (lycopene, beta-carotene, zeaxanthin, lutein) and the full vitamin E complex, especially beta, delta, and gamma tocopherol. Food doses of vitamin C (found in the white spongy material in red peppers and citrus, and other vegetables and fruits) also work with other antioxidants.

To liven up your healthy meals, include foods rich in phytonutrients that also assist liver detox. These include citrus peel (make a citrus peel zest or a marmalade with honey), caraway seeds (grind them just before use), turmeric, ginger, garlic, and dill, just to name a few.

The liver detox pathways also require B vitamins, especially thiamin (B1), niacin (B3), and the folates. But avoid the synthetic forms because these have to be detoxed and eliminated through the liver too. Alcohol, in small amounts, may actually help liver detox. In moderation, alcohol is broken down in the liver (although the process starts in the stomach) but by a different mechanism that also requires B vitamins. But excessive alcohol taps into Phase II detoxification, where it can cause significant stress.

If you have a history of liver problems, you should avoid certain foods and drugs. These include iron from dietary supplements, alcohol, and products containing acetaminophen (including Tylenol, Excedrin, and other aspirin-free products). Any drug, especially those taken by mouth (after absorption in the gut, they go directly to the liver), can be a problem. These substances can add significant chemical stress to the liver. In addition, avoid the foods that you know you're sensitive to and be especially aware of caffeine. While the liver is a powerfully amazing part of us (if a piece is surgically removed it can even grow back), we often won't get signs or symptoms that it's not functioning well until a third or even half of its function is gone.

The liver makes bile to help carry toxins through the gall bladder and into the intestines for elimination. Dietary fats in the diet keep bile flowing properly, helping the liver do its job. These include olive oil, avocado, nuts and seeds, and other healthy fats and oils. Extremely low fat diets can reduce bile production and can be dangerous. Likewise, high fat diets can overwork the gall bladder. (A variety of natural foods will also contain sufficient fiber to help remove the toxins from the gut.)

Improving liver function is a key to helping the entire intestine function in a normal healthy way, especially the large intestine. The ability to detoxify many chemicals made in our body and taken in via the air, water, and food is one of the liver's important functions. This contribution to improved fitness and health is another way athletes can improve athletic performance.

## The Kidneys—Helping Maintain a Healthy Acid-Alkaline (pH) Balance

A healthy diet does more than provide us with many important nutrients. Through digestion of food, an important biochemical acid-alkaline balance occurs, which significantly helps maintain our overall health. In addition to food, the kidneys play a vital role in this pH balance, and require sufficient water for their action. A healthy diet also provides many vitamins and minerals used by the kidneys.

The kidneys are bean-shaped organs, about the size of a fist, located just below the rib cage in the middle back, one on each side of the spine. Like the liver, the kidneys also filter the blood—about 200 quarts a day. From this, the kidney's filter out about 2 quarts or more of waste products, including extra water which becomes urine. The kidneys also produce hormones: EPO (erythropoietin), as previously discussed, stimulates the bone marrow to make red blood cells; rennin helps regulate blood pressure; and calcitriol continues the process of vitamin D production which began in the skin with sunlight.

The positive aspects of lactic acid production in muscles and the appearance of blood lactate were previously discussed, especially in relation to energy production. Higher levels of lactate also coincide with the lowering of pH—increased acidity. This shift in pH, which occurs during exercise, especially during hard training or racing, can adversely affect metabolism and muscle function. Consuming sodium bicarbonate in an attempt to counteract this shift in pH and reduce fatigue during racing is a decades-old idea. However, the consensus is that its use is without success. Nonetheless, this has given rise to new, hyped products to control pH. It is well known that the diet, however, can regulate body pH in significant ways.

In athletes, this lower pH comes from hard training and racing, but a poor diet actually can do the same. Certainly an imbalance in our acid-alkaline state can seriously disrupt our health, adversely affecting many metabolic functions. And, it can adversely affect training and racing because it's associated with fatigue. But the simple act of eating a healthy, balanced diet accomplishes this pH control and helps the kidneys function better than any so-called miracle product (ten times the cost of real food). There are dietary supplements made from natural foods—vegetable-based products—that can help those with acid-alkaline problems, but these too are not meant as a primary therapy—that's the role of the diet.

For almost all of human existence, our diet has been slightly alkaline, which is considered to be optimal for our body's brain, muscles, and metabolism. With the agricultural revolution of the past 5,000 to 10,000 years came a dramatic rise in processed grain consumption, which significantly added more acid-producing foods to the diet, disturbing the balance. Grain foods also replaced many vegetables and fruits in the diet, which were primarily those needed to maintain our healthy alkaline state. Today, most "Westernized" diets are full of highly processed grains, especially wheat, which contribute to an over-acid state. Excessive animal protein intake can also make the body more acidic.

Most food in our diet produces either an acid or alkaline residue. This affects our whole body via the bloodstream. For athletes in particular, maintaining proper pH is vital because of the many systems affected by it. Many aspects of metabolism and muscle activity will function better when pH levels are normal.

*The most potent foods that improve pH balance are vegetables and fruits, and to a lesser degree nuts and seeds.* Below is a list of the key foods associated with pH balance. Acid-producing foods, which lower pH, include:

- All grains, whether whole or refined
- Milk products, cheese, and all dairy
- Meats from all animals, including fish
- Eggs
- Salt

Alkaline foods, which raise pH, include:

- Vegetables
- Fruits
- Nuts and seeds

(Fats and legumes are neutral.)

These foods are not meant to be a list of "good" and "bad" but rather, a way to relate to your diet. For example, if your meals are typical of many athletes—high in bread, pasta, cereal, rolls, and other grains—it can obviously be a problem for acid-alkaline balance. By eliminating refined carbohydrates and replacing them with vegetables and fruits, you'll quickly be on the way to better pH balance.

Eating too many acid-producing foods can result in a general body-wide imbalance—a state of chronic acidosis. This can cause bone and muscle problems, such as fractures, osteoporosis, muscle weakness, and even muscle wasting. As athletes age, this increases the risk of falls, fractures, and disability, and also leads to the loss of independence, all of which contributes to increased mortality rate and reduced quality of life. Many other problems can develop too, such as kidney disease, high blood pressure, poor mineral balance (with significant loss of magnesium), asthma, cardiovascular disease, and other conditions. In addition to being a better athlete now, maintaining proper pH will assure better athleticism in your later years, along with improved health.

The answer to the problem of acid-alkaline imbalance is not to create an opposite imbalance by over-consuming a high alkaline product or eliminating all acid foods. Such is the case when high-quality animal protein is eliminated from the diet (which can actually worsen bone and muscle problems). Rather, establishing balance in the diet is a key to an optimal acid-alkaline state. It means eating sufficiently from both the healthy acid and alkaline food groups. For many athletes, this means eating more fresh vegetables and fruits—ten servings a day for adults. It also means eliminating refined grain products. And, to give your kidneys an easier time at doing their job filtering the blood, sufficient water intake is necessary. As discussed previously, this means maintaining an almost clear color of urine, avoiding the yellow color indicating mild (or even severe) dehydration.

The liver and kidneys, like the brain, are often a forgotten part of building endurance. By eating a healthy diet, avoiding the marketing hype, and drinking sufficient amounts of water, better detoxification and pH control will contribute to your overall plan for better fitness and health, and optimal training and racing.

# CHAPTER 22

# THE TRAINING TABLE—
## Healthy Recipes, Shopping Guidelines, and Cooking Tips

**M**any endurance athletes insist that they'd rather be outside training than stuck indoors cooking. But your kitchen can be a great training ground. That's because what you eat will significantly help determine how far and fast you can push your body, how well you recover, and how effectively your aerobic system can develop. It's wrong to assume that a prepackaged meal or quick stop at a fast food restaurant will provide a shortcut to eating well. In fact, just the opposite can occur—your training could actually start to fall off due to improper diet.

I often had patients come into my office who said they hated cooking and so they were stuck in a bad dietary rut for years. Most showed signs and symptoms of insufficient nutrition. But when they were finally convinced to eat better, they trained and raced better—and became healthier too.

One of my most common recommendations for these athletes was to start with the basics—to eat real food. This begins with shopping. If you only buy real food, while avoiding unhealthy items so prevalent even in so-called health food stores, you're much less likely to eat unhealthy meals. Proper meal preparation means taking these basic food ingredients—fresh raw vegetables and fruits, fresh meats, whole eggs, and others—and turning them into a tasty, healthy, satisfying meal. However, you don't need to be a graduate of the Culinary Institute of America to accomplish this daily task. There are plenty of simple-to-prepare recipes that will bring out your inner top chef—that's the point of this chapter, to offer an appetizing list of healthy recipes that are easy to whip up.

With few exceptions, most of these recipe ideas don't come with exact measurements and precise cooking instructions. I like to keep instructions simple, which also provides you with the potential to create variations that suit your tastes and needs. From salads and dressings to sauces and entrees—and even desserts—healthy recipes should be easy to make and delicious. Choose the recipes that are appropriate to your own needs and taste buds. For example, if you're not tolerant to dairy products, avoid recipes that include dairy, or substitute non-dairy sources such as coconut milk or oil instead of cream or butter.

Because athletes often dream of dessert during training—like a well-deserved reward—let's start with that.

# Desserts

### Pecandy

Heat 1 cup pecan pieces; ½ cup ground almonds; ¼ cup coconut flakes; 2 tablespoons butter, coconut oil, or pure cocoa butter; and ¼ teaspoon salt until very lightly toasted. Add ¼ cup honey and continue heating until simmering. Remove from heat. Add ¼ cup ground sesame seeds or tahini. Flatten and spread in pan or dish and cut into squares.

Options: Heat cocoa bits with butter and pecans for a chocolate cookie; toast shredded coconut before adding butter and pecans to have a crunchy coconut taste; stir in chopped dates; vary the type of nuts (walnuts, pistachios, hazelnuts).

### Irish "Potatoes"

Mix together 4 ounces cream cheese, 1 teaspoon vanilla, ¼ teaspoon cinnamon, ¼ cup honey, and ½ cup finely shredded coconut. Form into small balls and sprinkle with cinnamon. Serve chilled.

### Coconut Snowballs

Mix 1 cup unsweetened shredded coconut, ½ cup egg-white powder, 2 tablespoons honey, a dash of vanilla, and 1 to 2 tablespoons heavy cream (or enough to make sticky balls). Roll in toasted shredded coconut. (To toast coconut, place in a dry skillet on medium heat and stir frequently until slightly browned.)

### Butternut Squash Pie

This is tastier than pumpkin pie, and better for you too! Steam quartered butternut squash until tender; let cool enough to remove peel. Blend about 2 cups of butternut squash, 4 eggs, ½ teaspoon salt, 4 ounces cream cheese or ½ cup coconut milk, ⅓ cup honey, and ½ teaspoon pumpkin pie spice or favorite blend of cinnamon and spices. Place in buttered baking dish (and place baking dish in ½ inch of water). Bake at 350°F. Allow to cool for about 10 minutes before serving. Serve plain, with whipped or sour cream, or top with chopped nuts and dates.

### Almond Biscotti Cake

Grind 1 cup almonds (with some course pieces remaining). Mix in 5 eggs, a pinch of salt, ⅓ cup heavy cream or coconut milk, and ⅓ cup date sugar or honey. Pour into buttered dish and bake at 350°F for about forty minutes.

### Fried Bananas

Peel and slice small ripe bananas. Sauté in coconut oil until slightly brown and caramelized. Place in a bowl and sprinkle with coconut and a pinch of date sugar (or coconut sugar).

Options: Keep bananas whole; drizzle with cherry sauce; top with whipped cream; combine with other favorite fruit—mango is especially nice.

### Creamy Avocado Pudding

Blend until smooth 1 large avocado, 3 tablespoons sour cream, 2 tablespoons honey, 2 to 3 tablespoons lemon or lime juice, and a bit of zest. Top with slices of mango, sprigs of cilantro, and lime peel.

### Very Berry Sauce

Heat frozen blueberries, raspberries, strawberries, or other berries. Some prefer to press raspberries through a strainer to remove seeds. Add honey to taste. Use on desserts, healthy waffles, or other foods.

### Crepes de Frutas

Beat 1 egg per person with ½ teaspoon honey per egg and a very small amount of cream. Melt butter or olive oil in a small skillet on low temperature and add a thin layer of egg mixture. Slowly cook until surface is slightly sticky but firm. Remove from skillet, spread a thin layer of sour cream, and roll into logs. Top with Very Berry Sauce, fresh fruit, whipped cream, yogurt, or some other healthy topping of your choice.

### Coconut Pound Cake

Melt 1 stick butter, mix in 4 egg yolks, ½ cup honey, 1 teaspoon vanilla, and ¼ teaspoon salt until creamy. Add 1 cup coconut flour and 1 cup water or more until it's a smooth consistency. Whip 4 egg whites until stiff and fold into batter. Bake at 350°F for 20–30 minutes. Top with cherry sauce, Very Berry Sauce, or lemon-honey mixture.

### Banana Bread

Melt 4 tablespoons (½ stick) butter or coconut oil and stir in ⅓ cup honey and 4 beaten eggs until smooth. Add 1 teaspon of vanilla and 3 mashed very ripe bananas. Add 1 cup finely ground almonds, ½ teaspoon cinnamon, and ½ teaspoon salt. Add water if needed to make a smooth cake-like batter. Option: mix in ½ cup chopped walnuts. Bake at 350°F for 45 minutes.

### Cashew Chews

Mix well: 2 tablespoons cashew butter, 1 tablespoon sesame butter, 1 tablespoon egg-white powder, 1 tablespoon honey, and 2 tablespoons dried coconut. Roll into bite-size balls and push a small date (or half a large date) into each center. Sprinkle with additional coconut. Option: Add unsweetened cocoa bits.

### Mission Fig Mousse

Blend ripe mission figs with honey and heavy cream. Serve alone or on top of cheesecake, brownie, or other healthy dessert.

Variations: Cut top of fig and carefully scoop out the center. Blend with 2 tablespoons of cream and about 1 tablespoon of honey for six figs. Spoon the fig mousse back into the skins. Top with tiny strips of fresh sweet basil (cut strips with scissors). Sprinkle with date sugar and a pinch of salt. Option: A balsamic vinegar reduction decoratively poured over the top sets this off beautifully.

### Cheesecake

Blend well: 1 cup sheep or goat yogurt or cream cheese, 1 cup ricotta cheese, 4 eggs, ⅓ cup honey, 1 teaspoon vanilla, and pour into buttered baking dish. Place in another dish with an inch of water. Bake 30–45 minutes at 350°F until firm. This is wonderful hot or cold. Top with your favorite fruit, whipped cream, shaved almonds, fruit sauce, or other healthy topping.

### Mango Sorbet

Cut up 1 ripe mango and 1 or 2 small bananas and freeze until firm. Add to blender and mix well with ½ cup unsweetened coconut milk. Serve with colorful berries.

### Apple and Pear Crisp

Place 1 sliced tart apple and 1 sliced pear in a baking dish. Mix ¼ cup ground almonds, ¼ cup ground whole oats (optional), ¼ cup butter, ¼ cup honey, and ½ teaspoon cinnamon and sprinkle on top. Bake 45 minutes at 350°F.

### Fast Apple or Pear Crisp

Dice apples or pears and quickly sauté in butter until slightly browned. Place in serving dishes and sprinkle with cinnamon. Warm 1 tablespoon of honey and 1 tablespoon heavy cream in a sauce pan, mix well, and pour over fruit. Sprinkle with ground or chopped almonds. Option: Top with whipped cream.

### Phil's Fudge

Mix ⅓ cup unsweetened cocoa powder and ⅓ cup egg-white powder. Melt 2 tablespoons butter in a saucepan on low heat. Add ¼ cup honey to melted butter in pan, and mix in cocoa and egg-powder mixture.

The consistency should be like soft rubber. If it's too dry, add honey; if too wet, add cocoa or egg powder. Press into buttered glass pan and cut into squares. Keep refrigerated if you want them firm, or leave out to keep them soft.

Options: ¾ teaspoon of peppermint oil; almond, cashew, or peanut butter center (premix very small amount of honey with the nut butter and place between thin layers of chocolate); unsweetened shredded coconut—add to dry mix before blending. For white chocolate, use pure cocoa butter instead of butter and cocoa powder, and add ½ teaspoon of vanilla.

### Stuffed Majool Dates

Open date, remove pit, stuff with a small piece of blue cheese and butter, close date, eat, and enjoy!

### Flaxseed Crackers

Soak 1 cup of flaxseeds in 1 cup of water for 6–8 hours. Add salt and other favorite seasonings and mix well. The flaxseeds release a very sticky substance that holds the mixture together. Wet your hands to work with the mixture easily. Place 1 to 2 tablespoons of mixture on parchment paper and flatten out like a thin cookie. Dehydrate the crackers in an oven set at 180°F, outside in the sun, or in a dehydrator. Turn crackers over when top side is crispy. Dehydrate 4–8 hours until both sides are crispy.

# Salads

At least one salad a day is a good rule to follow for better health. Salads provide all-important raw foods, not to mention vitamins, minerals, phytonutrients, and fiber. A salad can be a great side dish to any meal, or it can be a meal itself. Making a daily salad need not be a time-consuming, tedious process. In fact, some of the best salads are very simple and easy to make: leaf lettuce, tomatoes, carrots, and other items can be clean and ready for the bowl. Add your favorite homemade dressing or just olive oil and balsamic vinegar and salt.

Here are some great salad ideas, followed by delicious dressings. Don't be afraid to experiment—adding or substituting just one healthful ingredient makes for an entirely new nutritional adventure.

### Apples and Beets

Shred green tart apples and raw peeled beetroots in a food processor or with a mandolin slicer. Mix together and squeeze in some fresh lime. Add salt to taste. Shred in carrots and ginger for a variation.

### Arugula and Pears

Mix fresh baby arugula and diced pears. Add pecans, salt, olive oil, and parmesan cheese, pecorino, or gorgonzola.

### Arugula and Roasted Grape Tomatoes

Roast grape tomatoes with extra virgin olive oil and salt in a single layer at 250°F for

4 hours. Allow to cool and add to fresh baby arugula. Add crumbled goat cheese.

### Asian Coleslaw

Shred carrots, daikon radish, cabbage, red peppers, and cucumbers in a food processor or with mandolin slicer. Make a dressing with raw sesame or olive oil, rice wine vinegar, salt, grated fresh ginger and garlic, fresh lime or lemon juice, and a bit of honey. Spice it up with cayenne pepper. Add cilantro or fresh basil for even more exciting flavors.

A note about peppers: Before they ripen, peppers are green. When ripe, they turn a particular color, depending on the variety. Ripe peppers are red, purple, yellow, or orange. Avoid eating green peppers as they are difficult to digest and not as tasty.

### Beets and Ginger

Steam or bake whole beetroots. Dice into bite-size cubes. Marinate in lemon juice, grated or finely chopped fresh ginger root, salt, and honey.

### Beets and Mache Greens

Dice cooked beets and add to fresh mache greens. Top with olive oil, white wine vinegar, and salt.

### Grapefruit, Avocado, Spinach

On a bed of fresh baby spinach, add grapefruit sections and diced avocados. Top with blended grapefruit sections, ginger, garlic, honey, salt, and olive oil.

### Grapefruit and Pomegranate Seeds

Simply mix grapefruit sections with fresh pomegranate seeds.

### Apples and Fennel

Thinly slice apples and fennel bulbs. Dress with apple cider vinegar, honey, and salt.

### Orange and Fennel

Mix orange sections with chopped fresh fennel. Sprinkle with unsweetened grated coconut. Add plain sheep or goat yogurt.

### Fresh Pickles

Slice cucumbers (the seedless, small ones are best) and add thinly sliced or diced garlic, fresh dill, salt, a small amount of honey, and white wine vinegar for the pickle juice. For a variation, include wheat-free soy sauce and sesame seeds.

### Herbs and Watermelon

Mix a variety of fresh herbs and baby greens (basil, mint, cilantro, tarragon, dill, arugula, chard, spinach, lettuce). Cut a small watermelon into cubes and add crumbled soft goat cheese. Toss with olive oil and salt.

## Dressings and Sauces

The flavors of many foods can be heightened with a good dressing or sauce. Following are recipes for my favorite healthful salad dressings and stovetop sauces.

## Phil's Salad Dressing

In a blender, mix 8 ounces extra virgin olive oil, 2 cloves garlic, 2 ounces or more apple cider vinegar, 1 tablespoon fresh or dried parsley, 1 to 2 teaspoons sea salt, and ½ teaspoon mustard. Options: Add 1 to 2 tablespoons sheep or goat yogurt, or cream. Blend in 1 avocado, 1 tomato, 1 mango, juice from half a lime (in place of the vinegar), or cilantro. Use 4 ounces of sesame or walnut oil for variation in taste. Once you find the best combinations, make a larger amount so you always have it available. Shake well before serving.

## Spicy Sesame Ginger Dressing

Combine rice wine vinegar, honey, sesame tahini, olive oil, miso, grated ginger, and chopped garlic.

## Basic Butter Sauce

The most basic of sauces is also the easiest to make—simply butter and sea salt. When you make your vegetables, put some "sweet cream" butter on the vegetables while still hot, along with some sea salt. ("Sweet" butter is made without salt—the cream used to make this butter is a higher quality and more tasty than that used for salted butter.) Even those who never liked vegetables will usually eat them with a butter sauce. Variation: sauté garlic or onions with or without some spices (tarragon works well) in butter and some olive oil.

## Ghee or Clarified Butter

Melt one pound of sweet (unsalted) butter and bring just to the point of low boil to allow separation of solids and fat. Skim off solids that rise to the top and add this to soup or vegetables. Use the clear butter (ghee) like any other butter. Ghee does not burn like butter.

## Basic Tomato Sauce

This is a quick and easy, tasty, and healthful all-around red sauce. Just put some chopped fresh tomatoes or whole canned tomatoes in an uncovered pot and boil (not simmer) until desired consistency. Add salt. When cooked down to a thicker sauce, tomatoes take on a unique taste all their own. Even without adding any spices you'll have a great-tasting sauce. You can also freeze it in small glass containers. Once you have the basic sauce, add garlic, parsley, basil, turmeric, or your favorite spices.

## Basic Cream Sauce

The fanciest basic sauce is the cream sauce, simply made from heavy cream, butter, psyllium, and salt. Use just less than the same amount of cream as the amount of sauce you want. For example, for about 2 cups of sauce, use a bit less than 2 cups of cream. Heat the cream to just before it simmers. In a separate pan, melt about a half-stick (4 tablespoons) of sweet butter on low heat. With a whisk, slowly stir in about ½ teaspoon finely ground psyllium into the butter. Slowly add the hot cream while continuously stirring over low to medium heat, bringing to a simmer for 5–10 minutes. Add sea salt to taste.

Once you can make a good basic cream sauce quickly and easily, you can make a variety of different sauces almost as easily. For example, adding some chopped onion or garlic, a bay leaf, tarragon, or other spices to the cream, after heating it, makes a different sauce. For a cheese sauce, add any type of cheese to the basic cream sauce.

## Soups

Almost any food can be the base for a delicious soup. And it need not be a lengthy or difficult recipe. Use or freeze vegetables in your refrigerator that are getting too old to serve fresh: salad greens and other vegetables, meat bones, chicken and turkey carcasses, and other flavorful foods that you might normally discard. Lightly sauté vegetables and meat scraps in oil or butter, cover with generous amount of water, and add salt and spices as desired. Strain the broth when cool and store in glass quart-size jars. If freezing, allow at least an inch of space from the top of the jar. If you are making a vegetable soup from wilted vegetables, try blending the cooked vegetables with broth, salt, and other seasonings for bisque-like soup.

### Shabu Shabu

This Japanese-style soup is fun and delicious. Mix shredded cabbage and carrots, chopped green onions, fresh basil leaves, kelp noodles, finely sliced mushrooms, garlic, and ginger, and set aside in a bowl. Make a beef broth with trimmings of steak while you are slicing paper-thin steak (best done when steak is still slightly frozen). Add wheat-free soy sauce and sesame oil to sliced beef and marinate at room temperature for about thirty minutes. Strain broth and place in a pot that can be heated at the table (either a candle warmer or electric hot plate). Keep the broth near boiling during dinner. Add some of the vegetables and noodles to the broth and then dip pieces of beef into broth, picking up veggies and noodles with the beef. Keep adding vegetables and noodles throughout the dinner. When finished eating the beef, serve the remaining vegetable soup in bowls.

### Zesty Cold Tomato Soup

Blend until smooth: about 12 ounces of fresh or canned peeled whole tomatoes, 2 carrots, 1 to 2 cloves of garlic, ½ small onion, and fresh basil leaves. Add salt and spice to taste. Serve with a topping of sour cream, diced avocado, and sprigs of fresh cilantro.

### Cold Cucumber Soup

Peel off the skin from 1 to 3 cucumbers (and/or zucchini) with the mandolin slicer to make julienne strips. Set aside for a separate salad. Blend remaining whole cucumbers with olive oil, fresh garlic, sea salt, and fresh dill. Top with sour cream, fresh dill leaves, and/or slices of avocado.

### Raw Carrot Soup

Blend well: carrots, vegetable broth, ginger, small amount of stewed tomato, peeled cucumber, curry, and sea salt. Serve cold. This recipe also works well with cooked carrots and may be served hot.

### Mushroom Soup

Sauté favorite mushrooms in duck fat (see Roast Duck below), olive oil, or butter, with onions or leeks. Salt to taste. Blend until desired consistency, chunky or smooth—you may need to add broth. Top with thin slices of fresh mushrooms.

### Lentil Soup

Soak dried lentils for two days, rinsing thoroughly twice daily. Cook for thirty minutes or until just tender. Sauté onions, garlic, ginger, and carrots in olive oil, and season with curry, cardamom, chili, and cayenne pepper to taste. Add lentils and ½ cup unsweetened coconut milk, and simmer until flavors are richly mixed. Serve with fresh cilantro, grated coconut, chopped walnuts, and fine-chopped dates.

### Butternut Squash Soup

Cut butternut squash into large pieces, removing the seeds. When tender, cool and remove the skin. Puree in blender with unsalted butter and some of the remaining water to desired consistency. Add sea salt to taste. Variations include using coconut milk and curry or other spices such as cayenne pepper or cinnamon. Top with cilantro leaves or fresh parsley, tarragon, toasted shredded coconut, browned thin slices of garlic, or caramelized onions.

### Egg Drop Soup

Heat chicken broth in a wide saucepan or skillet to just before boiling. Turn off heat and slowly drop in raw eggs (whole or lightly beaten) while slowly mixing the soup (use 1 or 2 eggs per serving). Serve in a bowl with chopped fresh spinach. Top with Parmesan cheese and salt to taste. This also makes a wonderful wintertime breakfast.

### Chicken or Turkey Soup

Simmer your favorite whole bird in salted water until almost done. Cool and remove bones and strain unwanted debris. Add chopped onions, zucchini, kale, spinach, carrots, peas, or other available vegetables and simmer until done. Season with salt and your favorite spices. Try cinnamon, cloves, cayenne pepper, and so forth. Stir in some sour cream or yogurt for a creamy variation.

### Pork and Ginger Soup

Brown ground pork with chopped ginger, garlic, and cabbage until done. Season with a bit of wheat-free soy sauce and salt to taste. Top with sesame seeds, cilantro, spring onions, or scrambled egg. Fresh mung bean sprouts add a terrific crunch to this flavorful Asian-style soup.

## Vegetables

Vegetables should be the bulk of most meals. From a simple dish such as steamed broccoli to fancy fare such as spinach soufflé, vegetables should be a healthy and delicious part of meals and even snacks.

### Acorn Squash

Carefully cut squash crosswise, scoop out seeds and trim ends slightly to create a flat bottom. Bake in a pan with large end down with about a ¼ inch of water at 350°F for about 15 minutes. Turn over, add a small amount of butter to the squash, and continue baking until soft. Option: Fill with sautéed diced apples, raisins, walnuts or pecans, and cinnamon in butter.

### Artichokes

Select large bright-green artichokes with the leaves tightly held together. Cut the thorny tips off with scissors. Slice down the center and through the stem, or boil whole in water and olive oil until leaves easily tear off. Serve hot or cold with garlic, salt and butter, and olive oil as the dip. (The thorny inside hairs of the artichoke heart can be easily scooped out with a spoon.)

### Asparagus

Buy in season or frozen; otherwise this vegetable can be very expensive. Spears should feel crisp and not limp. Cut or snap off the white ends (they tend to be woody and tough). Steam lightly and serve with a butter sauce. Or brush with olive oil and place a single layer on a baking sheet and broil until bright green. Leftover asparagus is great in soups or chopped egg dishes.

### Bok Choy

Baby Bok Choy is most tender and is becoming very popular and inexpensive in some Asian supermarkets. Remove the white tough stem from the green leaves. Sauté the chopped stem at a low temperature in olive oil, then add the chopped green leaves and stir until just barely wilted. Bok Choy is also great in soups.

### Broccoli or Cauliflower Soufflé

Cut or peel the tough broccoli stems and steam (or, cut a head of cauliflower in quarters and steam). In a blender, combine 4 eggs, salt, and 2 to 4 ounces of white cheddar or Swiss for the broccoli (or soft goat cheese for cauliflower). Pour into buttered pan and place in another pan of water to prevent browning. Bake at 350°F for 30–45 minutes.

### Broccoli

Buy heads that have tight florets and are bright green. Cut off heads, lightly steam, and serve with a butter sauce. They're also great with a garlic sauce or cold in salads. Save the stems and peel for soups by dicing them (like celery or potatoes). Leftover broccoli can be chopped and used in an egg frittata, soups, or other dishes.

### Brussels Sprouts

Clean and halve brussels sprouts (or keep the smaller ones whole). Lightly steam until just tender. Serve plain or with a butter sauce. Option: make a dressing of raw sesame oil, wheat-free soy sauce, grated ginger, and garlic, and sprinkle with raw sesame seeds.

### Butternut Squash

Cut lengthwise and remove the seeds. Steam until tender and remove skin. Mash with butter as vegetable side dish.

### Cabbage

Thinly slice or shred cabbage. Use raw for salads or toss with apple cider vinegar and salt for coleslaw (marinate for a day or two in refrigerator). For a side dish, sauté on low heat with olive oil and add ground caraway seeds, butter, and sea salt.

### Cauliflower Mashed "Potatoes"

Lightly steam cauliflower, mix in food processor with a small amount of butter, heavy cream, and sea salt. It can also be mixed by hand. It should be the consistency of mashed potatoes. Top with chopped chives or parsley, sour cream, or cheese.

### Eggplant Dip (Baba Ghanoush)

Cube eggplant and sauté in olive oil, whole garlic, and salt until soft. Blend with 2 tablespoons tahini, 1 tablespoon lemon juice, and basil (dried or fresh). If too thick, add more olive oil. Eat as is, use on flax crackers, as a sauce for meat, or with salads. It's delicious warm or cold.

### Grilled Eggplant

Slice the neck of the eggplant crosswise in quarter to half-inch slices, salt, and dehydrate in a covered strainer for a couple days. (Save the seedy section of the eggplant for other dishes, such as baba ghanoush.) Brush both sides with olive oil and sprinkle with salt. Grill to desired doneness. Serve hot off the grill or cold the next day. For a side dish add crumbled goat cheese and olive oil, or top with tomato sauce and ricotta cheese. It's also great as a base for lasagna in place of pasta.

### Green Peas

Frozen organic tender peas can be used for many dishes. They can be quickly warmed and served with butter, or served with mashed cauliflower (above). Leftover peas can be added to salads. Cooked peas can be whipped with olive oil for use in a soufflé. For an Indian dish, combine cooked peas with unsweetened coconut milk, ginger, garlic, and curry.

### Kale and Garlic

Steam chopped kale and set aside. Sauté thinly sliced garlic in coconut oil until crispy. Pour over kale and salt to taste.

### Leeks

Buy leeks with fresh-looking green tops. Thinly sliced leeks are incredibly versatile and can be caramelized in butter or olive oil, added to soups, and served alone or on the side of baked chicken or other meats.

### Mushroom Paté

Sauté mushrooms, onions, and whole garlic in duck fat (or butter) until soft. Remove from heat. Add coarsely ground pecans, cashews, and/or walnuts, sea salt, and favorite herbs. Blend in food processor to desired consistency and store in a pan refrigerated. This is great warm and cold.

### Roasted Fennel

Buy fennel that is firm and not wilted. The tops are great cooked in soups and raw in salads (see above). The bulbs of fennel can be sliced thin and served raw. For roasted fennel, cut the bulb into quarters, lightly steam, and then slow roast in a pan with olive oil and salt. For an Italian-style dish, serve roasted fennel with roasted red peppers, cherry tomatoes, and grilled eggplant or zucchini.

### Snap peas

Buy in season. They should be crisp and without brown spots. Snap peas are great raw in salads. They can also be slightly steamed or very quickly sautéed in olive oil.

### Spaghetti Squash

Cut crosswise, remove seeds, and steam until just slightly tender. Larger squash may have to be quartered. When cool, use a fork to gently pull out the spaghetti-like threads. This is great just with butter and salt. Or use like spaghetti as the base for a tomato or meat sauce, or in any other dish.

### Spinach

Baby spinach is best as a salad served with crumbled boiled eggs and thinly sliced onions. Or try it with strawberries, apples, or pears, with walnuts or pecans. Larger leaves of spinach can be chopped, lightly steamed, and served with a butter sauce. It's also great in soups, made into a soufflé (below), and used in many other dishes.

### Spinach Soufflé

Steam about 1 pound of fresh spinach, drain (save the water for soup), combine with 2 eggs, salt, 2 ounces mozzarella or cheddar cheese, and blend well. Bake in buttered dish (placed in another dish with small amount of water) at 350°F for 30 minutes (or until solid).

Option: Combine with a carrot soufflé. Follow the same recipe except substitute 2 medium carrots for spinach and add curry powder. Pour carrot mixture into dish first then carefully pour the uncooked spinach soufflé on top. Bake as above until firm.

### String Beans

Buy crisp young string beans. Snap or cut off ends. Flash sauté in olive oil keeping them crisp. They go well with toasted pine nuts, sautéed onions and garlic, a dash of sesame seeds, and very lightly tossed in raw sesame oil.

### Turnips

Young small turnips may be peeled, sliced, and served raw as part of a salad. Cooked turnips may be whipped and served like mashed potatoes. Roasted turnips are great with a pot roast, along with carrots and other root vegetables.

### Watercress

Fresh watercress is great raw in salads. Watercress is delicious when lightly sautéed in olive oil with a dash of salt. It makes a great dish with sliced roast beef.

## Zucchini

Choose smaller-size zucchini for dicing or julienning. Use larger zucchini for stuffing, baking, or grilling. Flash sauté julienned zucchini and then add a mixture of beaten eggs and cheese to make a delicious frittata. Turn once and lightly salt. Diced zucchini is also great when added to lightly sautéed chopped onions and garlic. Slice larger zucchini in long flat strips to grill outdoors or on stovetop iron grill. Align across the grooves in the grill to create dark stripes going across the length of the zucchini. Brush lightly with olive oil. Very large zucchini are great stuffed and baked. Cut lengthwise, scoop out center, and mix with sautéed onions, garlic, and ground meat or cheese. Replace the stuffing in the center of the zucchini boats and bake at 450°F until tender. (If the zucchini is very hard it should be slightly steamed before baking.)

# Breakfast Ideas

## No-Crust Quiche

Beat 12 eggs and 1 cup heavy cream until foamy. Stir in 1½ cups raw sheep or goat cheese, ½ cup cherry tomatoes halved, 1½ cup spinach, and season with sea salt. Pour into well-buttered pie plate and bake 30–40 minutes in a preheated oven at 350°F or until middle is set but still moist; do not overbake. Serve warm or cool. Add less cheese, more vegetables, or other variations.

## Wheat-Free Oven Pancakes or Waffles

In a good blender, place ⅓ to ⅔ cup ground almonds, 3 to 4 eggs, 1 medium apple, ½ teaspoon of psyllium powder, ½ teaspoon salt, and blend until smooth. Pour into buttered pan and place in 400°F oven for 25 minutes or until firm. Option: Top with berries or sliced fruit before baking. For waffles, simply use a well-buttered waffle iron. These waffles store well in the refrigerator or freezer.

A note on maple syrup: Avoid it. It's a very high-glycemic sugar. If a mild sweetener is needed, use a small amount of honey or prepare your own "syrup" by mixing honey with blueberries or other fruit. Or combine honey and berries with a very small amount of water in a saucepan and heat briefly.

# Lunch and Dinner Entrees

## Fish Marinade

Cut fresh wild salmon or dark tuna in ½-inch strips or keep whole. Marinate overnight in rice-wine vinegar, grated ginger, sesame oil, wheat-free soy sauce, and sliced scallions. Lightly sauté the fish and serve on a bed of greens.

## Baked Ocean Perch

Place ocean perch (or other small white fish like wild trout) in baking dish with crushed garlic, sliced lemon, and olive oil, with a very small amount of water. Cover and bake at 450°F for 10–15 minutes.

### Vegetable Spaghetti

Squash can be a great addition to a healthy meal, and it can be used in place of pasta. Below are some recipes that can include zucchini, yellow, and spaghetti squash.

### Wild Salmon Alfredo

Cut slightly cooked salmon (steamed is easy) into small pieces, or use smoked salmon. Add a few tablespoons heavy cream. Slowly heat to a simmer. Pour on top of cooked spaghetti squash or raw spiral-cut zucchini or yellow squash. Sprinkle with Parmesan cheese. (If you use smoked salmon, do not add salt.)

### Vegetable Spaghetti with Tomato Sauce

In a spiral vegetable slicer, prepare raw zucchini or small yellow squash. Or use cooked spaghetti squash. Lightly salt and top with hot tomato or meat sauce. Sprinkle with grated hard cheese. Option: add sliced pimento green olives.

### Zucchini or Grilled Eggplant Lasagna

In a buttered baking dish, add sliced medium-size zucchini or eggplant (both should be grilled or steamed). Add a layer of tomato or meat sauce, then ricotta, another zucchini/eggplant layer, and top with tomato sauce and grated cheese. Bake at 375°F for about 20 minutes or until desired tenderness. Very nice when baked and served in individual-size baking dishes.

### Lamb Patties

Combine fresh ground lamb with chopped onions, walnuts, mint leaves, and salt. Form into small patties and sauté over medium heat. Remove the lamb patties from the pan and mix 2 teaspoons sour cream into the pan to make a gravy topping. Options: cucumber-yogurt topping. Lamb patties are also great grilled or steamed. For a great wrap, serve patties in steamed cabbage leaves or crispy Romaine lettuce. To steam cabbage leaves, cut cabbage in half, remove the core, place flat side down in a covered pot with about a ½ inch of water, and steam until tender. Sliced tomatoes, grilled Haloumi, mint leaves, and even kiwi slices are terrific in this tasty combination of flavors.

### Grilled Lamb Tenderloins

Lightly grill lamb, then serve topped with mint pesto made by blending fresh mint leaves, garlic, olive oil, lemon juice, walnuts, and salt.

### Roast Duck

Pierce the duck's skin all over with a sharp knife and salt generously. Place in large pot with 1 to 2 quarts of water (covering about half the duck). Boil 90 minutes to 2 hours depending on size. After boiling, remove duck and save water. Place duck in oven and roast for 90 minutes at 350 to 400°F or until skin is brown and crispy. Serve with cherry sauce or cilantro and toasted pine nuts.

### Seared Tuna

Marinate tuna in wheat-free tamari, ginger, wasabi, green onions, and honey. Sear tuna lightly on grill. Serve with sautéed ginger and onions.

### Turkey

Follow the recipe for Roast Duck, but do not pierce the skin before boiling.

### Meat Loaf

Thoroughly mix freshly ground beef with about 1 cup finely chopped vegetables (zucchini, kale, spinach, carrots, etc.), 3 to 4 stewed tomatoes, 1 chopped yellow onion, and 4 eggs. Bake at 350°F for about 60–90 minutes. (This is a very moist meat loaf and looks pink inside, so check temperature to make sure it has reached 180°F.)

### Shepherd's Pie

Use the Cauliflower Mashed "Potatoes" and Meat Loaf recipes listed above. In a shallow baking dish cover cooked meatloaf with a layer of mashed cauliflower and top with Parmesan cheese. Bake until hot and cheese melts and browns slightly. (Single-serving baking dishes work great for this recipe.)

### Crispy Cheese Shell

Shred or thinly slice organic mozzarella cheese. Spread it out on a buttered flat pan, in whatever shape you want. Broil until it starts to brown. Let cool slightly and cut into chips or use as a taco shell (it will become solid if allowed to cool completely). Option: use a large lettuce leaf as a wrap, adding the cheese shell on the inside with guacamole, meat, tomatoes, salsa, and others.

## SHOPPING TIPS FOR HEALTHY EATING

The most important first step you can take for better dietary habits is to learn to properly shop for the food items that will bring about the greatest health. Bad food has less of a chance of getting into your body if it never gets into your grocery cart. With a little thought, planning, and effort, you can make sure only healthy items get into your home.

Taking the time to plan a few days or a week's worth of meals is necessary. Plan your shopping trip before you leave home to prevent multiple trips to the grocery store. And shop only after you have eaten a healthy meal, so your blood sugar is optimal and you're not craving sweets. Make a list and decide where you will shop. If you are limited to one stop, pick the store that reliably has the most items on your list. Many cities have health food supermarkets and even many of the larger chain grocery stores carry higher-quality foods, such as organic produce, meats, and eggs.

In most grocery stores, the healthiest items are found on the store's perimeter. The first stop is the produce section. Choose a variety of fresh greens, vegetables, fruits, and avoid starchy potatoes and corn. Once again, look for organic produce, especially if you are buying apples, bell peppers, celery, cherries, imported grapes, nectarines, peaches, pears, raspberries, spinach, and strawberries, as these crops have consistently been shown to harbor higher pesticide levels. The produce that consistently has the lowest levels of pesticides includes asparagus, avocados, small bananas, broccoli, cauliflower, kiwi, mangos, onions, papaya, and sweet peas.

Minimize the high-glycemic fruits such as pineapple and large watermelon. A traditional athlete's food is bananas, but avoid the large ones, as they are also high-glycemic. Instead, find the smallest bananas and eat them only when ripe (no longer green, with small black speckles). Always choose a variety of fruits: apples, grapefruits, and especially phytonutrient-rich berries. Always try to buy smaller quantities of a large variety of fruits and vegetables. Fill your grocery cart with a rainbow of colors—eggplant, blueberries, purple onions and cabbage, red peppers, radishes, tomatoes, butternut and yellow squash, carrots, zucchini, cucumbers, herbs, dark greens, and so forth. The more color, the more nutrients.

Your athletic body needs protein, so the next stop is the meat, eggs, and dairy section. Seek out organic animal products, or those that are truly "natural"—indicated by a label that says the animals were not given antibiotics, growth hormones, or animal by-product feeds. Organic grass-fed beef and lamb, pasture-raised pork, free-range poultry, and wild-caught ocean fish are the best choices. Many of these foods are now available organically in bulk through mail-order outlets. In general, avoid any processed meats and fish since many contain sugar, additives, and preservatives such as BHT and sodium nitrite. Most stores now carry organic eggs. They cost a little more but are still a protein bargain. Minimize the use of dairy products. If you use them, then select organic heavy cream, whole milk, sheep or goat milk products, unsalted butter, and unprocessed cheeses.

If you stick to the perimeter of the store, avoiding the bakery section, you'll find that you only rarely need to venture up an aisle for food items. The exceptions may be extra virgin olive oil, raw unfiltered honey, beans, nuts, nut butters, and spices. Buy as few items in packages as possible. If you do buy items in packages, always be sure to read the label and study the list of ingredients and nutritional facts. If you can't identify or pronounce the ingredients, chances are high that these packaged foods should be avoided.

# TIPS FOR HEALTHY COOKING

How you cook your healthy food is important, since even the best-tasting, healthiest ingredients can be ruined through improper kitchen practices. The biggest problems are overcooking, using too-high heat, and overheating certain types of oils. Consider the following guidelines:

- Meats, fish, and poultry can be oven- or pan-roasted, quickly grilled, and often cooked in their own juices. Fish is especially healthy when lightly steamed or poached and, when fresh and wild, can be eaten raw. Less oil or butter is needed for pan-cooking meats because they often contain their own fats. It's also important to avoid using high heat for too long. For instance when grilling a steak or lamb, trim off as much fat as possible and turn it every minute or so to prevent the excess formation of chemicals that can be harmful to your health. When you are grilling vegetables, turn them often as well. Ground meat should be bought fresh and cooked thoroughly as soon as possible. Many meat departments grind meat in the morning, so buy ground meats early in the day and cook or freeze them right away.

- The worst method for cooking is deep fat or high-heat frying using vegetable oils. While many healthy foods may be lightly sautéed in butter or olive oil, deep-frying overheats the oil and can be very dangerous to your health. In addition, the high heat may destroy other nutrients in the food itself. Coconut oil or organic lard is also acceptable when medium to higher heat sautéing.

- Vegetables can be steamed, stir-fried in olive oil, roasted, baked, or grilled. Cook vegetables minimally to avoid destroying nutrients—they also taste better when not overcooked. If boiling or steaming, use as little water as possible to avoid the loss of nutrients through the water. Slow-cooked vegetable stews will contain much of the minerals and heat-resistant vitamins in the liquid while some heat-sensitive vitamins will be lost. Don't throw out the water from your steamed vegetables. Either drink it or use it for a soup base or in a smoothie.

- Eggs can be soft- or hard-boiled, or cooked sunny-side up, over-easy, poached, or lightly scrambled. Letting the yolk remain soft is not only tastier but is healthier because heat-sensitive compounds are retained. Make sure the egg white cooks slightly because it's better for the intestines.

- Use monounsaturated and saturated fats for cooking as they are not sensitive to heat. Coconut oil and butter are the safest fats for cooking, followed by olive oil, lard, and duck fat; the last three contain some polyunsaturated fats so care should be taken to not heat too high. Most other fats are high in polyunsaturated oils and very prone to oxidizing when exposed to heat, producing free radicals—avoid corn, safflower, sesame, peanut, and canola oils.

## TIPS FOR EATING OUT OR WHEN TRAVELING

Dining out can be very enjoyable, and for many athletes is quite common. However, these meals should be as healthy as the ones you prepare at home; otherwise it is not worth it. Avoid restaurant chains as most use high amounts of processed and prepared foods. Don't hesitate to ask the appropriate questions about what's in the food—the oils used, any added flour or sugar, and so on. It takes more time, but you're more likely to get the food you want and avoid the food you don't want. Ask for vegetables instead of the starches or bread and fresh fruit for dessert.

While you may plan ahead and take care to have healthy meals, there's a real possibility that in the course of life you may get caught somewhere in your travels and need to find something to eat. Instead of a fast-food place, look for a grocery store or deli where you should be able to find ready-to-eat fruit, salads, carrot sticks, nuts, and the like. For some athletes, going without food until getting home may be more stressful than eating bad food but there should be options almost anywhere.

Many times, unexpected delays or changes in schedules force you to make this unsavory decision. Here are some travel tips for eating:

- Plan ahead. If you think about lunch the evening before you find yourself hungry and driving past "fast-food alley" you'll know where you're going to get a meal—from a small cooler of food you've packed.
- For a long drive or a day on the road, bring food in your car, on the train or plane, or whatever you are traveling in. An appropriate-size cooler is important.

- If you're going to a familiar location, know where the healthy stores or restaurants are located. Keep a log of these locations if you plan on visiting the same place again. Get a take-out menu from the restaurant and keep it in your car or at home for easy reference.
- If staying in hotels, choose those that have a refrigerator (ask when making your reservation). Bring your own food or buy it when you get there.
- If you find a healthy restaurant, order more than you'll eat and bring leftovers back to your room for later snacks or meals.
- Have some basic utensils in your suitcase at all times: plastic forks, knives, and spoons. Or, order room service the first day and rinse and save the utensils. Travel with plates and bowls as needed, or find hotels that have cooking facilities. Always carry a pocketknife.
- A coffee pot is not only useful for coffee and tea but also for heating food.
- Carry water with you. If you're on the road for more than a day or two, bring a small portable water filter to replenish your water bottle. Many stores carry bottled water.

# PERSONAL NOTES

*Photo credit: Timothy Carlson*

# The Importance of Self-Care and Injury Prevention

# CHAPTER 23

# ANATOMY OF AN INJURY—
## Physical, Chemical, and Mental

**E**very athlete's worse nightmare is to become injured. And yet many athletes believe injury is part of the game. While this may be true in contact sports such as football and boxing, this type of trauma typically does not occur in most endurance sports. Serious bike accidents are a noticeable exception, but usually, for endurance athletes, an injury means something went wrong with their body. As such, most injuries are preventable.

The big picture begins with the simple question, what really is an injury?

Most of us have grown up with a very simplistic view of an injury; you overwork part of your body and it gets hurt. For the endurance athlete, an injury should never happen. Even twisting an ankle on a rugged trail run may occur because of some preexisting imbalance in your physical, chemical, or mental fitness and health.

I categorize athletic injuries as three basic types: physical, chemical, and mental injuries. While they overlap most of the time, I will discuss each separately. Let's dissect a typical injury to find out where injuries come from.

# The Physical Injury

You wake up and prepare for your morning workout, and as you bend down to put on your running shoes you feel a little twinge in your right hamstring. Nothing more than that and you think little of it. But several days later, there it is again, now a bit more prominent. And that evening, the twinge has become more than an annoyance and is now beginning to hurt. The next day's workout is hindered, and by the following week, you are feeling real pain. Now your hip doesn't seem to move right and your knee is throbbing. After another week, all the pain has settled around the knee. You recall no trauma, your shoes seem good, and you've not changed training routines.

This "domino effect" takes place regularly in millions of athletes throughout the world. An injury begins from some seemingly benign event and evolves into real impairment. But there's logic to your body. A progression such as the one just described is not random. An injury is, with some exceptions, simply an end result of a series of dominoes falling over. One little, innocuous problem affects something else, and the dominoes start to tumble. After a half-dozen or so dominoes have fallen, a symptom—pain, dysfunction, feeling of lost power—occurs in response.

Let's go back to our "typical" pattern of injury and use knee pain as the end result. This is one of the most common injuries in endurance athletes. From a professional standpoint, there are two views when confronted with a knee problem.

## Traditional Injury Philosophy

The traditional view, and in recent decades the more popular approach, attempts to name the condition. If the pain is more lateral and especially a bit above the knee joint, it may be called "iliotibial band syndrome." If it's just below the knee and in the front, especially in a younger athlete, it may be called "Osgood-Schlatter." And if the pain is more medial, on the inner side of the knee, it may be referred to as a meniscus problem. While these conditions, especially the latter two, are real and serious, and sometimes do occur, even when these conditions are ruled out, their names are sometimes still casually used. This senseless attempt to name these symptoms tells nothing of how the problem occurred (what caused it), how to correct it, and how to prevent it from returning once it is corrected.

This approach also assumes, for example, that each "bursitis" is exactly the same, or every "tendinitis" is identical. Furthermore, modern medicine too often has an off-the-shelf treatment for each name—from rest to stretching, heat to cold, from anti-inflammatory drugs to surgery. (The exception, of course, is when you are in a "first-aid" state, such as from a serious fall. In this case, none of what I'm discussing applies. Instead, I am referring to the more common chronic injury that most endurance athletes develop.)

The most indefensible aspect of this cookbook approach is the fact that many professionals know what they're going to do to you and your injury before they even see you. They merely come up with, or look up, the name of your problem to find your remedy. It's a classic case of treating the symptom and ignoring the cause—not to mention the athlete.

### The Holistic Philosophy

The alternative view is to look at the whole athlete. And much like a detective, it's important to piece together the circumstances that led to the injury and accompanying symptom(s). A variety of clues may provide vital information on how the problem was created, and therefore how to avoid it in the future and how to correct the real cause of the problem. With this approach, each athlete is seen as a unique individual with specific needs that are most appropriate for his or her precise condition. Anything less tailored to the individual is an insult to the human body.

So just how does the symptom of, say, knee pain in a runner evolve? Of course, the same knee pain in a dozen runners could easily have a dozen different patterns. But let's go back to the example of the runner putting on his shoe in the morning. That twinge in the right hamstring muscle is not the beginning of the problem. The first domino fell, perhaps, long before this first manifestation, possibly months earlier.

Perhaps it was the left foot—the opposite side of the eventual symptomatic knee—that underwent micro-trauma due to the shoe not fitting properly. This common problem results in biomechanical stress in the left foot and ankle. While this produced no symptoms, it did affect, in a very adverse way, the mechanics of the left ankle. As is often the case in the body, this type of physical stress causes the brain to sense the problem and adapt to it. In this situation, perhaps compensation takes place through the bones and muscles in the pelvis. Specifically, the pelvis tilted to modify its movement so that weight bearing decreased on the side of stress to help it heal and increased on the opposite side—where the symptom will eventually take place. But not yet.

The increased weight bearing on the right side—something that is usually measurable by standing on two scales—may cause some of the muscles in the thigh to become overworked. This compensation is also associated with the gait change resulting from the tilt in the pelvis. Due to the shifting of body weight and the physical stress in the pelvis, the quadriceps muscles may, through an unsuccessful attempt at this compensation, become abnormally inhibited, or weak. And finally, related muscles on the back of the thigh—the right hamstrings—compensate for the quadriceps problem by tightening. Bending forward to put on the right shoe requires the hamstrings to stretch. But when these muscles are too tight, even a normal stretch can cause trauma resulting in slight micro-tearing. This is what produces that slight twinge.

So what could we propose as therapy for our knee-pained athlete? Anti-inflammatory drugs? Ice the knee? The answer is obvious now that the whole picture is apparent. Find and correct the cause of the problem. In this particular case, the first domino to fall was an ill-fitting shoe on the left foot. (Of course, this doesn't mean that all knee problems are the result of shoes.) Whether all the dominoes will line up on their own if you pick up the first one depends on the athlete and how much damage was done. Generally, the body has a great natural ability to heal itself. And in many cases, especially in those who are more healthy, this is just what happens when the cause of the problem is corrected—all the dominoes line up and in a very short time the pain is gone. This means the muscle imbalances improve, the weight-bearing problem is eliminated, and any secondary inflammation is removed because now proper muscle balance allows the joints to move properly.

### Prevention

How can you avoid problems before they begin? Consider that many athletes, when questioned about their injuries, often comment about clues such as their shoes not fitting or something just not feeling normal in the foot or ankle. It may be a passing thought, a subconscious note. But it's there. In my years of private practice, conducting a careful and adequate oral history was one of the most important aspects of treating and training an athlete.

Learning how to accurately read your own body comes with time, but it is worth the effort. More importantly, when your body provides an obvious clue that something is not right, such as a hamstring twinge, it's time to stop and assess what's going on. If you don't take that first step, it may soon be too late. Waiting until you're physically unable to train—the point at which your body forces you to stop—just results in more unnecessary damage and wasted time.

At the same time, you don't want to become obsessed with every little feeling, real or not, that your body produces. It's important to consider the fact that many of the symptoms you feel, including those related to some significant imbalance, are self-corrected by your body, often before you realize it. Being able to observe this process and intervene at the appropriate time is an important part of self-care.

Physical injuries are also associated with chemical factors. The complex interaction with various body chemicals that control inflammation and anti-inflammation is one example. This is sometimes the primary injury, and so in addition to physical injuries, many athletes have chemical types.

## The Chemical Injury

You spend a significant amount of your time training and racing, plus juggling work, family, and your social life with your sport. Going for a ride is as common as going to bed at night. But now it's getting harder to get through the day due to fatigue. Training no longer energizes you like it used to. You're more irritable than ever. The few pounds you've gained, the first in some time, are probably due to your increasing appetite, which includes constant cravings for sweets. And you're on your fourth cold this year. If you could only sleep as well as you used to. "Luckily I'm not injured," you tell your training partners.

Well, my friend, you are injured. You have a chemical injury.

Chemical injuries typically don't produce pain like their physical counterparts, although some chemical imbalances associated with inflammation can be painful. More often, and by far the most common characteristic, a chemical injury makes you tired. Fatigue is a common complaint from athletes. Either the cause of the problem, or the fatigue itself, may in turn produce other chemical symptoms, with a pattern of falling dominoes like that described above. In addition to fatigue, our chemically injured athlete has irritability, increased weight gain, excessive hunger, frequent colds (chronic infection), and insomnia.

As with any injury, the first step is to rule out more serious conditions, such as anemia, serious infections, or immune disorders. This is often easily done with the help of a healthcare professional who might perform blood tests, take a proper history, and perform a physical exam.

Once serious problems or diseases are ruled out, more conservative methods can be considered after reviewing lifestyle and training factors. Perhaps the problem originated when the training schedule became too busy. It wasn't just the training log but all of life's time commitments that pushed this athlete over the edge. Our athlete was squeezing too much activity into an already too busy schedule. For many individuals, this upsets the body's ability to properly recover—not only from training but from all the day's activities. And as the months go by, a recuperative deficit builds up. Perhaps a better word is "stress." The body's adrenal system is designed to adapt and compensate for all this stress but sometimes the load is just too great.

So, let me piece together the possible events leading to this athlete's chemical injury. Perhaps it was some early success in racing that led our athlete to increase training for longer competitions. Undoubtedly, total workout times were not only increased but so was the intensity. With that came the added stress of rushing through meals and dashing from the office to a workout, then from the workout back home. Almost all athletes can relate to this scenario.

Initially, the adrenal glands tolerated the increased stress. After all, that's their job. But like a long event you're not trained for, the vicious cycle of work, family and social life, training, and racing got faster and more difficult to maintain. Soon, there was less time to do the things that needed to get done, and recovery was hindered. And because our athlete attempted to keep up with life's busy schedule, eventually the adrenal glands became less effective at dealing with all the stress. At this point, the training equation (Training = Work + Rest) is no longer balanced. Waking in the middle of the night with difficulty getting back to sleep, not an uncommon sign of adrenal stress, further reduces recovery.

With the adrenals not able to keep up, many other bodily functions begin to decline. The blood sugar becomes unstable, which may produce symptoms of fatigue. Also, as the brain is deprived of the sugar it needs, cravings and increased hunger follows. And not only is the brain sensitive to relatively small changes in blood sugar but the whole nervous system is affected. As such, irritability and mood swings may follow. Because of the influence the adrenal glands have on other hormone systems of the body, the athlete's metabolism can fall. This is due to elevations in the stress hormone cortisol, which reduces the hormones DHEA and testosterone. High levels of cortisol can wake you in the middle of the night, and cause your body to shift fuel usage by increasing sugar burning and reducing fat burning. This can result in more stored body fat, and perhaps weight gain, and coincide with decreased endurance. Now our athlete has to work harder to keep pace even in training. And race results become even more frustrating, contributing to more stress. Inevitably, hunger intensifies—typically for sugar and caffeine—and fatigue worsens; and the vicious cycle continues to maintain, and worsen, the chemical injury.

Excess adrenal stress is frequently accompanied by decreased immunity. With the body's defense system suppressed, colds and flu, and even allergies or asthma, become more common. Telltale signs include colds that last much more than three days or those that recur a month or two later.

Like any problem you encounter, correction first involves finding the origin. While many people seek relief of symptoms—such as consuming more caffeine to help get through the day—the real cause may linger unless you or a healthcare professional determines the cause.

By avoiding symptom treatments and addressing the cause of the problem, the resolution of a chemical injury is usually not far off. Additional nutritional support for our athlete may be necessary. This might include vitamin A for the immune system or zinc for the adrenals. But if the lifestyle schedule, which may have created the original stress, is not modified, any nutritional remedy won't be successful, as problems can continually recur somewhere in the person's chemistry—either the same set of symptoms or a gathering set of new ones.

In addition to all the signs and symptoms associated with this athletes' chemical injury, these imbalances may cause other dominoes to fall that lead to secondary physical symptoms. They could even trigger a series of problems much like those described above for the physical injury. A common example of a combined chemical and physical problem is chronic inflammation. Joint pain is typically the combination of a physical muscle imbalance not allowing the joint to move normally, and the eventual chemical response to that impaired movement—inflammation. Hence, because both chemical and physical injuries enlist the actions of the brain and nervous system, there's a risk that these problems will also affect one's mental state.

## The Mental Injury

A physical or chemical injury can easily trigger a mental or emotional impairment of some type. When we think of mental problems, visions of psychological tension and emotional instability come to mind. But we should distinguish the mental state from the psychological and realize that many athletes struggle with mental and emotional distress but are psychologically stable. Stress affecting the brain, from the chemical or physical aspects of the body, can easily cause a mental injury. The problem is not uncommon in the athletic community.

Unlike a physical injury such as an aching Achilles tendon or sore knee, a mental injury is often invisible. Moreover, athletes will talk freely about their aches and pains, but when it comes to discussing their true mental or emotional state, they tend to stay mute. It's like some kind of unwritten law within the athletic community. The social stigma is that athletes are tough, and immune to mental and emotional harm. (This is especially true of the word "stress," which, according to some, implies mental weakness. I've been asked by professional athletes, and sometimes even by team management honchos, to not use the word "stress," especially with the media, because it imparts an image of lack of self-control on the part of the athlete.)

All these ideas of mental and emotional stress being a sign of weakness, of course, are myths. In fact, athletes are as vulnerable to stress and to mental and emotional injury as anyone else. What makes an athlete tough and able to endure is optimal balance of fitness and health.

Let's consider the case of a former patient of mine whom I will call Robert. A talented twenty-nine-year-old triathlete, he was in his third year of great racing. His training never felt better, and in a triathlon he was nearly unbeatable. Always full of energy, and without injury, Robert was climbing the ladder to national success.

But then Robert became increasingly anxious about competition. He dreaded showing up on race morning. He had not only lost his desire to train or race, but his personal life was being affected as well.

What was happening to Robert in the absence of disease? He was experiencing a functional imbalance in the brain's chemistry—a subtle yet noticeable change in certain neurotransmitters that can chemically modify the way one thinks, feels, and acts. Fortunately for Robert and others, with few exceptions, these problems are reversible and, more importantly, preventable. Normally, when you think a thought or perceive a sensation from the outside world, it's the result of major chemical reactions in the brain. Billions of messages are sent throughout the brain and body on a regular basis by chemicals called neurotransmitters. Different neurotransmitters in the brain make you feel certain ways: high, low, sleepy, awake, happy, or sad. Sometimes the brain may have too many of one type of chemical or not enough of another. As a result, you may feel too high or too low, agitated or depressed.

There are dozens of types of neurotransmitters in our brains and elsewhere in our bodies, especially the intestines. These neurotransmitters are vital for relaying messages throughout the brain and body. Some of our important neurotransmitters are made in the body from amino acids derived from dietary protein, and once produced, they are often influenced by the amount of dietary carbohydrates we consume via the hormone insulin.

Two important examples of neurotransmitters that can significantly influence our mental and emotional state are serotonin and norepinephrine. Serotonin is produced with the help of the amino acid tryptophan and functions with the help of insulin. This neurotransmitter has a calming, sedating, or depressing effect in the brain. A high-carbohydrate meal, such as pasta or oatmeal, or eating sweets, results in more serotonin production. An individual who is overactive may benefit from a natural high-carbohydrate meal, but the same meal in those who are a bit mentally low may get worse, even to the point of depression. Sweets are traditionally thought of as providing energy, but for the brain they are sedating. Go to a nice hotel and you'll find some type of sweet treat on your pillow— that's because sugar usually helps you sleep. (Sometimes, sweets may give the feeling of a pick-up but that is very short-lived.)

In Robert's case, the overproduction of serotonin—a common problem even in athletes—may have helped establish his mental injury. This would have corresponded to his high intake of refined carbohydrates, and as he progressed into his mental injury, his craving for more sugar further worsened his problem.

Norepinephrine is another neurotransmitter produced with the help of the amino acid tyrosine—but only in the presence of normal levels of insulin. A high-protein meal with little or no high- or moderate-glycemic carbohydrates will provide the brain with increased norepinephrine levels. This neurotransmitter has a stimulating effect on the brain. The person who needs a mental pick-up or is depressed could often benefit from more of this brain chemical. If you're taking a class, have an important meeting, or are driving your car, you want more of

## DRUGS AND DIET FOR MENTAL INJURIES

Certain drugs are sometimes recommended for patients with chemical imbalances because they manipulate brain chemistry in an attempt to balance neurotransmitters. The depressed athlete may be given medication to enhance or block certain neurotransmitters. Prozac, Wellbutrin, Effexor, and Celexa are examples of antidepressants that affect the balance of serotonin and norepinephrine, thereby changing the way you feel. (Tranquilizers, such as Valium and Ativan, function other ways through different neurotransmitters.)

Most people don't need antidepressants. But these drugs are among the most prescribed in the United States, with well over 100 million prescriptions a year! That's even more than drugs prescribed to lower cholesterol and blood pressure. In those patients who are considered for antidepressants, conservative measures should be tried first; improving diet and lifestyle factors can often resolve a mental injury.

But with drug manufacturers openly advertising antidepressants, which results in many patients asking for antidepressants, and too many health-care professionals

this neurotransmitter and less serotonin so your attention is high and you don't doze off. A protein meal or snack without refined carbohydrates can be key. But the relationship between food and neurotransmitters is very sensitive—even eating a single meal of high carbohydrates can quickly change your brain chemistry in the wrong way, resulting in dozing off after lunch or getting sleepy during a long drive.

An imbalance in serotonin and norepinephrine—with a shift toward the former—may produce more feelings of depression. Perhaps Robert was eating too many sweets and other carbohydrates, which increased serotonin and made him more depressed. Upon careful questioning, he noted that he became very sleepy after lunch and couldn't concentrate on his work very well.

Fortunately, most people do not need medication, and Robert succeeded without it. His first step toward eliminating his mental injury was the Two-Week Test. In fact, after the first few days, he reported an 80 percent improvement in his mental state.

In addition to the way he ate, Robert's training, may also have contributed to his mental injury. Especially if he was overtrained, which can result in undue stress on his brain and emotional instability.

not taking the time to properly evaluate patients, the dramatic rise in the use of these drugs continues, and too often without success.

In 2010, *The Journal of the American Medical Association* published a study that called into question the efficacy of antidepressant drugs. While the research team, led by Jay C. Fournier and Robert J. DeRubeis of the University of Pennsylvania, acknowledged that the drugs make a positive difference in cases of severe depression, the study found that for most patients—those with mild to moderate cases—the most commonly used antidepressants are generally no better than a placebo. "The message for patients with mild to moderate depression," Dr. DeRubeis told *The New York Times*, is that "medications are always an option, but there's little evidence that they add to other efforts to shake the depression—whether it's exercise, seeing the doctor, reading about the disorder, or going for psychotherapy."

For those athletes with mild or moderate depression, especially those with symptoms associated with other mental injuries, making the right diet and lifestyle changes can often rapidly change the brain with dramatic improvements in mental health. If the diet can affect the mental state, then clearly certain nutritional supplements can

Overtraining is frequently preceded by too much anaerobic work. While we're familiar with the importance of lactic acid and anaerobic exercise, most have not heard of its adverse effect on the mental state. For a long time, scientists have known that increased lactic acid—more specifically, lactate—in the body may provoke depression, anxiety, and phobias. (Even the production of very high amounts of lactate by relatively normal subjects can produce anxiety, depression, and panic.) Given this, either Robert's high level of anaerobic activity produced too much lactic acid from training and racing, or he didn't have sufficient levels of nutrients for proper regulation of lactate.

Yet, was Robert training beyond his ability? Was he racing too much? More often it's a combination of actions. By sitting down together, Robert and I were able to assess each aspect of his life. Being objective was the hardest part for him. Accepting that there really was a problem was a difficult hill to climb. Making the appropriate changes, whatever they may be, can often result in a speedy remedy. In Robert's case, decreasing the amount of sugar and other high-glycemic carbohydrates in his diet, and increasing protein foods and balancing his training, helped get him out of his funk. Within a couple of weeks, or sooner, Robert was feeling significantly better, and within a do the same. That's because specific vitamins and minerals, along with the appropriate amino acids tryptophan and tyrosine, are required for the brain to make both serotonin and norepinephrine. Some of the more common ones include vitamin B6, folic acid, niacin, iron, and vitamin C. All these nutrients—except for tryptophan—are available over the counter. (Tryptophan was banned by the FDA in 1990 due to contaminated sources that made some people ill.)

However, before taking a dietary supplement, improving the quality of the diet is the first step, as this usually provides these nutrients.

The bottom line: Taking too many serotonin-precursor nutrients, including a high-carbohydrate diet, may contribute to a mental injury. Or another way to view the problem is that consuming a diet not very well balanced in these nutrients can cause an imbalance of neurotransmitters.

month his training also became noticeably improved. Two months later, his first race was dramatically better, and he would continue improving.

Injuries in the physical, chemical, and mental body can occur in any combination in any athlete. Sometimes it's a physical problem that appears first, and at other times a hidden chemical injury triggers a physical or mental one. In some, all three injuries are evident, the result of many dominoes falling throughout the body and brain—this is something that commonly exists in chronic overtraining.

In the vast majority of athletes, the resolution of an injury—fixing the problem—is relatively quick once the cause is found and properly addressed. The actual time frame of recovery depends on many factors, including whether one is seeing a health-care professional, addressing the problem oneself, and whether many changes are needed such as with one's diet, training, and stress management. Overall, most athletes should be resuming training and seeing improvements within a week or two once the problem is found, sometimes even after a day or two. At times, longer care may be needed, such as in the case of an athlete who is chronically overtrained or one who needs three months of aerobic base building.

# SUMMARY OF PHYSICAL, CHEMICAL, AND MENTAL INJURIES

## Physical injury:

- Physical impairment, such as muscle or joint problem.
- Common signs and symptoms include pain and loss of muscle power.
- Typical cause is muscle imbalance.

## Chemical injury:

- Impairment of body chemistry, including hormone and nutrient imbalance.
- Common signs and symptoms include fatigue and frequent illness.
- Typical causes include metabolic problems, especially hormone imbalance and poor diet.

## Mental injury:

- Impairment of brain function.
- Common symptoms include feelings of depression, reduced initiative, poor concentration.
- Typical causes include imbalance in brain chemistry (neurotransmitters) and excess carbohydrate intake.

# CHAPTER 24

# REHABILITATING AND SELF-ASSESSING YOUR PHYSICAL INJURY

**I** have never actually kept count of the number of athletic physical injuries I have treated in thirty years of private practice. That number is certainly well into the thousands. From my personal experience, the most common causes of injury are these three: over- and improper training, over-supported and improper footwear, and muscle imbalance. Fortunately, the majority of these injuries could be successfully treated, often with positive results of immediate relief while the athlete was still in my office. Other times, recovery took several days or weeks. I found that when a patient addressed certain lifestyle, fitness, and health needs, he or she would typically mend more quickly.

There are at least three ways the body can mend itself from a physical injury:

The first remedy is by the body itself. This occurs often and without you even consciously being aware of a problem or the body's correction. It could be that the problem is relatively minor and early in the process of a particular injury. This ongoing routine of healing yourself can be helped greatly by being as healthy as possible, enabling the body to best accomplish self-correction.

The second way to fix your own problem is by consciously taking some specific action based on clues by the body informing you that there's a problem—an aching joint, a painful muscle, or any number of signs and symptoms the body creates. These clues are very important to consider.

A third way to correct an injury is with the help of a health-care professional—the subject of this book's final chapter.

## Heal Thyself

The concept that the body can fix itself dates back to ancient times. From Chinese medicine to Hippocrates to modern science, it's well known that the body is continually repairing itself. Something as minor as a bruise, cut finger, or other common injury usually heals up quickly without need for medical assistance—unless it gets infected. The healthier you are, the better and faster you heal. This is another reason to not only be fit for better performance but healthy so your body takes better care to correct and prevent injuries and ill health, including better day-to-day recovery.

### The First Step

It's simple: Don't treat the name. Too often we want to affix a label to a symptom or condition. And then with that information, we rush to have the "name" treated instead of looking at underlying causes. This approach often comes up short because up to half of initial diagnoses are incorrect. In fact, assuming the serious medical problems have been ruled out and there's no need for first-aid care, such as surgery for a meniscus tear or a cast for a broken bone, most endurance-related problems are relatively minor and easy to correct. And they often don't have a name to attach except for what really is the cause, such as muscle imbalance.

While most injuries—95 percent or more—are of the less serious nature, there are still significant imbalances causing them. This also doesn't mean a minor problem won't cause pain or keep you from training—it can. Even a relatively minor muscle imbalance, for example, can be debilitating, and if not corrected by your body or a health-care professional, can potentially end your athletic career. Yes, even minor problems can lead to serious consequences—a common cause of frustration in athletes who sometimes go from one health-care professional to another without obtaining relief from a very painful condition.

Most injuries are *functional*, meaning that the problem is much less serious than say, a torn ligament, because the injury is without significant damage. For this reason, even extremely painful conditions can be resolved very quickly—sometimes during one visit to an appropriate healthcare professional. Or just changing shoes, when that's the primary cause of serious knee pain, can return the body to pain-free function by the next day. An analogy is your car not starting. It just might be due to a faulty battery contact or a spark plug that needs replacing. A good mechanic can make a repair in minutes; you certainly don't need a new engine. (This is not to say that all injuries can be corrected with one magic treatment by some sports doctor—they can't.)

Functional problems can often be soft-tissue injuries, such as simple muscle imbalances. These types of problems can be cured with more conservative measures and quite often by the athlete. Let's discuss what you can do to help your body correct its own problems. After all, that's what your body is supposed to do. And you will be pleased to know that most injuries also have simple remedies.

One problem with an injury is that it can restrict your training. Aerobic activity is very therapeutic: it improves blood flow and immune function, and significantly helps support bones and joints. Consequently, being unable to train can prevent your injury from self-correcting. So the first consideration is to find an aerobic activity that does not aggravate the problem, and do it. Walking is a great remedy if it doesn't hurt. Running in a pool is also effective—the shallow end of a pool will provide some but not too much gravity stress. Stationary equipment, such as a bike, sometimes works well, but it's important to make sure it's set up or adjusted to fit your body.

There's no need to spend the same amount of time performing these activities as your previous schedule; just maintain some level of activity that does not aggravate the injury—when in doubt, do less. This *active recovery* is powerful, so don't underestimate the benefits. Even a twenty-minute jog in the pool or a half-hour easy walk can stimulate the aerobic system providing many benefits for the body to correct problems. Consider these activities as a workout, and perform a warm-up and cool-down each time—even if the entire workout consists of warming up then cooling down! It's also most important to avoid stretching during this period, as discussed in section I. Many injuries are the result of over-stretched (weak) muscles, with tightness developing as a secondary problem. The combination of both is muscle imbalance.

If you are experiencing pain, use that uncomfortable sensation as your guide. Ask yourself: Does the workout lessen the pain? Not affect the pain? Worsen the pain? The best rule to follow regarding pain is that if it lessens as your workout progresses, it's generally a good sign. This is what will often happen if you already have a great aerobic base. (Of course, having a great aerobic base is one of the best ways to avoid injuries.)

If the pain isn't exacerbated following the activity—immediately or the next morning—that's a good sign, too. But if the pain gets worse with activity, avoid it. In this case, you can try another activity, one that is easier and lower in stress. This might include swimming.

An effective option is to take three days off and try to work out again. Occasionally, whenever an athlete could not get to my clinic, I would recommend that he or she take three days off as therapy. Most often, this "rest" approach is done before an injury has become extreme, especially during its early stages. This gives the body a chance to recover and possibly correct its own problems. Resumption of training should be cautious for about a week or two to make sure the problem does not recur.

I can't emphasize enough that both warming up and cooling down have significant therapeutic effects on your entire body—from your muscles to your metabolism. In many cases, lengthening your warm-up and cool-down time can also greatly help.

Keep all your workouts strictly aerobic until your injury heals. Be even more conservative with your exertion; train below your maximum aerobic heart rate. Avoid all weight lifting, anaerobic intervals, and other hard workouts, and of course competition.

## When Injury Strikes, It's Time to "Cool It!"

The therapeutic use of cold is called cryotherapy. It is a form of counter-irritation, where the skin and the areas below are slightly stimulated with cold temperatures in order to trigger a healing process by reducing inflammation and muscle tightness. However, though ice can be very helpful when properly applied, it can do harm when used incorrectly. Ice should never be applied directly to your skin. Instead, use a moist cloth or towel on the skin with the ice placed on top of it. A moist towel helps transfer the cooling benefits whereas a dry one can partly insulate your

skin from the cold. In this way, the cooling effect can reach all areas, including some bones.

The ice can be placed in a plastic bag, with smaller pieces of ice working better than large ice cubes. A package of frozen blueberries or peas, or other items in your freezer, may also work just fine. Or you can use a freezer gel pack, but be sure the gel pack is not leaking, as that can be irritating to the skin.

Applying ice to your body produces four stages of sensation you can easily feel. First, as the area becomes cool, you will feel the cold effect immediately. Second, you will feel a prickling or itchy sensation, sometimes described as a burning itch. Following this sensation, you will get an achy feeling—in some cases this can become painful, which signals it's time to remove the ice. The last stage is numbness, and one to avoid. If you feel numbness, immediately remove the ice.

Usually, the numbness stage takes up to twenty minutes. When it doubt, remove the ice earlier. The therapeutic effects occur in the early and mid stage and risk of soft tissue damage increases in the later stage. You can apply the ice again once the skin temperature has returned to normal, although once every hour or two is sufficient for most situations.

### When and Where to Avoid Ice

Many areas of the body are not well endowed with sufficient muscle or fat, such as the foot, ankle, kneecap, and elbow, and the use of ice has greater potential to cause harm in these areas. Some of these regions also contain large nerves. The overenthusiastic use of ice can literally freeze these nerves, along with the skin and small blood vessels, causing additional serious injury. Essentially, cryotherapy can result in frostbite unless ice is applied with caution. Also avoid ice on areas of reduced sensation, which may exist as part of an injury, because you won't know the ice is hurting if left on too long.

In some individuals, ice should be avoided because it can cause further damage. Those with rheumatoid arthritis, Raynaud's Syndrome, or any type of paralysis should not use ice.

A small number of people have cold allergies, and ice can cause adverse reactions. Most people already know the condition exists because of previous adverse reactions to cold, including pain and skin rash. Those with high blood pressure should also be cautious when using ice as it can raise blood pressure.

Care should be taken in using ice boots or other strap-on ice packs because these are often used for too long. They are frequently used for convenience allowing the person to be active during cryotherapy—itself a reason to avoid them, since rest is most often what is required. Do not put these devices on before going to sleep as they can over-treat the problem.

For acute injuries, especially during the first twenty-four hours, ice is the preferred therapy, but certain remedies should be avoided. These include the use of heat in any form, whether a hot bath, heating pad, or heating gel. Heat can aggravate inflammation. An aggressive massage can also create heat and should be avoided. Differentiating between the need for heat or cold is relatively easy: *If an area of injury is warmer than the rest of your body, cool it; if it's cold, heat it.* In general, cooling is the best therapy for acute problems.

### Cold Compresses

The benefits of cold need not always come from ice. An excellent alternative is to use a towel soaked in very cold water with the excess water rung out. When not in use, place the towel in the refrigerator to keep it sufficiently cold. This can have a very good therapeutic effect, especially if a five- to ten-minute application is all you require. Don't underestimate the benefits of this approach.

### Cool Bath

Another method of cooling the body is a cold bath. This is also a safer and more effective form of cyrotherapy, and is often more therapeutic than using ice. A large bucket or small foot tub works well for areas such as the foot or hand. For leg, knee, hip, and other areas, a bathtub may be necessary. Add enough ice to prevent the water from getting warm. However, do not fill the tub with ice. Depending on the temperature of the water, you can keep your foot, leg, or other body area immersed between five and twenty minutes, with less time in colder water. A deep cold bath that cools the muscles is often one way to improve muscle imbalance, and can be more therapeutic than ice placed only on the area of discomfort. In warmer weather, you might want to stand or sit in a cold stream, river, or large body of water. Even if you're not injured, a cold bath is a great way to speed recovery from long or hard training and competition. If you're going to take a hot shower in this situation, end the shower by cooling the injured area with cold water.

## Self-Assessment

The most important aspect of an injury is that it should teach you something about your training, competition, equipment, and lifestyle. Once you've learned this important lesson, you'll become more sensitive to your body's needs, especially with injury prevention and enhanced training and racing. This self-assessment process is one of the features I've regularly seen in better athletes.

Self-assessment is not the same as diagnosis. A diagnosis pertains to disease or serious conditions such as a bone fracture. Since most injuries are functional in nature, a proper assessment requires the gathering of important information about your body and its function.

An assessment can come in the form of questions you ask yourself, such as your workout and race history or various signs and symptoms. For example, the questions below about a new injury are not unlike the ones I used when treating an athlete.

*1. Did the problem begin soon after a new activity?*

Some athletes develop an injury soon after modifying their training, typically increasing volume and/or adding anaerobic work. If a change in activity is associated with the onset of a problem, it may be that the activity is too much for your body to handle, that some previously silent muscle imbalance exists, or that you created one. The remedy: Return to your previous schedule to allow the body to heal.

*2. Did the injury begin soon after new or different equipment or technique was used?*

A new bike position, pair of running shoes, or change in swim stroke can be physically stressful. Once again, the cure is simple: Go back to your previous gear or technique until you feel better. Easing into these types of changes may be most important.

*3. Does the problem get better or worse with movement or rest?*

If your problem feels better with movement, it's generally a good indication that it's a less serious problem. As you move about, the muscles warm up and are able to function better. A proper warm-up can help balance muscles. Sometimes an adequate warm-up takes more than fifteen minutes, and some problems may feel better only after this period of time. But if you feel worse with any type of workout, stop. Don't push yourself if the pain persists. If a problem worsens during activity, especially after you've had time to warm up, it usually means you should be resting to give the body a chance to heal. It may mean there's a more serious problem, but it could simply be that the body needs more recovery time because of muscle inhibition. Pushing yourself in this situation often makes the problem worse and could lead to a chronic, recurring type of problem. The remedy: Reassess your training schedule, take three days off, use cold if indicated, try walking as a therapy, or use combinations of these methods to help the body self-remedy the problem.

*4. Does your injury feel better or worse at the end of the day?*

Generally, if your problem feels worse at the end of the day, physical activity, or even just weight bearing, such as prolonged standing, is an aggravating factor. In some cases, you may have accumulated fluid in your foot, ankle, and lower leg by the end of the day. The solution is to reduce training or take three days off and reassess these factors. Spend more time without shoes through the day. Use cold as indicated. If problems that are worse at the end of the day are not easily remedied, they may need further input from a health-care professional.

*5. Is the problem better or worse in the morning?*

After being off your feet all night, most physical problems feel better in the morning because your body has had time to recover without the added stress of standing, moving, or training. This may not happen if the aerobic system is poor or there is significant muscle imbalance. If these problems are not better in the morning, it may point to other complications.

Certain types of joint pain in those with arthritis may not feel bad in the morning until they get out of bed to stand and start walking, but gradually feel better after movement for an hour or so. This pattern of pain may indicate metabolic problems associated with diet or nutrition, in particular due to the regulation of calcium. In this case, too much calcium may deposit in the painful areas during the night, making movement initially more painful in the morning. The remedy varies with the individual.

*6. Does the area of injury feel different or the same on the other side of the body?*

If you have a problem, say, in your knee, feel all around the area. Then feel the same area on the other knee. Both areas should normally feel about the same. While the body is not perfectly symmetrical, both sides should be very similar. Many people become overly concerned—even obsessed—about how a specific joint, muscle, or other body area looks or feels.

### Look for Clues from Your Training Diary

One of the athlete's best sources of self-assessment clues should come from the training diary. Look for notes on subtle clues about some abnormal physical feelings, such as too rapid a change in training volume, the onset of working out with a group of athletes, and, most importantly, your MAF Tests.

**Question:** Do you recommend easy walking or jogging if you have a strained Achilles tendon? Will this aggravate matters? I've been climbing the walls for the past several weeks because of this nagging injury that refuses to go away. I had been running thirty miles a week. Will biking help or hinder the tendon?

**Answer:** Maintaining fitness during an injury is a key part of recovery. By losing fitness, which you easily can do over several weeks of not working out, you're creating more problems—not only are you getting out of shape, but your injury may also not be corrected. Find some aerobic activity that does not hurt your Achilles, such as biking, swimming, or jogging waist-deep in a pool, and maintain that while figuring out how to resolve your injury. This might include finding a health-care professional if you can't do it yourself with some self-remedies described in this book.

In the process of self-assessing, be on the lookout for *signs*, such as skin rash or increased joint swelling, because they are more objective indications. *Symptoms* are more elusive and difficult to measure objectively. Pain may be the most common of all symptoms (see chapter 26).

Some injuries are acute, meaning they are a recent occurrence, taking place within a couple of weeks. Problems referred to as chronic have been present for a longer period, including recurrent problems such as a chronic ankle sprain or lower back pain. These are more than two weeks old. Many problems are considered recurring, but these are usually chronic problems that have symptoms that come and go.

Overall, many physical problems are directly or indirectly due to muscle imbalance. Even in cases of blunt-force trauma, such as a fracture, muscle imbalance can play a key role in both cause and recovery. Most imbalances you develop are silent and self-corrected by the body. Others that cause various signs or symptoms provide important clues that can enable you to fix your own problems. In some cases, however, obtaining help from an appropriate health-care practitioner is necessary.

# MUSCLE BALANCE AND IMBALANCE

The popular image of the ideal athlete immediately suggests big bulging muscles. This belief, or rather myth, implies that more muscle mass leads to better athleticism. This, of course, is not necessarily true, especially in endurance sports where power is not the key factor in long-distance training and racing.

Your body's muscles are, however, a vital part of overall fitness and health. Our muscles are the body's largest organ, and they aren't just for lifting, pushing, carrying, moving, or sprinting across the finish line. They are responsible for helping to pump blood through the body's miles of blood vessels, for immune function, and for burning body fat.

There are three different kinds of muscle in our body, each with different functions:

1. Smooth muscle makes up the walls of the arteries to control blood flow and surrounds the intestines from begin-

ning to end to regulate the movement of food during digestion. These muscles are controlled to a great extent by the autonomic nervous system (sympathetic and parasympathetic function).

2. Cardiac muscle is unique to the heart. While it's influenced by the brain and nervous system, hormones, and stress, the heart also contains its own intrinsic mechanism allowing it to beat on its own.

3. Skeletal muscle comprises the bulky muscular images we're so familiar with in

sports. Most muscles in humans are comprised of a variety of different fibers, primarily the aerobic and anaerobic types. While their basic movement is under conscious control from our brain (with many other actions taking place we're not always aware of), we can also influence skeletal muscles significantly through training, diet, hormones, and therapies.

This chapter is a more in-depth discussion of skeletal muscles, how they function and what happens when they get out of balance. It's important to note that muscles work because the brain and nervous system control them; as such, we should refer to a *neuromuscular system*, which includes the brain, spinal cord, nerves, and muscles.

In addition to their physical attributes, skeletal muscles influence many areas of metabolism, including fat stores, the liver, and the brain. Skeletal muscles also play a significant role in immune function because of their antioxidant capabilities; they are essentially home to much of our antioxidant protection, given a healthy diet. Muscles are even a major source of blood and lymph circulation. This occurs mostly in the red aerobic muscle fibers, which are well endowed with many miles of blood vessels.

## The Full Spectrum of Muscle Function

Muscles move bones and allow us to use our body for standing, walking, running, and every other physical action. Muscles can and will take on many different degrees of function and, when they don't work properly, it creates dysfunction. In general, the full spectrum of muscle function can range from very loose muscles (gross weakness) with no perceivable contraction to the other extreme of hypertonic or very tight, spastic muscles. Between these two extremes are a number of other important states.

### Normal Muscle Function

Normal muscle activity is a combination of contraction and relaxation, technically referred to as *facilitation* and *inhibition*, respectively. When running, for example, contraction and relaxation occur continuously throughout the body. When muscles contract, they get tighter and provide more work, and when relaxed they work with less force and allow their opposite muscle to contract better.

The best way to explain normal muscle function is for you to feel it yourself. Let's use the biceps muscle on the front of the upper arm and the triceps muscle on the back of the arm. The contraction and relaxation of these two muscles, which usually work together, can provide an accurate view of how muscles normally work throughout the body. Let's try this experiment:

First, in a relaxed, sitting position, with your left hand feel your right biceps muscle on the front of your upper arm. Then feel the right triceps muscle on the back of your upper arm. At rest, they should both be relatively relaxed—firm but neither tight nor too loose.

Next, place your right hand under your thigh, then pull upward as if trying to lift your thigh; in doing so you contract the biceps muscle. Now feel the biceps muscle again with your left hand, and it should feel noticeably tighter. This is how a contracted muscle (one that is normally facilitated by the brain) feels.

While continuing to lift up on your thigh, now feel the triceps muscle on the opposite side of the arm. This should feel much looser than the biceps and even a bit looser (depending on how much you pull up on your thigh) than when at rest. This is how a muscle relaxes itself more to allow the opposing muscle to contract. The biceps muscle is contracted (or facilitated), and the triceps is in a state of inhibition. In fact, without this extra relaxation (inhibition) by the triceps, the biceps could not properly contract.

During a run, this same facilitation and inhibition takes place constantly in opposing muscles, just like the biceps and triceps. It occurs in the quadriceps (front of the thigh) and hamstrings (back of the thigh), the anterior tibialis muscle (front of the leg) and calf muscles (including the gastrocnemius and posterior tibialis), the pectoralis muscles (upper chest) and latissimus (middle of back), and so on.

Normal muscle function is the optimal state of the neuromuscular system. It provides the best balance of the physical body—with the right combinations of inhibition and facilitation during physical activity.

## Abnormal Muscle Function

Understanding the normal function of muscles can also give you a better idea of the abnormal. The most common abnormal muscle condition in athletes is muscle imbalance, which occurs when two or more muscles don't contract and relax as they should. Using the example above when you contracted the biceps and the triceps got looser, imagine if the biceps remained tight and the triceps remained loose even after you released your grip on your thigh. This is very much like the condition of muscle imbalance—except both muscles are in an abnormal state.

A muscle that stays too relaxed is referred to as *abnormal inhibition* and sometimes called "weak" (although this is not true weakness, which refers to the lack of power). This muscle imbalance can be relatively minor causing minimal impairment, or in some cases extreme to the point of causing severe pain in a joint controlled by that muscle. More importantly, in most cases, this inhibition causes an opposite muscle to become too tight, a condition called *abnormal facilitation*. These abnormal muscles—muscle imbalance—can adversely affect the joint(s) they control, the tendons they're attached to, and other muscles, ligaments, and body areas all over. Most physical injuries are caused by muscle imbalance, whether the pain or problem is felt in the joint, ligament, tendon, or muscle.

The full spectrum of muscle function goes from extreme weakness to extreme tightness, with normal in the middle (see chart on page 374). The extremes are usually due to a brain or spinal cord injury; those with cerebral palsy, multiple sclerosis, or who've had a stroke typically have this type of muscle weakness.

Muscle imbalance, the combination of abnormal inhibition and facilitation, is a very common problem in endurance athletes. Here's what happens:

The inhibited muscle is abnormally lengthened, and is often the starting point for many common physical injuries that are not induced by trauma such as falling off your bike or twisting an ankle on the trail. This muscle weakness itself is often silent. However, you might feel the lack of function produced by it, such as something not right in the knee joint or difficulty in maintaining a proper running gait. And, when the muscle doesn't properly control the movement of a nearby joint, it causes that body part to become inflamed.

The other side of abnormal muscle inhibition is tightness (abnormal facilitation). This tight muscle is often noticeably uncomfortable and sometimes painful, and it can impair movement by restricting flexibility. Tight muscles are shortened, making them candidates for mild, slow stretching; however, in most cases this would be treating the secondary problem as the cause is usually the weak (inhibited) muscle. In addition, in attempting to loosen the tight muscles through stretching, you risk weakening the inhibited muscle more (because it's already over-stretched).

It should be noted that muscles attach to bones through tendons. So when a muscle is not functioning properly, the tendons don't either. Most tendon problems are secondary to muscles that don't work well. Likewise, ligaments connect bones to other bones. And muscles have an important support relationship with both ligaments and bones, both directly and indirectly. So when a ligament or bone problem exists, there is usually an associated muscle imbalance as well.

The cause of muscle imbalance must be addressed if normal muscle balance is to be restored. Often, the body can accomplish this on its own, especially when it's fit and healthy overall. In fact, the body is always self-correcting problems because normal wear and tear of endurance training can cause minor muscle imbalances. Even without knowing it, the body is always working to restore balance. During the process of correcting its own problems, the body may show relatively minor symptoms, and often none at all. When your body can't fix a particular problem, that's when symptoms appear and an injury develops.

## Evaluating Muscle Function

Muscle imbalances can't be easily evaluated using X-rays, CAT scans, or other high-tech devices. Electromyography (EMG) equipment can help determine some of the imbalances discussed above, but it's not

| Full Spectrum of Muscle Function | | | | |
|---|---|---|---|---|
| Gross weakness (little/no movement) | Abnormal inhibition (so-called "weakness") | Normal | Abnormal facilitation (tight) | Gross tightness (hypertonic or spasm) |

sensitive enough to find the more subtle imbalances seen in athletes. Properly done, manual muscle testing can effectively evaluate muscle function and can eliminate the need for EMG and other tests, many of which are much more expensive. When working with athletes to assess their muscle function, I would study the posture and movement or gait on a treadmill or track. I also performed manual muscle testing to evaluate individual muscles. This was in addition to other assessment procedures such as physical exam, questions about training and racing, and reading their training diary.

I found that the history of a person's injury usually provides a significant amount of information regarding which muscles are imbalanced. Today, taking a patient's history is a lost art, with many health-care professionals no longer talking much with their patients. This is unfortunate since athletes unknowingly provide many clues by talking about their symptoms, and a good question and answer session may be the best assessment process. Simply listening to athletes talk with one another before or after a race can often help determine what is causing their physical problems.

Observing muscle imbalance is relatively easy. One just has to watch the runners at the end of a marathon, long bike event, or triathlon to see the more exaggerated forms of imbalance: irregular movements, and, in runners, even the erratic sounds of shoes hitting the pavement. However, the more common and subtle muscle imbalances in athletes are often only observed by those trained to see them. I recall my days as a student, learning about muscle imbalance and which muscles perform which movements, and which imbalances cause slight irregularities in gait. Some of my classmates and I would go to an indoor mall and watch people walk by, assessing them with our newfound observations.

In addition to gait, evaluating standing or sitting posture is important, especially in cyclists. And the swimming stroke also provides many clues about muscle function. Muscle imbalances are represented by deviations in posture—curving of the spine, tilting of the head or pelvis, rotation of the upper body, or other distortions; some very subtle, others not.

Most importantly, when the proper therapy is applied and muscle imbalance is corrected, gait and postural irregulari-

# CRAMPS, SPASMS, AND SIDE-STITCHES

A muscle cramp is a tight, suddenly contracted muscle that is over-facilitated. It usually occurs during activity, but waking in the middle of the night with foot or leg cramps is not uncommon. The exact cause of muscle cramps is often not fully known and may be very individual (one person's cramp may be caused by something different than another's cramp). A muscle cramp usually involves a single muscle or group of muscles. Possible causes might include dehydration, low levels of sodium or magnesium, an overworked muscle, or side effects from a prescription drug. Muscle cramps generally last a relatively short time (unless you're having a bad one like a calf cramp in the middle of a bike ride; then it feels like a long time). The terms "muscle cramps" and "spasms" are often used interchangeably as their definitions are somewhat scant. True muscle spasms occur most often in people with neurological diseases such as multiple sclerosis and cerebral palsy and those with severe spinal cord injury.

Side-stitches refer to pain typically in the side of the upper intestinal area; these usually occur during running. They may be directly or indirectly related to either the skeletal muscles such as the abdominals or the smooth muscle of the intestines.

Side-stitches are also not well understood by physiologists but they often appear to originate from the diaphragm or the intestines, and usually just after fluid or other food is consumed. They can not only be painful but also reduce your physical activity, often causing you to slow or stop during competition. Bending forward while tightening abdominal muscles or breathing through pursed lips with increased lung volume can help reduce these painful stitches. During activity, the most success I've seen is with deep breathing associated with a specific foot strike, swim stroke, or pedaling cadence. For example, while running, breathe in during three foot strikes (right, left, right) and out during the following four foot strikes (left, right, left, right). During faster running, inhaling on two and exhaling on three foot strikes is effective.

ties should noticeably improve very quickly (along with the patient's pain patterns or other symptoms). That's because many therapies change the neuromuscular system and the effects are immediate. This is unlike the effects of weight lifting to improve strength, where a certain amount of time is required for an increase in muscle strength.

### Manual Biofeedback

Among the many tools I used to help train and treat athletes are various forms of biofeedback such as heart-rate monitoring. Manual biofeedback is another procedure I developed, which helps improve muscle imbalance by correcting muscle weakness—abnormal inhibition—whether from local muscle problems, or brain or spinal cord injury. It's a safe and effective, and relatively easy approach for use by most health-care professionals (and even lay people), usually producing a rapid response. Manual bio-feedback is useful for virtually all athletes, including those who have obvious physical injuries, and those who appear injury-free but may have subtle muscle imbalances that can adversely affect performance.

Most people who have injuries associated with muscle imbalance fall into at least one of two categories:

- Local muscle injury is the most common cause of physical problems, and is often associated with trauma to the muscle itself, such as the result of a fall, a so-called pulled muscle, a twisted ankle, or other injury. Micro-trauma is even more wide-spread; it's the accumulation of minor physical stress in a muscle or joint, often unnoticed while it's happening, eventually causing a more obvious muscle problem. Endurance training produces significant wear and tear on the body's mechanics—a stress that most athletes should adapt to well. But often, this stress is not compensated for and muscle imbalance develops. Non-athletic activity can also be a problem: too much sitting, repetitive motion injury, or walking in poor-fitting shoes often leads to micro-trauma, which in turn ultimately causes muscle problems. Local muscle injuries can result in anything from minor annoying ache to a serious or chronic debilitating condition.

- Brain or spinal cord injury can occur at any age, even before birth, and usually milder forms can be found in athletes. Trauma, infection, or reduced nutrient supply can easily cause brain or spinal cord damage resulting in poor muscle function. An athlete involved in a bike crash can often sustain a brain or spinal cord injury with or without a helmet.

Manual biofeedback can help promote and restore muscle balance, and in doing so help improve overall physical movement. Increased movement is a powerful therapy in itself; it not only helps locomotion and posture, but the brain as well, including speech, vision, balance, memory, and even intellect. And because muscles have other important functions, such as energy production, circulation, and immune activity, increasing physical movement can improve overall health.

While traditional EMG (electromyography) biofeedback uses computer equipment, including mechanical sensors and electrodes attached to the skin, manual biofeedback does not use any equipment. Instead, manual bio-feedback uses another person's neurological sense (the practitioner's) in the biofeedback process. This is a more personalized approach, recruiting more brain-body stimulation with verbal, visual, tactile, and other sensory cues, that further enlists the person's participation and motivation. Like many forms of biofeedback, manual biofeedback relies on muscle testing.

# Breathing Muscles

Of all the vital muscles necessary for optimal endurance, perhaps the most important one is the diaphragm. This breathing muscle is located on top of our abdomen and under our lungs. The large, flat muscle allows us to breathe by pulling in oxygenated air and expelling unwanted carbon dioxide. In well-trained endurance athletes, the breathing mechanism may be the weak link in good performance. In this case, less air enters the lungs and the blood does not receive the proper amount of oxygen. Moreover, poor exhalation does not eliminate the necessary amount of carbon dioxide, which can also reduce endurance.

All athletes can incorporate the actions of normal breathing into their training program—not necessarily during training, but most especially during rest or down time. This can help recovery and actually help repair muscle and other imbalances.

## Normal Breathing

We take breathing for granted, until we experience a breathing difficulty. But some people breathe improperly and don't even realize it, while many others could improve their breathing to further help their endurance and overall health, especially through controlling stress. Normal breathing is associated with proper muscle movement—the most important being the abdominal muscles in the front and sides of our abdomen and the diaphragm muscle. These muscles work together allowing us to efficiently breathe in and out. Without normal breathing, the abdominal and diaphragm muscles may work improperly, and even cause other muscles to not work. In this scenario, body movement—posture and gait, for example—can become impaired, oxygen can be reduced, and other problems can occur.

The abdominals also help physically support our body structure—the spine, the low back, pelvis, shoulders, and even the neck. The abdominal muscles help us run, bike, and swim more efficiently. In some cases, improper breathing is the beginning of a complex set of imbalances causing an injury to the low or middle back, hip, shoulder, or almost any other areas.

Given the importance of the abdominal and diaphragm muscles, let's look more closely at the two components of normal breathing—inhalation and exhalation.

During inhalation the abdominal muscles relax and extend outward, while the diaphragm muscle moves downward. This movement allows air to enter the lungs more easily and is accompanied by a slight whole-body backward extension, especially of the spine.

# MORE ON MANUAL MUSCLE TESTING

Manual muscle testing is a form of biofeedback, and is commonly used for the evaluation of muscle imbalance. The first textbook on manual muscle testing appeared in 1949 to evaluate muscle weakness in polio patients, and gradually, muscle-testing techniques were improved for the evaluation of a full range of muscle dysfunction in all types of individuals. Today, manual muscle testing is used by tens of thousands of health-care professionals worldwide. The objective of muscle testing differs considerably among its users, with most using it as a form of assessment. For example:

- Neurologists perform muscle testing to help evaluate brain function.
- A physical therapist may use muscle testing to rate a patient's level of disability.
- An athletic trainer may use muscle testing to assess a particular athletic injury.
- Chiropractors, osteopaths, and other medical doctors may use manual muscle testing as a form of assessment for all these and other reasons.

During exhalation the abdominal muscles contract and tighten, and are gently pulled inward; the diaphragm muscle "relaxes" with an upward movement. This helps push air out of the lungs, with a slight whole-body flexion.

By watching another person's breathing, especially the belly moving out on inhalation and in on exhalation, one can often tell if it's correct. You can also evaluate your own breathing by feeling the muscles move. So try this quick experiment:

- Place the palm of one or two of your hands on the abdomen (over your belly button).
- Slowly breathe in and feel the abdominal muscles expand outward. Your belly should get bigger during inhalation.
- Slowly exhale and feel the abdominal muscles tighten and be pulled inward. The belly is more flat on exhalation.

- During normal breathing, most movement occurs in the abdominal areas, and only slightly in the chest, which expands more with much deeper breathing.

Those who breathe improperly often move their muscles opposite that of normal. In other cases, the chest is quickly and fully expanded and the abdominal area doesn't get a chance to move properly. These poor patterns of breathing can be caused from stress, the stigma of not showing a big belly, and yes, even over-exercising the abdominal muscles—typically with sit-ups or crunches—making them too tight to relax.

One important note: Be aware of your breathing during times of stress, which is often when normal breathing can switch to abnormal breathing as we hold more tension in our abdominal and pelvic muscles. This

While the purpose of manual muscle testing is widely varied, there is one common feature among all the professionals using it: manual muscle testing is an important form of biofeedback used to help evaluate physical body function, especially in helping to determine muscle imbalance.

Manual muscle testing involves physically evaluating individual muscles. This is accomplished by first positioning an arm, leg, or other body part associated with a particular muscle's action. In this position, the practitioner applies force against the athlete's force. If the athlete cannot properly maintain resistance, it may indicate abnormal inhibition ("weakness"). In addition, a muscle that functions well does not do so only because it is powerful or strong.

Even a very powerful weight lifter can have abnormal muscle inhibition, and the frailest, most out-of-shape elderly person can have muscle facilitation.

can even occur during training and especially during competition, when mental stress is high. In particular, I have seen many athletes not breathing as well: not inhaling fully, exhaling fully, or both.

If your breathing is not normal, it's important to immediately retrain the breathing mechanism. This can be done using respiratory biofeedback (see chapter 28). The procedure is simple, using the steps just outlined above for normal inhalation and exhalation.

## How Muscles Affect Bone Health

In general, by maintaining proper muscle balance and by being healthy and properly trained, you can significantly reduce the risk of bone problems, the most common one in endurance athletes being stress fractures.

Should you have a stress fracture, healing occurs much more rapidly if you have better muscle balance and are healthier overall. Of course, many stress fractures occur due to muscle imbalance interfering with weight bearing, gait, and other movement.

Stress fractures are usually less severe than most other bone problems, but can significantly interfere with training and racing. While some occur from simple trauma—a bike crash, for example—others occur from repetitive overuse or a sudden increase in activity. In some cases, metabolic causes are evident, such as in female athletes with amenorrhea (the lack of a normal menstrual period), which is associated with hormone imbalance affecting bone strength, or due to osteoporosis in either sex. While the bones in the legs (tibia and fibula) are common sites of stress fractures, they can also occur in the foot's metatarsal and navicular bones, the bones of the pelvis, and many other bones.

Pain from a stress fracture typically improves with rest and worsens with activity. There is often some swelling in the area, but sometimes it's not noticeable. The swelling around the site of fracture may prevent a proper diagnosis by X-ray if taken within the first two weeks of injury. Only after some healing has taken place will the X-ray show the problem. In these situations, a bone scan may help locate the stress fracture when the X-ray can't.

Most stress fractures will heal well in a healthy person without major therapy. Rest, cooling the site of fracture, cessation of weight-bearing exercise, and hard-soled flat shoes are often sufficient, but each case must be treated individually. Aspirin and other NSAIDs must be avoided as they can delay bone healing.

Just as important is the fact that something caused a stress fracture to occur; and that something—some imbalance in muscles, hormones, diet, or often a combination of problems—must be found and corrected. If this does not happen, the athlete is vulnerable to future fractures.

A low-fat diet may be associated with a higher incidence of stress fractures—statistically more in female athletes. Fats are important for many aspects of health, with certain fats helping to carry calcium into bones (and muscles). Bone health is related to more than just calcium: zinc, vitamin K, and many other nutrients, including protein, are also very important for bone health—all factors that a healthy diet provides. Vitamin D may be the most important nutrient for bones and our most important source is from the sun.

Surprisingly, the importance of muscle function in bone health is often not discussed, but it may be the most important contributing factor in stress fractures. In addition to muscle imbalance, which can cause reduced support and increased stress on specific areas of the skeleton, reduced muscle mass is associated with reduced overall health, including nutritional and hormone imbalance, making the bones vulnerable, too. Low muscle mass also physically reduces bone support, especially when the aerobic muscle fibers are not well developed.

And while we often discuss the negative aspects of excess physical stress, too little physical stress can also be a problem. Those who don't regularly perform gravity-stress-related exercise may be more at risk for bone problems. Endurance athletes in general don't have this problem, but if you're a swimmer, and don't perform any other workouts such as walking or running, the gravity stress on your body may be less than optimal. In some cases, even cycling can result in significantly less gravitation stress on the body than running or even walking. In these instances, cross-training can be very helpful Athletes who are fit and healthy dramatically lower their risk of stress fractures, along with other injuries.

# CHAPTER 26

# THE PAIN GAME AND HOW TO CONTROL IT

The symptom of pain is a subjective yet important part of endurance sports. It's an emotion our brain relies on for survival, helping us get to the finish line, or telling us there's a problem somewhere in the body. While pain is felt in the brain, the body parts that produce it may have either physical or chemical causes.

Pain is how our body tells us to slow down or rest so it can repair itself. While pain is often the symptom associated with muscle imbalance, the gut can produce pain from cramping, a common problem in athletes. Pain medications, which only treat the symptoms, not the cause, are among the best-selling prescription and over-the-counter drugs worldwide.

Pain's many cellular chemical compounds are even triggered by certain substances that are directly associated with the balance of fats. Too many omega-6 fats, including some saturated ones, can promote the production of more pain-producing chemicals. The same mechanism promotes excess inflammation. With acute pain, these changes are an important, healthy part of the healing process of recovery from easy workouts to hard events. But pain can become chronic, which is not normal or healthy.

There are at least three possible causes of chronic pain:

- The problem that caused the pain is unresolved. For example, a muscle imbalance causing stress in the knee joint can cause inflammation and pain. Until the cause of the problem is corrected, inflammation and pain will continue.
- Even when the physical cause of the problem is corrected, the chemical imbalance associated with poor fat balance may still be present. Until this problem is corrected, pain-producing chemicals (including those of inflammation) can continually be produced.
- Certain types of brain cells, called glia, can become overactive following some injuries that have caused pain. These cells can continue to stimulate the pain in the brain even after the original cause of pain has resolved. And certain pain medications, especially morphine, seem to actually worsen this process. What triggers the glia to become overactive and act in this fashion is not well understood by scientists. Some substances can potentially turn off the overactive glia. These include THC, the active component in marijuana, and stronger prescription drugs (immune suppressant drugs such as etanercept and narcotic receptor blockers such as naloxone).

Pain starts in nerve endings found in the skin, blood vessels, nerve fibers, joints, and coverings of bone. These nerve endings send messages through the nervous system to the emotional center of the brain (called the limbic system), where we interpret the feeling as pain. Call it an emotion, a feeling, or a mental state—it's simply an interaction between the body and brain. This is why pain is relatively subjective, with no two people feeling it the same. If pain were a true sense, like smell, taste, vision, or hearing, it would be much more difficult, if not impossible, to control it with physical measures (applying cold), chemicals (taking aspirin), or mental measures (through hypnosis).

Once pain messages reach the brain, the brain sends messages back to the source of pain in order to release natural analgesics such as endorphins. The spinal cord, comprised of nerves that go from the brain to the body, is the relay station for pain perception. This is one reason that "spinal blocks" can reduce pain.

The cause of a problem that produces pain is usually located where the injury occurred. But many times pain is associated with problems elsewhere in the body, or with problems that don't produce symptoms. To those with non-traumatic pain in or around the knee, the physical cause of the pain is likely due to muscle imbalance in the foot or ankle—and is often silent (asymptomatic). This is one reason so many knee problems never get fully corrected and become chronic; the true cause remains undetected and only the symptom is treated.

The gradual development of knee pain is a phenomenon I have seen and heard from countless endurance athletes who limped into my office. The chronology of a typical patient history went as follows: slow onset of knee pain, then, after several weeks, more severe pain. Aspirin and other non-steroidal anti-inflammatory drugs (NSAIDs) improved symptoms by reducing pain and inflammation somewhat, but the pain kept returning and restricted training. Running typically made the pain worse, so biking and other activities such as swimming were used to maintain active-recovery fitness. Racing only worsened the pain, and in time, competition was restricted or eliminated altogether. Several other remedies were tried, including various therapies applied to the knee—the usual ice, creams to dull the pain, rest; therapies for feet, including orthotics; trying different running shoes; and others administered by various health-care professionals. Some of these approaches appeared to help temporarily, but the pain soon returned. In some cases, the pain disappeared only to show up in another location around the knee or even in the hip joint.

As simple as this may sound, I've seen many hundreds of athletes with just this type of injury. Often, it marked my first encounter with them. My comprehensive evaluation of the athlete usually revealed an imbalance of some of the muscles of the foot and ankle, causing mechanical instability of the ankle and stress in the knee. Correction of the foot problem through the use of biofeedback would often quickly resolve the knee pain and the athlete was happily able to return to normal training and competition.

More importantly, a positive outcome often affected the athlete in another positive way—he or she learned to look at the big picture such as diet, stress, training, and other lifestyle factors.

Unfortunately, some athletes I've helped overcome a significant injury could not relate well to the big picture. While they relied on me to fix their physical problems, they would not improve their diet or training, and when another injury cropped up, they would visit me again for repair. I would expend significant energy trying to educate them—explaining that injury means they're not training well, eating well, or have other problems that need correcting. I also told them that by fixing their injury, I was simply treating symptoms and they were basically not allowing me to correct the true cause of the problem. For those few who could still not understand or were unwilling to comply, I would reluctantly decide that I could not see them, since there were many other injured athletes on my waiting list who wanted to see me.

One benefit of pain, however, is that it informs us there's a problem. By doing so, it can help the body compensate by using other muscles or changing the running gait to avoid further stress on a particular joint that's inflamed. It can also prevent us from continuing activities that should be avoided. Different types of pain such as throbbing or swelling have particular meaning. For example, physical pain can be associated with increased pressure, such as a swelling, typically from trauma. This type of pain is often described as "stabbing" or "knife-like." Or if it's associated with blood vessels, sufferers experience it as "throbbing" or "pounding."

Chemical pain often comes from inflammation and muscle fatigue. This type of pain is often described as "burning" or "hot." Thermal pain from extreme cold or hot temperatures can also produce pain. This may be due to an ice pack left too long on the skin or sunburn. In fact, sunburn pain can come from all three types: thermal stress (hot sun), physical damage to skin, and chemical inflammation.

Songwriters and novelists have longed portrayed the extremes of emotional pain, like losing a loved one. Athletes are not immune, of course, to grief and sadness. Studies show that an athlete's response to a season-ending injury or dropping out of a major race can be emotionally traumatic.

Emotional pain may be experienced in the same brain areas as physical pain. In addition, emotional pain can be stressful enough to adversely affect training and racing. This can occur due to the brain's relationship with adrenal function. While training usually helps those trying to cope with emotional pain, overtraining may worsen it.

## Nonsteroidal Anti-inflammatory Drugs (NSAIDs)—How They Work and Hurt

Aspirin, ibuprofen (such as Advil), naproxen (such as Aleve), and other nonsteroidal anti-inflammatory drugs (NSAIDs) are commonly used for pain relief. If taking NSAIDs lessens your pain, it probably indicates your fats are not balanced.

It is no secret that endurance athletes take various types of painkillers and other drugs, especially NSAIDs, before races in hopes of improving their competitiveness. The fact is, it doesn't work, and these drugs most often cause more stress on the whole body. While most of these drugs are not banned in competitive sports, they usually can cause much more harm than many of the drugs that are banned, in part because they disrupt the normal balance of fats, reduce recovery, and have harmful side effects.

Be forewarned: NSAIDs can cause significant health problems in athletes, reduce fitness, and can be deadly. Refer to the list on page 266 that explains the health problems associated with NSAIDs.

NSAIDs can also increase the risk of heart attack. In fact, some COX-2 inhibitors, including Vioxx, have actually been recalled due to their risk of causing heart attack, stroke and even death in some patients. Because of these and other problems, Merck recalled Vioxx in 2004. In 2005, the U.S. Federal Drug Administration asked Pfizer to recall its drug, Bextra, due to similar side effects.

## Other Muscle Pains

In addition to pain caused by muscle imbalance, other types of muscle pain are common in athletes. There are three general types of pain associated with muscles:

## REFERRED PAIN

Athletes less commonly experience another type of pain pattern, neurologically different from, say, knee or foot discomfort, and this is known as *referred pain*. Referred pain is experienced in one location on the body while the cause is located elsewhere. One of the most common referred-pain patterns is in the case of a heart attack, where pain is felt in the lower neck, shoulder, and arm usually on the left side, while the problem is in the heart. Or, pain in the middle of the spine may come from an irritation in the stomach. Referred pain occurs because signals from the heart, for example, and those from the skin in the arm (the referred-pain area) "cross" in the spinal cord, and when the message gets to the brain it's impossible to differentiate between the signals' origins. That's why it's critically important to differentiate between arm pain that's due to a skeletal muscle problem and that from a heart attack.

- Pain experienced during or immediately after physical activity may have a chemical origin. Lactic acid does not cause pain directly, but may be responsible for pH changes in the blood, associated with pain. Reduced blood flow may also be linked to this type of muscle pain, which will subside quickly once activity is stopped.

- Delayed-onset muscle soreness usually develops within twenty-four to forty-eight hours after activity, with a peak in discomfort between forty-eight and seventy-two hours. This pain is usually associated with muscle damage. Diminished ranges of motion accompany this pain pattern, and muscle dysfunction often continues long after pain has resolved.

- Muscle cramps may be due to some type of imbalance. Proper hydration and the use of sodium or magnesium may be helpful in correcting and preventing muscle cramps; rarely is potassium or calcium needed. Proper breathing can help prevent and treat diaphragm problems associated with the common "side-stitch"-type spasms.

## Natural Pain Remedies

Home treatment of pain associated with physical activity is best accomplished with cold stimulation—soaking the body area(s) in cold water for ten to fifteen minutes can be miraculous. Ice is not always needed; cold tap water works great and sometimes ice can cause excessive irritation by freezing the skin. Use cold stimulation two or three times the first day, once or twice the second. In most cases, this will significantly and quickly improve pain.

The use of heat for pain is a common remedy. However, it can do more harm than good. Inflammation can be worsened with the application of heat. Unless you're quite sure an area is not inflamed, avoid using heat. Most areas of pain, including the joints associated with muscle imbalance, are accompanied by some degree of inflammation. Inflammatory pain occurs when fat imbalance produces more pain chemicals—balancing dietary fats helps prevent chronic inflammation.

Low-fat diets can worsen pain and increase the risk of other muscular injury.

Many people drink alcohol when pain is present, but this can just as easily amplify pain. The pain-reducing ability of alcohol occurs with high intake, something that also creates fat imbalance ultimately increasing pain.

Simple gentle rubbing of the skin, called tactile stimulation, can also control pain. This is accomplished by lightly stroking the skin at or near an area of pain. If you bump your head, you probably subconsciously rub the area. This stimulates large nerve endings in the skin that can help block pain sensation in the brain (the same mechanism as electrical nerve stimulation devices).

## Other Types of Pain Drugs

In addition to NSAIDs for pain control, a second type of drug used for pain relief includes acetaminophen. These drugs, mostly non-prescription ones such as Tylenol, don't act by reducing inflammation, and therefore are less likely to interfere with healing and recovery. It's not entirely clear how these drugs work, but liver stress is among the side effects;

the body needs to break down these drugs in the liver, which requires large amounts of the amino acid cysteine (best obtained in the diet from whey consumption).

Narcotics, such as opiates, are another type of pain reliever. These act in the brain to reduce the sensation of pain and don't affect inflammation. However, they are easily addictive, and their use as a pain reliever wears off as the brain cells become desensitized. Common narcotics prescribed for pain include morphine and other opioid drugs such as codeine and oxycodone (OxyContin).

Yet another pain-relieving drug is THC, the active component in marijuana, which controls pain by stimulating certain receptors in the brain, similar to those that opiates act upon. THC can stimulate the brain's natural opiates, like endorphins. The only prescription form is the product Marinol, although many states now have medical marijuana laws.

As common as pain is for endurance athletes, living with pain is an unacceptable consequence of endurance training and racing. Eliminating pain begins with finding the cause and addressing it. Too many athletes fear the loss of fitness, and therefore train through pain. Another misguided notion—"no pain, no gain"—encourages athletes to train with pain, This just worsens the problems that cause the pain, often sending athletes on a downward spiral of injury, further pain, and poor performance. The most sensible remedy is to find the cause of the pain, correct it, and prevent it from coming back.

# CHAPTER 27

# FIT BUT UNHEALTHY—
## Why Death Is the Ultimate Injury and Measures to Prevent It

**T**ragically, an undetected injury can sometimes lurk as a ticking time bomb inside an athlete's body. At the 2008 U.S. Olympic marathon trials, Ryan Shay, one of America's best runners at age twenty-eight, collapsed and died about five miles into the race. New York City's chief medical examiner said that Shay's death was caused by "cardiac arrhythmia due to cardiac hypertrophy with patchy fibrosis of undetermined etiology. Natural causes."

"Natural causes?" There's nothing natural about a twenty-eight-year-old, exceptionally fit athlete's heart stopping in the middle of competition. Shay's irregular heartbeat stemmed from an abnormally enlarged and scarred heart.

Media coverage of athletes dying in sports as diverse as basketball, football, triathlon, and running is not uncommon. While we take physical injury in sports as an intrinsic part of competition, we're bewildered when a seemingly healthy and young athlete drops dead. Through the looking glass of our sports culture, spectators and participants alike, we tend to view knee, back, shoulder, and other injuries as the normal "wear and tear" of supposedly giving 110 percent. But when the "injury" occurs in the heart, we are perplexed—and wonder why. The fact is, only about 2 percent of young athletes—under thirty years of age—who die suddenly are reported to show normal cardiac structure on standard autopsy examination. For the rest, there's typically some form of heart disease present.

## Triathlon Deaths

Sudden cardiac arrest is the primary cause of death in triathlon; it usually strikes during the swim. In the span of three weeks in 2008, three male triathletes suffered fatal attacks during the swim. Their ages were sixty, fifty-two, and thirty-two.

There have been nearly thirty deaths in triathlons since 2004, as recorded by the national governing body USA Triathlon. Close to 80 percent of these fatalities occurred during the swim. The average age of those who died was forty-three years.

Medical researchers have no definitive explanation for this phenomenon because in a few cases, autopsies revealed no blocked arteries; instead, researchers have several theories. "The combination of apparent good health and a negative autopsy suggests a fatality caused by abnormal heart rhythms," Dr. Pamela Douglas, a Duke University car-

diologist who has studied triathletes, told the *New York Times*.

Another researcher, Dr. Michael Ackerman, a cardiologist and the director of the Windland Smith Rice Sudden Death Genomics Laboratory at the Mayo Clinic in Rochester, Minnesota, told the *Times* that swimming may trigger a certain type of cardiac arrhythmia caused by a genetic condition called *long QT syndrome*. About 1 in 2,000 people is born with a heart condition that causes a glitch in the heart's electrical system, and the most common of these is called long QT syndrome, after the telltale interval on an electrocardiogram. The long QT heart recharges itself sluggishly between beats, and that delay sets up the potential for a skipped beat.

So what causes the skipped heartbeat during the first leg of the triathlon? Is it caused by the adrenaline rush of racing? Inexperience in open water? An accidental kick to the body from another swimmer?

"It's not that swimming is horrendously dangerous and running is not," according to Dr. Ackerman. "It's really a perfect storm that needs to happen. It requires a second hit, something to irritate it, and we know that swimming is one of those triggers, but it's not going to be the absolute trigger." An expert could detect most cases of long QT syndrome on an electrocardiogram, Dr. Ackerman said.

Dr. Kevin Harris of the Minneapolis Heart Institute Foundation and his colleagues presented a paper at the American College of Cardiology 2009 Scientific Sessions that reported that the risk of sudden death in the triathlon was 1.5/100,000 participants, a "not-inconsequential" risk that is nearly double the risk of sudden death in marathon runners. Comparatively, a study by Dr. Donald Redelmeier (University of Toronto, Ontario) of more than three million marathon runners showed the rate of sudden cardiac death to be 0.8/100,000 participants.

Harris told the media there was no significant difference in the death rates in the different triathlon distances. But he added something of particular note: "Maybe what's going on is that you're getting less well-conditioned athletes or more novice athletes, although what's interesting is that we know of only a couple of athletes where this was their first triathlon."

By the time a triathlete suffers a heart attack in the mass frenzy of the swim, it's often too late to save him or her, even with nearby lifeguards. So it's up to the individual to decide if he has signs or symptoms that might trigger sudden cardiac arrest, such as a family history of heart disease. A checkup before participating in a triathlon makes perfect sense.

And therein lies the irony: triathlon's popularity is driven by a continuing revolving door of new participants who are eager to prove to themselves, family, friends, and colleagues at work that they are "fit." Yet there's something markedly wrong with this scenario. First, the meaning of health is self-lim-

iting and wrong if one only considers fitness as its sole criterion. One cannot be healthy while diseased. Additionally, neither youth nor middle-age athleticism automatically confers health. Death comes when something goes wrong—some problem causes the heart to stop, a blood vessel clogs, or some other pathology causes death. Second, most of these problems are preventable. Third, we must differentiate between those young athletes who die in their twenties, teens, and younger, and those in their thirties, forties, and older age-groups who make up the majority of competitive endurance athletes. Fourth, whenever the issue of fatality surfaces following a sudden death in a race, the lifestyle habits of the person are almost never mentioned as a possible cause—especially those factors that can contribute to heart disease, including diet, stress, and even overtraining.

## Fitness versus Health

Our society views highly trained athletes as the healthiest of all people. This is one reason for the confusion when a young, seemingly healthy athlete dies during competition. These athletes, and those of all ages, who break down with a heart attack are clearly more fit than 99 percent of the general population, but obviously they are not healthy. So let's separate the definitions of fitness and health for a clearer perspective.

*Fitness* can be defined by athletic ability, with the level of fitness associated with the levels of training and competition. But *health* is very different; it's the optimal function of all the body's systems—muscles and bones, organs and glands, heart and lungs, nerves and brain. It is very common for athletes to be fit but unhealthy. They can be world champions or "back-of-the-pack" joggers; many are even injured and sick more than the average out-of-shape person. And sometimes they die in the course of their chosen passion, often due to an injury of the heart.

Many athletes, including weekend warriors, spend much of their time getting fit but don't pursue health with the same vigor. Many others can actually become less healthy as a result of pushing and sacrificing their bodies beyond some imaginary limit. In doing so, they induce significant stress from training, or overtraining, poor diet, or other factors, rendering them less healthy. The result is an injured knee, recurrent respiratory infections, chronic fatigue, and other health problems considered part of the game. But it's not part of healthy training. These problems are indicative of an imbalance between fitness and health. One can have both good health and achieve very high levels of athletic performance.

Of course, most people don't exercise at all, nor do they focus on their health. When a person in this group dies at a younger age, we say it was due to neglect. The fact is, being an athlete doesn't convey health benefits any more than being healthy makes you a great athlete if you don't train.

## Preventing Death

It is obvious that preventing death in sports should be our prime concern. About 30 percent of the deaths of young athletes are due to a heart condition called hypertrophic cardiomyopathy (HCM). In the United States each year, several dozen young athletes die during training or competition from this problem (with another 6,000 non-athlete deaths among the more than 600,000 people with HCM). Prevalence of HCM is significantly higher in dark-skinned individuals, and in men, although African American female athletes have a relatively high incidence. These conditions are considered congenital, acquired before birth during heart development.

About half of the young athletes who die have some other type of unhealthy heart condition, which is also preventable. These include coronary artery abnormalities, abnormally enlarged ventricles, myocarditis (inflammation of the heart), and coronary artery disease. A smaller number, probably less than 2 percent, die from asthma, with prescription and recreational drugs representing about 1 percent of the deaths.

Accidental death of young athletes not associated with disease occurs in about 20 percent of cases. These are mostly due to blunt force trauma to the chest, which can immediately stop the heart. This occurs when the chest is hit by a ball or other object, or by another person, at a very precise point in the cardiac cycle. The incidence of death by blunt force trauma can be reduced by adhering to specific rules in every sport.

Electrocardiograms (ECGs) are simple and inexpensive tests that can help diagnose many potentially fatal heart problems. Abnormal ECGs are present in 40 percent of trained athletes, including those without detectable disease, are twice as common in men, and are more prevalent in endurance athletes such as runners, swimmers, and cyclists. Most cardiologists would consider these heart abnormalities related to so-called normal physiological changes from training. However, in some highly trained athletes, the abnormal ECGs are identical to non-athlete patients with heart conditions such as HCM and other abnormalities. Whether these changes are due to overtraining, poor lifestyle, or are actually normal may be determined by further evaluations.

The changes observed in the hearts of most athletes are considered to be training-induced and not unique to some genetic factor. While genetics always plays a role in our development, the hearts of these athletes are primarily associated with non-genetic factors; in addition to training, these include body size and surface area, type of sport, gender, and age.

Most deaths in those with heart problems can be prevented. A discussion of this issue becomes an ethical one as well. Both the International Olympic Committee (IOC) and the European Society of Cardiology (ECS) have advocated that all young competitive athletes be screened routinely and completely (including an extensive history, physical exam, and 12-lead ECG). But the latest guidelines of the American Heart Association do not make this recommendation, saying there is no law in the United States defining legal requirements of sports governing bodies and educational institutions with regard to the screening of competitive athletes. However, in some European countries, local law requires cardiovascular screening, and physicians are considered criminally negligent if they improperly clear an athlete with an undetected cardiovascular abnormality that ultimately leads to death. These strategies have been successful, with about a 90 percent reduction in death from heart disease in competitive athletes.

Many athletes fear cardiovascular screening because if a problem is found they can be banned from competition. Twenty-three-year-old college basketball superstar Hank Gathers died during a game in March of 1990; the cause appeared to be myocarditis. Writing in the *New England Journal of Medicine*, Dr. Barry Morano of the Minneapolis Heart Institute Foundation, and an expert in this field, stated: "It is possible that had Gathers been withdrawn from competitive sports, his heart disease might have resolved within six to twelve months, permitting him to return safely to competition."

For athletes in their mid-thirties or older, at every level of sport, sudden death is primarily due to atherosclerotic coronary artery disease—also known as clogged arteries. What's so remarkable here is that this preventable condition can develop through a less-than-healthy lifestyle that begins during youth. These health problems include poor diet, excess stress, and overtraining.

One reason the cause of death changes in athletes over their mid-thirties is time; these individuals have been alive longer and therefore have more time to develop disease. While in young athletes, screening is the measure that can rule out diseases that kill, in older athletes, prevention refers to slowing the aging process that typically causes a buildup of plaque in the blood vessels—this can be remedied with a healthy lifestyle.

## Lifestyle Factors

A healthy lifestyle can contribute significantly to good fitness and health. Heart disease is a leading cause of death in the Western world and, like most other chronic illness, is a preventable condition. Both improved health and prevention of disease can be accomplished with the help of a healthy diet, and the moderation of stress, including not overtraining. (Even in those with so-called genetic predispositions, lifestyle factors can "turn on" or "turn off" the gene for heart disease.)

In addition, stress in its broadest definition can be a significant contributing factor in the development of heart disease. Stress can come from an imbalanced diet, from trying to squeeze too much training into a day also filled with work and family obligations, and from mental pressures, including competition.

Overtraining is a significant and common stress in athletes. In addition to causing an imbalance in the brain, nervous, and hormonal systems (through increased sympathetic activity), it can increase chronic inflammation as well. Any of these problems can contribute to heart disease and increased risk of death. Stress and abnormal cardiac changes can be measured in overtrained athletes, even in the early stages. These include peripheral vascular resistance, high blood pressure, high cortisol levels, and abnormal heart rate variability.

Overtraining in its early stage, just beyond the normal overreaching aspect of training, can produce abnormalities; ironically, this can result in short-term improvements in athletic performance. Many athletes who experience this phenomenon continue pushing themselves, mistakenly thinking their training is successful. Continuing on this path brings further ill health, including clearer indications of overtraining. For example, abnormal blood markers (such as plasma cardiac troponin T and I) have been found in triathletes and marathon runners following long races. These tests are indicative of a transient myocardial problem—a heart injury. Experts say they are still unsure about the seriousness of this problem. Immune markers are also distorted in many athletes following competition, and during periods of hard training, even following a single, long training session.

This is associated with an increased frequency of upper respiratory illness in athletes. Some have severely compromised immune function making them vulnerable to more serious health problems. Overtraining ultimately results in declining performance.

The acceptance of poor health, by both athletes and even their coaches, is well documented in all sports. This has led to an epidemic of physical injuries. There is even a name for athletic cardiac changes: "athlete's heart." Other overtraining outcomes have special names, too, and are often glorified: runner's knee, swimmer's shoulder, and runner's anemia.

Can countries with higher death rates of young athletes, such as the United States, mandate more effective screening? The International Olympic Committee and European countries already do this to reduce the number of deaths during competition. Many oppose such a requirement, saying it's impractical. The American Heart Association's report in 2007, "Recommendations and Considerations Related to Pre-participation Screening for Cardiovascular Abnormalities in Competitive Athletes," states that, despite being able to detect heart disease in young athletes, "A large population pre-participation screening initiative for U.S athletes that mandates a 12-lead ECG, such as that proposed by the ESC and IOC, is probably impractical and would require considerable resources that do not currently exist."

While there are clear ethical considerations, the responsibility also rests with the athlete or, in the case of minors, the athlete's parents. Consider that many athletes, even weekend warriors, are more than willing to place themselves at high personal risk for the thrill of competition.

Should the government impose restrictions on sports because of potential health problems? Can we prevent a young, talented athlete from fulfilling his or her dreams because an ECG shows abnormal readings? How many of those tests are false positives (meaning the test shows a problem but none really exists), leading to unnecessary testing, anxiety, and removal from a potentially rewarding career? There are obviously more questions than adequate answers. We do, however, treat athletes differently because we put them on a pedestal, and from an early age. This includes the media, who write about them, colleges, universities, and professional teams who recruit them, companies who sponsor them, and the public who glorify them. But does this special treatment include making a different medical decision regarding their health? Most health-care professionals would say no, but the problem continues.

Until many of these ethical and legal issues are sorted out, one important factor is clear: Each person is responsible for his or her own health. Should we choose to put a marathon or triathlon ahead of our health, we must also be responsible for the outcome, win or lose. Most importantly, we must teach ourselves the importance of health and that it's an important part of building fitness.

# CHAPTER 28

# BUILDING A BETTER ATHLETIC BRAIN

*What is the brain?* The simple act of reading those four words requires the work of hundreds of millions of brain cells (called neurons). Though the brain weighs less than 5 percent of total body mass, it controls nearly every bodily function, from holding this book to going up a flight of stairs. The brain uses between 20 and 50 percent of the oxygen we breathe. Our everyday tasks are achieved with the brain's arsenal of more than 100 billion neurons and 100 trillion interconnections—greater than the number of stars in the universe—existing between those neurons. The brain is more complex than the greatest supercomputers, and this makes the organ truly magnificent, almost beyond our comprehension.

For endurance athletes, there are three important factors to consider regarding the brain. The first is the brain's overlooked role in training and racing. The second is how to improve brain function through biofeedback stimulation—a simple process that you can perform on your own. Third, a variety of lifestyle habits will help you develop and maintain a better athletic brain.

## Brain-Body Chemistry

Physical activity is intricately related to ongoing brain development. This process begins at the earliest age when a child's first movements stimulate brain growth, and continues throughout life unless one stops being active. This activity increases levels of a family of natural protein-based chemicals in the brain called neurotrophins. Perhaps the most researched chemical includes brain-derived neurotrophic factor (BDNF), which promotes cellular growth and repair in the brain and body. BDNF improves brain function by helping cell-to-cell communication, important for learning, memory, and overall cognition. BDNF also stimulates the production of new brain cells—a process called neurogenesis—and protects cells from degeneration, associated with a decline in brain function with age. Physical activity also stimulates BDNF to help mobilize gene expression, switching on many of the genetic benefits programmed within the body while turning off the bad genetic profiles. Even an easy workout can benefit the brain in another way, by promoting plasticity—the ability to improve overall brain function at any age. Those individuals with depression, Alzheimer's disease, and other brain disorders often have low levels of BDNF. Even those with high body fat, diabetes, and other conditions are low in BDNF.

BDNF also affects our muscles by helping them function more effectively through improving contraction and fat burning for energy production throughout the body. And BDNF is considered a key chemical for overall human survival—something we don't think much about these days, but a long endurance event is just that: a test of survival that relies heavily on optimal brain and muscle function.

Which workouts are best for brain health? The answer is any training that promotes overall health, especially those that are aerobic. This can even include an easy walk, regardless of one's level of fitness.

For endurance athletes, the brain's most important job is to preserve the body's delicate physiological mechanisms to prevent injury, ill health, and possible death in the extreme circumstances of tough endurance races. Even during competition, when one's more rational thoughts sometimes get lost in the heat of the battle, the brain will pick up the slack. If you consciously decide, for example, to keep up with the lead pack in a cycling event, despite a usual finish in the middle of the pack, your brain will prevent that attempted high level of effort—subconsciously slowing you down by reducing muscle power. This natural decrease is ultimately for your benefit.

Another common way the brain protects athletes is through its ability to help the body physically compensate for problems such as muscle imbalance. Our eyes play a key role in this physical balance. (The brain also relies on the inner ear's delicate nerve endings to control balance by sensing body motion and adjusting muscle activity.)

Our eyes, which are part of the brain controlled from within, can influence the muscles throughout our body and even change our running, cycling, or swimming form for better or worse. Here's an example. Normally, vision is very high up on the brain's list of priorities; the brain dedicates a significant amount of neurons and energy to visual activity.

Through visual input, the brain will maintain body balance even at the expense of muscles in the neck, shoulder, lower back, and legs. Here's why. It's important that the normal position of both eyes resides in a horizontal plane for optimal function. If muscle imbalance in the neck causes the head to tilt, the eyes may not maintain their normal horizontal position. This is because muscle imbalance can cause the head to tilt slightly to one side, causing the eyes to lose their normal horizontal balance. When this happens, the brain must immediately compensate in the easiest and best way to bring the two eyes back to balance. If the problem muscles in the neck can't be corrected by the brain, other types of compensation are attempted. The brain can do this by creating an opposite imbalance in other muscles, slightly tilting the spine and pelvis to accomplish this task. While this restores the eyes to their normal position, it's done at the expense of other muscles, which now don't function as well. Some of these muscles may be key to the process of running or biking, reducing our effectiveness and altering our form. In addition to slowing us down, it also increases the risk of additional secondary muscle problems and increases stress on joints and other mechanical areas such as ligaments and bones.

This example is very common; just watch marathoners approaching the finish line and you'll see some who are literally, physically twisted—wounded by the brain's compensation. But if the brain didn't act accordingly, the athlete may not have ever completed the race.

By remaining fit and healthy, one can usually prevent the original imbalance in the neck, which caused the eyes to become stressed, thereby eliminating the need for the brain to make such dramatic compensations.

## Racing Through the Brain's "Eyes"

Poets have often written about how the eyes are the windows to the soul. For endurance athletes, the eyes are also a portal to the brain's inner workings. Using the example of a ten-mile road running race, let's take a journey through the eyes of a competitor's brain. The challenge for our fictional runner is to finish the race in just under eighty minutes, a decision based on his MAF Test results (data), course terrain (data), past race experience (memory), and overall general feelings (emotional).

Throughout the race, the brain will monitor the body's activity through messages sent by nerves informing the brain about muscle balance (physical capability), terrain (up and down hills), fat and sugar burning (energy availability), body temperature (a reflection of metabolism), foot stress (influence of shoes and road conditions), pain (emotion), and many other factors such as heart and breathing rate. These factors provide the brain with sufficient information to create a highly effective race strategy.

Even before the gun sounds, our runner's body and brain are continuously sending messages back and forth in preparation for the event. If he goes out too fast, his brain will make the appropriate changes to slow down, both consciously, when he hears the first mile split, and subconsciously (by reducing muscle power to slow him down).

After the second mile, the brain slows the pace because it has determined that the current speed is too difficult to maintain. As the gravitational stresses fluctuate with the uphills and downhills, continuous adjustments are made with pace, muscle function, and energy needs. Perhaps he is checking splits with a watch, consciously and subconsciously estimating a finishing time.

By mile five, the halfway mark, the brain assesses where he is in relation to the finish line and what it will take to maintain current pace. This includes reserving the energy and physical capability. But subtle muscle imbalance that previously existed is now worsening with the physical and metabolic stresses of the first five miles. The brain has been noticing these changes, and now knows it must make take action. It sends messages from the motor cortex down through the spinal cord to create the most effective compensation for the reduced power output of certain muscles by providing more contraction to other muscle fibers. This is accompanied by adjustments in fuel use, attempting more fat burning to conserve sugar. The result of these neurological adjustments is that the pace is slightly reduced.

By mile seven, the body's fuel gauges indicate a problem—there is still too little energy coming from fat and too much from sugar. This imbalance has caused a slight reduction in blood sugar with too much glycogen use. This complication resulted from trying to keep pace with nearby runners up a hill in mile six—an emotional situation the brain must now adapt to. Because of these metabolic changes, the mile seven pace must be adjusted downward. Also, dehydration has caused too much of an increase in body temperature and water must be consumed; our runner also pours water on his head for added cooling. As a result of these effective adjustments, he recovers and runs mile eight at a slightly quicker pace.

Now that the finish line is mentally within his reach, adjustments are made near mile nine. These include making conscious decisions to continue quenching thirst (which prevents too much dehydration and controls rising temperatures), factoring in pain tolerance (accepting the discomfort knowing the race will soon end), adjustment of breathing (a bit deeper), and slightly shortening stride length to cut down on physical stress. All this takes place while the brain continues adapting from moment to moment to all the other physical, chemical, and mental requirements, including muscle balance, energy production, and stress control.

During the last mile, if his brain and body coordination was successful throughout the race, he has an increased pace and finds himself crossing the finish in reasonably good shape, perhaps with a stronger kick at the end. If not, he becomes a wounded warrior, limping erratically through the final painful mile. Or worse, he collapses before the finish line because his brain has shut down the body to prevent serious damage. Consider Julie Moss in the February 1982 Ironman Hawaii race—she was forced to crawl those last few feet.

This continuous back-and-forth communication between the brain and body during the race comes with another interesting feature: trial and error. This is due to the brain's periods of "uncertainty" where it must make a particular physiological adjustment during a race, then wait to gauge the result. For instance, if, during mile seven the brain determines that the blood sugar levels are dropping too low, some physical adjustments are made—perhaps reducing muscle contraction to conserve sugar, which slows the pace, or converting more glycogen to glucose. Then the brain may have to wait again to see if these changes improved blood sugar; if not, it considers what other changes may be necessary, such as further slowing or even stopping at the water station. But while the brain is preoccupied with such activities, all this compensation can take away from better performance by using up more energy, ultimately slowing one's finishing time. Over the years, I have noticed that experienced athletes who are healthier physically, chemically, and mentally can maintain better pacing through a long event with less of the brain's trial and error periods, which can also increase wear and tear, contribute to injury, and slow recovery.

## Stimulating Brain Health

Just like with training, when we stress our muscles, we must use our brain by pushing it a bit to reach new limits, but not too much to hurt it. To paraphrase the great singer-songwriter Bob Dylan, if we're not busy being born, we're busy dying. This sums up the remedy for optimal brain function throughout life. This use comes in the form of sending a variety of sensations into the brain from the body. This can be accomplished through various means:

- *Physical stimulation.* Every step we take, each stroke we make, influences many different brain areas significantly. Even a physical massage can provide great stimulation for the brain, as can walking barefoot.
- *Auditory stimulation.* The best example is listening to enjoyable music, which may stimulate all the brain's areas.
- *Visual stimulation.* Even taking in the sights during a workout is a great exercise for the brain.
- *Avoid stressful stimulations.* Try to keep away from annoying sounds, sights, smells, and environmental factors (such as running or biking in a crowded urban setting, with all that traffic noise and vehicular air pollution).

Diminished brain function can result from too little or the wrong kind of stimulation. It's estimated that one in four people in the United States suffers from some form of mental or emotional disorder, also known as brain injury. Many more have diminished brain function, which is often temporary and can be corrected by providing the brain with sufficient stimulation. Human error is a common result of diminished brain function, and is the cause of the majority of cycling, automobile, airplane, rail, boating, and other tragic accidents reported in the popular press every day. Medical mistakes, which kill and maim millions of people, are also usually due to human error. Whether it's poor memory, such as not remembering that phone call you wanted to make, or getting lost in your own neighborhood due to a serious cognitive condition such as Alzheimer's, in most cases these problems are preventable through proper food and nutrition, stress regulation, and lifestyle. And the idea isn't just to avoid cognitive problems—you want your brain to function at a high level until you die!

### Brain Biofeedback

One way to improve brain function is to stimulate certain levels of consciousness—in particular, those that result in particular brain waves. This is accomplished with an important form of biofeedback I developed called *respiratory biofeedback*. The procedure is very similar to EEG (electroencephalograph) biofeedback, or neurofeedback, which helps improve brain function by increasing alpha wave production. Increases of this brain wave can not only help overall brain function but reduce unwanted stress hormones. Like with manual biofeedback (see chapter 25), respiratory biofeedback can also be performed without costly equipment.

All athletes can benefit from respiratory biofeedback, which not only helps the brain but the body as well. This biofeedback can reduce high levels of stress hormones to improve adrenal function and fat burning, control blood sugar, and other benefits such as correcting and preventing muscle imbalance. We can use it on ourselves as a quick, effective daily remedy to improve overall health. Respiratory biofeedback can also be performed before other physical therapies are used to help improve the efficacy of these remedies (and sometimes eliminate their necessity). For example, before getting a hands-on treatment from a chiropractor or osteopath, respiratory therapy can help prepare your body for these other therapies. In fact, some health-care professionals use respiratory biofeedback on their patients.

Respiratory biofeedback is associated with a number of significant health benefits that can also improve fitness:

- It can increase oxygen to the brain, potentially improving a variety of neurological imbalances. This is accomplished through more efficient breathing that brings more air into the lungs and more oxygen to the brain.

- Respiratory feedback can help restore and improve normal breathing. Improper breathing is often associated with brain and spinal cord injuries, and is sometimes a hidden problem even in relatively healthy athletes.
- It can help improve the function of the diaphragm and abdominal muscles. In addition to breathing, these muscles play a significant role in physical activity, improving posture and supporting the spine and pelvis.
- Because of its effect on the brain and nervous system, respiratory biofeedback can help improve the function of other muscles in the body as well, and help reduce pain—two reasons to perform this procedure before other manual biofeedback.
- It can help reduce harmful stress hormones, especially cortisol, balance the autonomic nervous system, and promote muscle relaxation—all very important features for a healthier brain and body.

### Respiratory Biofeedback Procedures

Once you have a better understanding of brain waves and normal breathing, you can then perform respiratory biofeedback. While it's important to relax the body as much as possible during this process, if this procedure is new, you may be a little tense as you go through each step. But soon, you'll be able relax and obtain the maximum benefits of respiratory biofeedback.

While each of the steps below can produce some alpha wave activity, combining all of them can be a very potent five-minute therapy. Here are the five steps for respiratory biofeedback:

1. It's best performed relaxed, in a lying position, although slightly reclined while sitting is also effective.
2. Place your hands or arms on the middle of the abdomen and keep them relaxed. This sensation and weight provide a biofeedback effect on the diaphragm and abdominal muscles during movement.
3. Close your eyes.
4. Listen to enjoyable, relaxing music—popular or classical. The tunes that are your favorites work best, especially if headphones are used, which keep out distracting noise.
5. Breathe easy and deep. Most people can comfortably, slowly inhale for about five to seven seconds; then, exhale for the same five to seven seconds. If five to seven seconds makes you feel out of breath or dizzy, adjust the time—try three to four seconds during inhalation, for example, and the same for exhalation.

Continue respiratory biofeedback for about five minutes.

Caution: It's very important that you do not fall asleep, or even start drifting into sleep, which produces delta waves. If you start getting sleepy after two minutes, perform respiratory biofeedback for just less than that time and gradually work up to five minutes—but always avoid getting sleepy. If you consistently get sleepy during respiratory biofeedback, there may be other sleep-related issues such as sleep deprivation or sleep apnea (often caused by carbohydrate intolerance).

As a powerful self-therapy, respiratory biofeedback can be performed once or twice daily, or more if necessary. It's also a great pre-workout and pre-race routine, helping to balance the nervous system and muscles. And by correcting muscle imbalance and improving the nervous system, it can also help control pain.

## Brain and Blood Sugar

Do you remember where you were when President Kennedy was assassinated? Maybe you weren't been born yet. How about when the space shuttle Challenger exploded? Or when the World Trade Center towers collapsed? Most people have vivid memories of where they were when these intense events occurred. At the same time, many people can't recall a friend's frequently called phone number or the name of someone they just

## OUR BRAIN WAVES

An important component of respiratory biofeedback is the production of healthy brain waves. The brain produces different frequencies and amplitudes of electrical waves depending upon our levels of consciousness. Sensation, attention (self-awareness), intellectual activity, and the planning of physical movement have distinct electrical correlates in the brain that can be measured using an EEG.

There are four commonly measured waves, and at least two others that have been observed:

Beta waves (12–32 Hz) are associated with full awareness and high cortical activity—typical of a busy brain, such as during a business meeting, planning a trip, or when mentally doing several things at once.

Alpha waves (8–12 Hz) are associated with a sense of "relaxed alertness" and high creativity—typical during meditation, listening to music, and when eyes are closed. The ability to generate alpha waves is associated with the self-regulation of stress and may contribute to an expanded state of consciousness.

Theta waves (4–8 Hz) are an awake but dreamy state common just before the onset of sleep; most prevalent in youth because the brain has not yet fully developed, they also occur during deep creativity and meditation in adults at any time.

Delta waves (0.5–4 Hz) are very slow waves occurring during most stages of sleep. It is abnormal for them to occur while one is awake, and may indicate a lack of nutrients such as glucose or oxygen, medication effects, or poorly functioning neurons.

Another brain wave type is gamma (30–80 Hz). Much less is known about this type of wave. It may be associated with more complex cortical function and higher levels of consciousness. A sensory motor rhythm (12–15 Hz) above the higher end alpha and entering beta has been associated with alert but muscle-relaxed states.

Our brains should make specific waves in certain brain regions at appropriate times. An abnormality might include a normal wave occurring at the wrong time. For example, delta waves that occur while driving to the pool for a swim workout are abnormal, leading to distraction and increasing the risk of a traffic accident. And the appearance of theta waves while on a long bike ride is abnormal and could account for getting lost or drifting into the rear wheel of the rider in front of you.

The ability to produce alpha waves is associated with an overall healthy brain and body, especially in relation to controlling stress. It is one reason people have, for thou-

met a half hour ago. The strong memory of traumatic events persists due to the powerful adrenal response—the fight or flight mechanism—that raises blood sugar to optimum levels. While the body utilizes both fat and sugar for energy, the brain is primarily dependent upon sugar. If the level of blood sugar rises too much, or falls too low, the brain has an immediately reduced capacity. This means you don't remember as well, don't respond as well to external stimuli, and can't learn as easily. Reductions in overall mental and physical performance can follow:

- High-glycemic carbohydrates, especially sugar and processed flour products, can reduce and impair brain function due to the effects of insulin.

- Blood sugar can be controlled exceptionally well by snacking on healthy items. By eating five or six meals daily, you can help stabilize blood sugar, allowing the brain to do its job properly.

- Stress can wreak havoc on blood sugar and reduce overall brain function.

## Mental Energy

When we consider mental energy, it's clear thinking and creativity we want, rather than that foggy feeling or depression. Too many endurance athletes set themselves up for anxiety or depression, which adversely affects physical performance. This can result not only from a bad race or the frustration of training, but from poor brain function.

sands of years, pursued meditation, the use of psychedelic or hallucinogenic drugs, prayer, and other activities that seek to promote the alpha state. Specifically, alpha waves can reduce high levels of the stress hormone cortisol and help balance the autonomic nervous system. These alpha waves can have dramatic effects on our whole body, such as improved memory, learning, and comprehension, better blood sugar regulation, improved gut function, and balanced hormones. When we're relaxed, creative, meditating, and happy, our brain produces large amounts of alpha waves. For these and other reasons, one main focus of respiratory biofeedback is the creation of alpha waves.

The inability to produce alpha waves signifies underlying problems. Inadequate sleep, overtraining, nutritional imbalances, and very high levels of stress hormones can impair the ability to produce alpha waves. Even certain structural problems, such as those in the jaw joint or neck muscles, can significantly reduce our ability to generate healthy alpha waves.

When you have a thought or feel a sensation from the outside world, it's the result of major chemical reactions in your brain. Diet can have an immediate and profound effect on brain chemistry, often as much as drugs, but easier to regulate and without unwanted side effects. A meal at dinnertime can influence your sleep, dreams, and how you feel during your morning workout. And what you eat, or don't eat, for breakfast can determine your overall human performance for the rest of the day.

Most of the forty or more types of neurotransmitters are made from amino acids derived from the protein in your diet. Certain vitamins and minerals are also required for their production, including vitamin B6, folic acid, niacin, iron, and vitamin C. There are many important neurotransmitters related to mental function. They include serotonin and norepinephrine—the two most commonly discussed substances.

## Drugs and the Brain

A variety of over-the-counter and prescription drugs can impair brain function. Many of these drugs won't signal obvious symptoms that the brain is adversely affected. Alcohol can depress brain function, although in small amounts it can improve social activity—this may be a great thing for the brain. Balance is key—even if it's only one small alcoholic drink, whether wine, beer, or distilled booze—if you don't feel right drinking, or feel the effects the next morning, avoid alcohol altogether.

Drugs are often prescribed to balance brain chemistry. Depressed patients are given medication to restore balance to the neurotransmitters. Prozac, Elavil, Buspar, Aventyl, Tofranil, and Zoloft are antidepressants that affect the balance of serotonin and norepinephrine. But these medications have side effects, including reductions in glutathione, the most powerful antioxidant, which protects the brain from damage and is important for the body's recovery from a workout or race.

## Brain and EPA

One of the most important brain nutrients is the omega-3 fat EPA (along with its related fat, DHA). Most people won't get enough from food, so supplementation is often necessary. The omega-3 fats are key ingredients for the development and repair of the brain, especially the eyes. Imbalances in essential fatty acids—particularly deficiencies in omega-3 fats—have been implicated in depressive disorders in adults and behavioral problems in children and adolescents, including Attention Deficit Hyperactivity Disorder (ADHD), difficulties with learning, impulsivity, hyperactivity, aggression, and anger. Athletes are not immune to these types of problems; I've helped many restore normal brain function and eliminate medication, often with the help of EPA. These brain problems often go hand in hand

with chronic inflammation; EPA not only can improve brain function but can also help balance fats so the body can make natural anti-inflammatory chemicals for recovery and injury prevention.

Researchers continue to identify the positive effects of EPA on the brain and also have established a direct link between an imbalance in fatty acids and depressive disorders. In fact, it appears that these fats regulate neurotransmitters in ways that mimic the effect of some antidepressant medications. These fats also coat the brain-cell membrane, serving a protective function when neurotransmitters are fired in the synaptic phase.

EPA and DHA have other benefits in brain function as well. They are most vital for the fetus and child during development of the brain. They may also help control the release of the stress hormone cortisol, resulting in improved brain and adrenal gland function. And they may help reduce the severity of degenerative brain diseases that lead to memory loss and dementia, including Alzheimer's disease.

## Other Brain Requirements

Any dietary inadequacy can potentially have a dramatic impact on brain function. Numerous studies show that many people with depression also have low levels of the nutrient folate. Consuming foods containing this nutrient can significantly improve depression in these people. For this reason, anyone considering antidepressant medication should first be screened for folate levels through a blood test for homocysteine, the best indicator of folate levels in the body. For depressed individuals who have low folate levels, adequate folate intake and use may be as effective as Prozac or other antidepressant drugs for treating mild, moderate, and severe depression. Folate is contained in green, leafy vegetables and fruits; in some cases, fruit, especially citrus, can be a better source than leafy vegetables. For many people, synthetic folate or folic acid, as from most supplements, may not be as effective or as well utilized as folate obtained from real food sources. In fact, up to 30 percent of athletes may be unable to make use of synthetic folate.

Other micronutrients are important for the brain, too:

- Sodium, potassium, magnesium, and calcium—the same electrolytes we need for optimal training and racing—are also important for sending messages through the brain.
- Zinc is important for growth and maturation of the brain, and is used for many chemical reactions in the brain, especially those related to behavior.
- Copper is also important for the brain. While copper deficiency has been associated with deterioration of mental function and physical coordination, too much of this mineral can have the same results.
- Manganese, like copper, is both important for proper brain function and has potential for adversely affecting the brain if taken in excess.

- Lead, arsenic, and mercury are all toxic to the brain and pose real health problems throughout the world. Lead poisoning has been known about for centuries. For years scientific literature has described mercury poisoning, which can happen through consumption of fish contaminated with accumulated methyl mercury (introduced to the food chain by industrial waste) or consumption of grain treated with mercury fungicide. The debate over dental fillings is still a concern to many in the scientific community.
- Vitamin B6 is another important brain nutrient and is used in the regulation of certain neurotransmitters. Because estrogen can reduce the levels of vitamin B6, this may be important for some women, especially those taking birth-control pills and estrogen-replacement therapy.
- Many athletes consume and even rely on caffeine to help the body train and race. Though caffeine isn't considered a nutrient, it is a drug with potentially significant brain effects. This is obvious to those who regularly consume caffeine. Don't think so? Try *not* drinking your daily brew for even one day! A key effect of caffeine is increased mental performance and alertness, though negative brain effects can appear soon afterward when the drug wears off and you crave more, especially if your healthy food intake is inadequate. The physical side effects of caffeine can be unhealthy for some while others can tolerate relatively small amounts of caffeine

each day. It's up to you to determine if your brain and body can tolerate caffeine and, if so, how much.

## Sports, Music, and the Brain

Currently, one of the hottest fields in medical science is research into the brain—how it functions, what consciousness and memory are, biofeedback, behavior modification, and biological self-repair. Music plays an especially key role in brain research and injury treatment. For athletes, this can be a godsend. Because being in the right mental state while listening to music can affect one's brain waves, which, in turn, can improve one's overall fitness and health.

In Dr. Oliver Sacks' best-selling book, *Musicophilia*, he investigates the profound relationship between music and the mind. In one passage, the well-known neurologist describes how he hurt his leg while mountain climbing and was able to get down the mountain before nightfall by singing "The Old Volga Boatman." He said that he "musicked along" and the rhythms and melodies made his mind forget the pain. Later, in the hospital, he repeatedly listened to a cassette of a Mendelssohn violin concerto. Then, after weeks of struggling to walk, he stood and found that "the concerto started to play itself with intense vividness in my mind. In this moment, the natural rhythm and melody of walking came back to me . . . and along with this [came] the feeling of my leg as alive, as part of me once again." This example of the healing powers of music is one every endurance athlete may benefit from.

The body's response to an injury includes a stress reaction but often, before an injury, there's also preexisting stress. And stress itself may contribute to or actually cause the injury. In either situation, the related high levels of stress hormones can interfere with our repair and recovery. Music can help reduce stress hormones, allowing the healing process to proceed more effectively and quickly. Music also helps coordinate the brain and muscle memory. Think about the power of music and muscle memory in complicated dance routines. Visualization is a practical application of this for any athlete. Listening to music while envisioning a successful workout, or especially a great race, is a wonderful way to add more training without adding miles. I've extensively worked with many people who had serious muscle problems and found that through biofeedback—by improving communication between muscles and brain—normal function can be restored even in those with strokes, spinal problems, and brain injuries.

When we listen to music, the brain focuses on all the sounds, which in turn affect other brain areas. The more sounds, the more involved the brain becomes. In a piece of music with just a guitar and vocal, like a simple folk song, the brain will "light up" all over; lyrics may trigger all kinds of memories; melodies affect other brain areas; and bass notes can awaken still other brain regions, and so on. A song about social injustice

## SLEEPY AFTER A BIG MEAL?

The reason many people get sleepy after a big lunch or dinner is usually due to too many carbohydrates, including sugar. In the case of a typical holiday meal, it's not the turkey but the bread (usually high glycemic), potatoes (including sweetened sweet potatoes), gravy (made with flour), cranberries (sweetened with sugar), and, of course, those extra servings of pie (there's always more than one type to taste). Throw in some alcohol and it's no wonder you're craving more than just one cup of coffee.

The carbohydrates cause a rise in the level of the brain neurotransmitter serotonin—this has a calming, relaxing, sedating effect on the brain, because the more carbohydrates you eat, the more sedating its action.

Sleepiness after any meal may be indicative of carbohydrate intolerance because of higher levels of insulin. This would also indicate that your body is burning more sugar and less fat, just the opposite state you want for optimal endurance. So if you often feel sleepy after meals, it's time to evaluate, or reevaluate, your eating habits. While sweets are traditionally thought of as providing energy, they are in actuality mentally sedating. Sometimes sweets may give the feeling of a pick-up, but that is very short-lived, until insulin lowers the blood sugar, resulting in more fatigue.

If you need a mental pick-up, try eating some protein. A protein-based meal with little or no carbohydrates causes your body to produce less insulin, and provides a higher amount of tyrosine and increased norepinephrine levels. This neurotransmitter has a stimulating effect on the brain.

might get the brain working more diligently than simple nonsense or pop lyrics. The act of listening to a full symphony orchestra playing a complex piece of music will let an enormous number of sounds enter the brain. In turn, this can increase blood flow to the brain, bringing in more nutrients to help brain function—including those areas that control our muscles, ranging from relaxation to power. As a simple experiment, spend a few minutes listening to Vivaldi's Four Seasons or Beethoven's Fifth Symphony—not while doing something else or as background music. Close your eyes and let the auditory experience take over your brain. Or, go to my Web site at www.PhilMaffetone.com and listen to the song "Rosemary" during your five-minute respiratory biofeedback session.

Music "therapy" is similar to heart-rate monitoring; it's just a different form of biofeedback. You listen and your body responds. This approach to brain biofeedback is basic and one I like using because the increased alpha waves can improve brain and body function (which regulates our exercise activities), improve oxygenation, balance the nervous system, and control stress. With music therapy, there is no need to pay for a series of expensive biofeedback sessions, courses to take, or lengthy learning curve. Using music during respiratory biofeedback helps make this technique even more powerful as a brain therapy.

Music as therapy is thousands of years old. Perhaps the first written therapeutic use came from Chinese medicine about five thousand years ago. About 2500 BCE, followers of Pythagoras developed a science of "musical psychotherapy." Today, the long winding road of music includes treatment for many types of patients, including those with depression, autism, learning disabilities, Alzheimer's, and others. But almost anyone can enjoy the music as well as its health benefits. In fact, music therapy has been making substantial inroads into contemporary mainstream health care. Music therapy is used at many medical facilities, including Greenwich Hospital in Greenwich, Connecticut, Beth Israel Hospital in New York City, and Children's Hospital at Vanderbilt Medical Center in Nashville, Tennessee. The University of Michigan Medical Center is among a growing list of schools that offer programs to certify music practitioners. The American Music Therapy Association has specific curriculum requirements including courses in research analysis, physiology, acoustics, psychology, and music and therapy. There are about six thousand certified music therapists in North America alone.

Music can even enhance mental visualization, which has long been an effective training technique in endurance sports. That's why music is often a part of the process—not only when learning a particular visualization but when putting it into practice.

While many athletes are familiar with visualization, other music-brain relationships are equally important. The musical beat or rhythm can also help improve certain brain areas such as the cerebellum, which acts as our internal metronome. Maintaining a continuous natural rhythm of running, biking, or swimming is something most athletes can relate to. You don't need to listen to music when working out, but encourage your brain to mentally play it. In a long workout, once warmed up, your body gets locked into that wonderful continuous rhythm, whether it's your feet hitting the ground or the repetitive circular motion of pedaling. This natural rhythm helps keep you going—it's the athlete's dance. Additionally, this movement involves communication between at least two brain areas—the cerebellum and motor cortex—to maintain steady, continuous, muscle activity. These actions can improve the economy or efficiency of our gait or stroke movement used during running, biking, or swimming. These benefits from the cerebellum occur because this part of the brain controls physical coordination and balance.

So which songs or type of music produces the best training or therapeutic response for endurance athletes? That depends on you and your circumstances. I could name hundreds of songs. But first let me explain something important here. Music can rev you up as easily as it can relax you. Thus, one key is picking the songs most appropriate for what you want. Most athletes need additional help with their rest and recovery, so soothing music—like the slower classical pieces—may be best. Sometimes, it's how we listen as much as what we listen to. When hearing high-energy songs that get us moving, it's often the drums and bass guitar that affect our nervous system and rev us up. The melody (in songs with words, it's the part that's sung) is what most people remember and can be a powerful therapy. Or, by listening for things you may not have heard before in a familiar song, such as one of the background instruments like a subtle piano or acoustic guitar, the brain responds.

Often, those who normally don't respond to music can't take their mind off everything else around them when the music is playing. Try a good pair of headphones (especially the noise-cancellation types) and close your eyes. In this state, the brain doesn't have to listen to anything except the music, and there are no distractions from visual stimuli, which turn on more of the brain than anything else. This gives the brain more "energy" to focus on the music, and often in this state you can hear things in a favorite song you may never have heard before.

Which songs do I like listening to? Ask me this question tomorrow and I'll have a different list. Virtually any Beatles song will work well, especially "Hey Jude," "Yesterday," or "Here Comes the Sun." I've used "Day Tripper" in measuring brain waves with patients. I also like "For No One." Most classical music works exceptionally well, too. Like many Beatles' songs, Mozart's modal music is great, but experiment—there is almost an endless supply. Some great pop picks include: "Chelsea Morning" by Joni Mitch ell, "Heart of Gold" by Neil Young, "Hey" by Red Hot Chili Peppers, "Hallelujah" by Leonard Cohen, "San Diego Serenade" by Tom Waits, "Time of No Reply" by Nick Drake, Dylan's "Like A Rolling Stone" or "Desolation Row," James Taylor's "Fire and Rain," John Lennon's "Imagine," Paul Simon's "Graceland," and Tom Petty's "Learning To Fly."

Music can also help you calm pre-race tensions. It could even be better than meditation because many people can't meditate successfully since it takes some training. Music, on the other hand, is right there, front and center, especially when you wear headphones and close your eyes.

Most athletes are generally smart about their own bodies, and incorporating music therapy is worth trying. It potentially offers a high return on a small investment and with virtually no risk. The results will speak for themselves, that is, if you listen carefully. There's nothing like listening to Mozart, the Beatles, or Cat Stevens to reduce stress or meditatively ponder life. There's a place for Chopin and Dylan in your training sched-ule—but not while biking! Match the music and your mood, and you're on your way. After a hard training session, relaxing and listening to some good music can help the brain and body—both can come together in a healthy way.

## BEAT THE BONK WITH YOUR BRAIN

Call it hitting the wall or bonking, but when your brain and body feel like shutting down, and you have almost no energy to continue moving, it means something is physically and mentally wrong. *Bonking is not normal.* Having helped endurance athletes avoid bonking throughout my coaching career, and having experienced this painful event myself early on in a marathon, I am convinced that with proper diet and training you can avoid the dreaded bonk.

You'll know when you're bonking—it typically occurs seemingly out of nowhere and fast. For marathon runners, it usually happens around the so-called wall at twenty miles, or for triathletes anytime during the run of an Ironman-distance event. The mileage is not relevant, but the time and intensity of your race is a key to when you may bonk. And in addition to the obvious physiological nature of the problem, which has a lot to do with the kinds of fuel you're burning (fat and sugar), the notion of a "wall" can be a psychological stumbling block for some athletes.

The signs and symptoms vary with individuals. You usually feel sudden weakness throughout the body (muscles seemingly not responding as they should). There's often a loss of normal mental function and reduced concentration. You no longer think about finishing the race, and stopping sounds like the best idea (although many try pushing themselves). Fellow competitors are flying right past. This further discourages you. Your own world seems to be going in slow motion. In extreme cases, you might collapse.

Bonking is caused by an inability to burn sufficient fat for energy. This source of sustained, long-term energy and stamina has deteriorated and without it one must rely mostly on sugar and its strict limitation to provide energy. In the process, one uses up too much of one's glycogen stores and now the blood sugar becomes too low, depriving not just the muscles but the brain of fuel.

Once you're out of gas, it's game over. Bonking actually prevents you from further damaging your body by trying to continue—at least in most cases.

Once you reach the point of bonking, it's difficult to escape this state in the course of a race, even if you slow down, consume carbohydrates, or even stop to cool off. The time to avoid bonking in a race begins long before, in your training, and continues through the implementation of a pre-race plan of food and race nutrition and pacing.

If you find yourself frequently hitting the wall (I believe once is too much), some self-assessment can help alleviate this condition. Ask yourself: "When does the sudden fatigue happen?" In shorter endurance events of one to two hours, the reasons are different than for longer races. A bonk that occurs during a shorter event often indicates one isn't using sufficient fat burning for energy. A well-trained endurance athlete with great fat burning can often race this distance without consuming any nutrients during the race except water, because his or her body fat provides so much of the energy.

Other athletes may need to consume nutrition during a shorter race; in addition to water, this can be some form of carbohydrate, such as a drink you previously determined in training works well for you. The use of carbohydrate during any endurance event is important, especially to help the body maintain fat burning and preserve glycogen and blood sugar.

Other problems that can reduce fat burning include starting the race too fast. This is not unusual in these shorter endurance events. When this happens, you begin racing much faster than your body can convert fat to energy (and much faster than you could possibly maintain for the duration of the race). This forces your body's metabolism to rely more on sugar and less on fat. The result is you use up your stored energy in the form of glycogen, and burn too much blood sugar—recovery from this debt early in a race is nearly impossible and can easily lead to a bonk.

Your pre-race meal is important and can also influence fat burning. This is not only breakfast the morning of the race but also dinner or an evening snack the night before. If these meals are made up of high-glycemic carbohydrates, it can raise your insulin too much, thereby reducing both glycogen stores and fat burning when the gun goes off. The result: a bonk.

Pre-race stress can also be a factor in reducing fat burning, with some people more vulnerable. This is particularly true in those with adrenal dysfunction, where cortisol levels are too high (or too low), typically in athletes who are overtrained. Combine this with pre-race tension and it could contribute to a bonk.

In addition to fat-burning problems, water regulation can contribute to a bonk. Given the right set of circumstances, significant dehydration can stop you quick. Causes can include not enough water intake before the race, not enough during the race, high temperatures, dry air, or competing at higher altitude. Other factors can also contribute to bonking in a shorter event: nutritional imbalances, extreme weather conditions, allergy or asthma, and a lingering cold or an oncoming flu. Many times, an athlete will bonk because more than one problem exists.

Many of the same factors can cause a bonk in longer events, such as those lasting more than two hours. But the main factor that makes these races different is the need for continuous nutrition throughout the event. This comes in the form of water to prevent significant dehydration and carbohydrates to help maintain fat burning. Most athletes in longer events need more fuel, with both protein and fat contributing to energy needs as well.

Once an athlete understands his or her needs during any endurance event, bonking should never occur. Being smart about training and racing begins by understanding your body's needs. The process of experimentation should take place during training, not racing. Once you find your optimal routine, including nutritional requirements, pacing strategy, stress control, and other physical, chemical, and mental factors that pertain to you, not only will you avoid bonking but you'll race better.

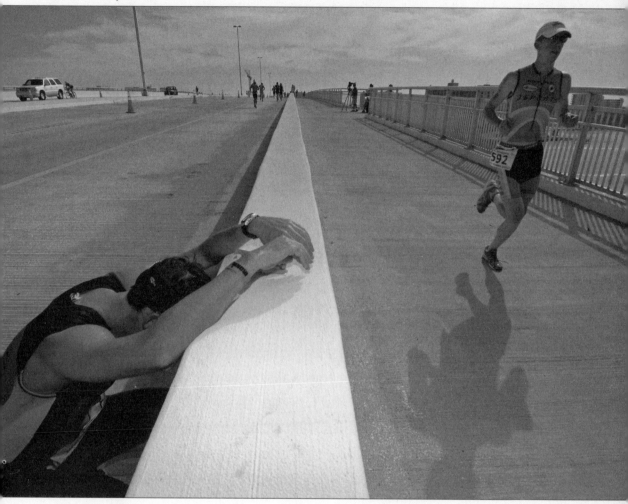

*The time to avoid bonking in a race begins long before, in your training.*

# CHAPTER 29

# BURNING OFF BODY FAT AND OTHER WEIGHTY ISSUES

The issue of body fat remains a sensitive one for endurance athletes. On one hand, many believe that with all the training they do, their body fat should melt right off. But the reality is something quite different: they don't see that happening; in fact, higher than expected body fat is common among multisport athletes. Diet plays an important role in burning off excess body fat, but using a heart-rate monitor and finding the correct maximum aerobic heart rate will turn your body into a fat-burning machine.

The problem of excess body fat often begins when athletes are in their twenties and thirties. This period marks a change in metabolism. The body no longer tolerates certain dietary imbalances, non-optimal training, and daily stress that one's golden youth once easily brushed aside. Once you are past the age of twenty, several physiological functions begin to diminish. These include maximum oxygen uptake, maximum heart rate, lung capacity, muscle mass, and strength. The rate of decline is dependant upon overall fitness and health, especially aerobic capacity. As these age-related changes take place, body fat content tends to rise. Studies have shown that for active endurance athletes, body weight

**Question:** From your own experience watching, coaching, and training endurance athletes, would you say there is an optimal body size for triathletes, like there usually is for cyclists and runners?

**Answer:** There are many fitness and health factors you can control, from building aerobic function and avoiding injury to controlling body fat and preventing most chronic disease. So obtaining your own personal ideal body by training and eating right for your needs should be your goal. Obviously you can't change your body type to some theoretical image for your sport. While we think about the ideal athlete for any given sport, it's really just an academic discussion for most people. Researchers use body size (mass), total surface area of the body, and other factors to calculate and compare measurements such as maximum oxygen uptake, power output, and other variables when performing experiments with groups of athletes (although physiologists disagree on just how to do this). Your genes dictated your body type—how it functions in sports is greatly dependent upon how you program it.

may remain the same with age, but body fat content can rise 3 percent each decade. But for an aging athlete who is fit and healthy, these typical declines in body composition—more fat, less muscle—don't occur.

Each one of us must address this issue individually, and for almost every athlete burdened with higher-than-normal levels of body fat, this chapter will answer the common question, *"How do I get rid of this extra body fat?"* While the short answer is that a heart-rate monitor can help burn off body fat when used to build an aerobic base, there are a number of issues to address, one of which is why, other than aesthetics, too much body fat is harmful.

## The Problems of Excess Body Fat

There are a number of important reasons why excess body fat is harmful to your health:

- It represents a combination of improper training and poor eating habits.
- Stored body fat produces inflammatory chemicals that are a serious threat, not just to injuries and recovery from training and competition but to overall health. Chronic inflammation is the first step in the development of various physical injuries.
- Higher body fat adversely affects athletic performance for most sports (with some

## THYROID TROUBLES

While most people with excess fat can lose it by fully developing an aerobic system and eliminating refined carbohydrates, some have true metabolic problems. Perhaps the most common is thyroid dysfunction. Low thyroid function is commonly associated with increased body fat. Other signs and symptoms include depression and skin problems (especially cracking around the heels and on the hands), hair loss, especially thinning of the lateral one-third of the eyebrow, and low body temperature.

If this is a potential problem, the first step is to evaluate thyroid function. Blood tests for the thyroid include free T3 and T4, and TSH levels. If these are not normal, thyroid antibodies should be evaluated. But blood tests don't always show the relatively

exceptions, such as sumo wrestling or long-distance cold-water swimming).

- As body fat rises, changes in body composition are associated with further age-related reductions in oxygen uptake and athletic performance.

- Higher levels of body fat are a source of extra—sometimes excess—estrogen, which could have adverse effects on overall fitness and health.

- Body fat content in athletes varies considerably. I'm not going to assign any numbers or range of percent body fat because they are not meaningful for athletes. Instead, those with obvious excess levels, including those who have gained body fat compared to previous years already know they are carrying around too much.

- The size of your waist is a good general indication of changes in body fat. The fit-

test period of my life was during high school and college sports. Today, I'm still about the same size in my waist. While my muscle mass may be a bit lower and body fat a bit higher—a normal pattern in optimal aging—it's still within a reasonable, healthy level. In many cases, athletes will see their waist size increase by two, four, or more inches—an indication that there is probably excess body fat. That's because that extra fat takes up a lot of room.

Measuring your waist on a monthly basis may be the best overall method of tracking body fat content. Do this at the level of the umbilicus, the belly button.

Most people consider excess body weight and body fat as synonymous. But this is simply untrue. Because we are a weight-conscious society, stepping on the scale each morning is minor functional thyroid problems common in stubborn cases. Saliva tests may be more important for these types of evaluations. You can also take your temperature—those with low thyroid function usually have low temperatures. Below-normal temperatures—less than about 98.6°F (37°C)—may indicate thyroid dysfunction. (Note that NSAIDs can also disturb metabolism and decrease body temperature.)

If you make the necessary corrections, whether it's improving your diet, building the aerobic system, or others (including the right combinations), your thyroid function should improve and fat burning should increase. This will be reflected in a more normal body temperature and any other blood or saliva tests. In some cases, you may have to find a health-care professional who can help you improve thyroid function.

a powerful ritual—and one difficult to break. A lot of the weight the scale measures is water, and most of this water is in the muscles and other body areas, not fat. Body fat weighs much less. However, body fat takes up much more space than water. In fact, many of the patients I helped lose body fat often didn't lose weight—and some actually gained weight while losing inches off their waist. The reason is that as body fat is reduced, muscle function and weight are improved.

There are varying ways to measure body size, and even percentage of body fat. And many weight-loss programs sell various gadgets for determining the amount. But in keeping with simplifying the stress in your life, my suggestion is to avoid the task of trying to focus on these more detailed measurements—and avoid the risk of creating a new obsession of weighing yourself. Reducing body fat should be done in a healthy way. Start with the Two-Week Test (see chapter 14).

## Problems of Calorie Restriction

Restricting calories as a means of losing body weight is the most common approach used in the weight-loss industry and by individuals, especially athletes. About 95 percent of those who go on a calorie-restricted diet will fail in the long run. Endurance athletes often count calories to reduce or avoid too much body fat. By restricting calories, runners, cyclists, swimmers, and others risk not supplying sufficient energy for optimal training.

Of those who lose weight initially with calorie restriction, most will gain it back—plus more—in the end. Moreover, most will not lose body fat. Much of this problem is due to the fact that by restricting calories, one's metabolism is adversely reduced, with the result of eventually storing more body fat.

By performing a computerized dietary analysis on almost every patient I've seen in practice, I noticed that most of them who restricted calories also restricted nutrients. This results in a loss of health and athletic performance. Dehydration, nutrient loss, muscle and bone loss, lowered metabolism that shifts to more sugar and less fat burning, and other health issues are most often the real result of weight loss from calorie restriction. In some, the result has been an eating disorder that can be even more difficult to treat.

### Heart-Rate Monitoring to Burn Fat

To a large extent, training for endurance is about fat burning. This is accomplished by building a great aerobic base. For those whose goals include reducing body fat to healthy levels, building an even larger aerobic base is the first step.

It's obvious that those with higher levels of body fat have higher respiratory quotients (RQ). This means they're burning too much sugar for energy, and too little fat. Studies have also shown that those with higher levels of body fat have higher numbers of anaerobic muscle fibers and lower numbers of aerobic fibers. Your goal in training, therefore, is to not only increase the fat-burning capacity of your aerobic muscles, but to increase the number of aerobic fibers in your muscles. This is accomplished by building as large an aerobic base as possible.

By increasing fat burning, you'll reduce body fat, have more energy, and create a powerful foundation to further your endurance goals. Take the MAF Test to make sure your body is increasing its fat-burning capability. As your MAF Test improves, your body fat content should reduce.

## Removing Fat-Burning Restrictions

A variety of problems can prevent you from building a great aerobic base, and therefore increasing fat burning. The three most common obstacles in relation to reducing body fat to healthy levels are carbohydrate intolerance, excess stress, and lack of good nutrition as supplied by a healthy diet.

### Carbohydrate Intolerance

As we age, we become more resistant to insulin, which causes us to be more carbohydrate intolerant. So, even if we eat the same amount of refined carbohydrates we could eat at a younger age without a problem, it now turns to fat. This is an oversimplification but a good example of how our body changes over time.

Most importantly, refined carbohydrates have played a significant role in the overfat or obesity epidemic of the past fifty years in America. A diet rich in highly processed, high-glycemic foods—wheat and other flours, sugar, potatoes, and others—converts to fat very easily.

## Excess Stress

Excess stress reduces fat burning, increases insulin, and causes other metabolic problems that promote the storage of fat. It's not just the amount of stress in your life but how your body adapts that's most important. An abnormal level of the adrenal gland's stress hormone—cortisol—is one of the best indications that your body is not adapting well to stress. This is best measured by testing the level of cortisol in saliva four times throughout the day (see chapter 7). This type of problem is often associated with increased belly fat, something you'll be alerted to as you regularly measure your waist.

## Healthy Diet

Natural carbohydrates, fats, and proteins are three important components of a healthy diet. For most athletes, low-fat diets, restricted calories, low protein, and other popular, unhealthy approaches usually fail to burn off excess body fat. In addition, water and fiber are vital. Also beware of so-called health food store items that are high in sugar and calories and are unhealthy. Organic junk food can make you fat fast.

In addition to macronutrients, all other nutrients are necessary for optimal health and fat burning. These include vitamins, minerals, and phytonutrients. Most are easily available from a healthy real-food diet, especially when about ten servings of vegetables and fruits are consumed each day.

# BODY FAT—LESS IS NOT BEST

The other extreme of having too little body fat is also unhealthy. Unfortunately, too many athletes seek to reduce their levels of fat at the expense of their fitness and health. Part of the problem is the ongoing myth that the lower your weight, the better you'll race. This generalization is untrue because weight loss typically involves loss of muscle, which will obviously make you race slower, as will dehydration (water being the primary number we see on the scale's weight).

For most athletes, the process of losing body weight causes a number of metabolic problems. These include the disruption of normal hormone balance, particularly with testosterone, insulin, and others, important for optimal training and racing. While hormone imbalances are often discussed in relation to female athletes who develop menstrual disturbances, men are also affected, with problems such as reduced muscle development and bone loss. Adverse metabolic effects of insulin can also be a problem for the generation of energy, in particular reduced energy due to diminished fat burning.

As the problem of low body fat develops, the brain attempts to compensate. But athletes who consciously choose low-fat foods (which are typically much higher in refined carbohydrates and other sugars) despite the brain's signals to increase dietary fat consumption create an ongoing vicious cycle between brain and metabolism, causing significant imbalances that can ultimately lead to poor training, injury, and diminished race performance. In an attempt to reduce body fat, athletes often sacrifice nutrients. These include essential fats for anti-inflammatory control and fat-soluble vitamins such as A, E, D, and K for many aspects of training and racing. Viewing dietary fats as the "bad" component of the diet often results in avoiding healthy foods with important fats needed to improve endurance. These include avocados, olive and coconut oils, egg yolks, and others.

The myth of "calories in, calories out" has been part of the confusion about weight loss and body fat. The concept is so simplistic that it creates lingering problems for many athletes. This antiquated idea claims that if we eat fewer calories than we burn during training, we lose weight. The problem with this notion is that it doesn't consider whether the calories taken in are from healthy foods or not. For example, two carbohydrate foods of the same caloric value can have glycemic indexes that are significantly different, making the low-fat food more detrimental in terms of body fat. In other words, a low-fat food can cause more body fat storage than the lower glycemic item, and it can reduce conversion of body fat to energy for training and racing. This is why a dessert made from refined white flour and sugar is worse than one made with almonds and honey, even though they can have the same number of calories.

When dietary intake and training are balanced, body fat will usually find the level that is ideal for you and your particular needs.

Furthermore, it's difficult to say what one athlete's optimal body fat level should be. Instead, if you focus on building great aerobic function, eating well and balancing nutrition, controlling stress, and addressing other issues related to your particular needs, your body fat levels should attain their optimal level. While this may be a logical explanation, it's not easy for many weight-conscious athletes to accept, as our society is fat-phobic and weight-obsessed.

I once had a patient named JR who was a better-than-average thirty-seven-year-old triathlete. He was an example of what many of my patients went through. JR first came to my clinic with a recurring injury, and through careful evaluations I determined it was caused by his drifting into and out of the overtraining syndrome each year. JR's diet was high in refined carbohydrates and low in fat and protein. With a predisposition to gaining weight easily, JR gained three to five pounds of weight each year and often had to reduce calories to control his weight. When asked about clothing sizes, JR said there was a steady increase in clothing size over recent years, especially in the waist—three inches in seven years. Among the recommendations I made to JR were to increase healthy fats and protein and improve fat burning by building more aerobic function. Over the course of the next six months, JR lost over two inches in the waist with corresponding losses all over. Not surprising to me, JR's scale weight did not change since body fat doesn't weigh much and as aerobic function improves it often increases muscle weight slightly. Now, with more energy, more leanness, and injury-free, JR began a long stretch of better racing.

# CHAPTER 30

# FEET FIRST—
## Understanding the Body's Structural Foundation

**W**hen competing in high school and college, I would sometimes race barefoot. This felt better on the "new" synthetic tracks that were smoother and easier on the feet than cinders. When I ran my first marathon in New York City in 1980, the running shoe industry was manufacturing many good shoes, but that would quickly change due to a change in marketing strategy. Running shoes became laden with all sorts of newfangled cushioning, thick waffle soles, shock-absorption, and rigid heel support. And the gullible running public pounced on this new "more is better" trend, buying shoes that, in reality, contained unnatural foot-bed support systems.

In my own private practice, I began seeing more patients with running injuries. It didn't take me long to figure out why. Running shoes were crippling runners. It was not unlike cigarette companies promoting "healthy" cig-arettes (which, by the way, Big Tobacco did in the '50s and early '60s).

I began discussing the running-shoe paradox in my lectures at races—while the shoes were hyped by companies as "injury prevention," they were doing the exact opposite. In these talks, I cited a variety of published medical studies that provided evidence that shoes often caused significant stress in the feet and legs. To demonstrate this concept to my audience, I would have an athlete run across the stage or up and down the aisle in his running shoes, pointing out the abnormal heavy heel strike that the cushioned shoe sole caused. Then I would ask the volunteer to take off the shoes and run barefoot. To the audience's astonishment, the athlete's stride transformed into a beautifully arched and light prance reminiscent of world-class runners.

I also began writing about this topic but encountered heated resistance, especially from running magazine editors. No one wanted to publish articles on the dangers of this new breed of running shoe. Once, I discussed this topic with a long-time editor at *Runner's World*; he just kept saying, "there's no proof, and the shoe companies do research too." What he didn't say, and what's obvious even today, is that running shoe advertisers help pay the bills for his magazine, and in doing so indirectly control editorial.

I never lost my love of barefoot running and would train that way for endurance runs on and off through the years, and especially when I lived near a flat, sandy beach. I also convinced more than a few athletes to run barefoot.

Recently, runners have taken notice of the harm caused by built-up running shoes and are taking the matter in their own hands (I should say feet). The best-selling book by Christopher McDougall *Born to Run* has influenced this consumer trend toward barefoot running and minimalist, low-tech footwear. Ironically, in 2009, *Runner's World* contacted me for a quote about barefoot running, but in its annual shoe review issue published several months after my quote appeared, the magazine featured page after page of new models of thick-heeled, well-padded running shoes. Sadly, the majority of these shoes will cause more harm than good.

While most athletes instinctually know the importance of good shoes, they often take their feet for granted—at least until they start to hurt. Only then do they realize that their shoes were not the best match for their feet. But one's feet don't even need to hurt to cause trouble. Subtle muscle imbalances in the foot and ankle, for example, can disturb the delicate biomechanics by putting undue stress on the knee, hip, and spine.

The more we understand about our feet, the better we can care for them and even fix them when their function goes astray. Our feet must last a lifetime. The feet are subjected to more wear and tear than any other body part. Just walking a mile, you generate more than sixty tons—that's over 120,000 pounds—of stress on each foot! Fortunately, and what's even more amazing, our feet are actually made to handle such natural stress. It's only when we interfere with nature that problems arise. Almost all foot problems can be prevented, and those that do arise can most often be treated conservatively through self-care.

From birth until death, our feet are very important in the development of overall fitness and health, but they may be one of the most neglected parts of the body. The feet are our structural foundation. They form the base of our body's physical stature, and any departure from optimal balance can have significant adverse effects not only locally in the feet but throughout the entire body. These problems are often transmitted through the ankle, an extension of the upper part of the foot. Anatomists technically consider the foot and ankle as two separate areas, but I consider the ankle as a vital part of the foot for ease of discussion. The ankle is a vulnerable area; approximately 25,000 Americans sprain their ankle each day.

While our skeleton is an important part of our structural health, it's the skeletal muscles that allow us to move. The same is true with the skeleton of our foot—muscle function is a key part of foot fitness and health. The early stages of most foot problems are associated with muscle imbalance. Bone problems, including joint dysfunction, are usually secondary to muscle imbalance. Trauma can cause injury to any component of the foot, including a muscle, bone, ligament, tendon, or joint.

Another important job of the feet is to help balance the whole body. The feet continuously communicate with the brain to regulate the rest of the body's daily movements, including standing, walking, cycling, running, and other movement. This is accomplished by powerful nerve endings at the bottom of our feet. These nerve endings are developed from infancy and their function is necessary throughout our life. Disturbances of these nerve endings due to trauma, disease, poor footwear, or neglect can lead to further health problems.

The nerve endings at the bottoms of our feet also become a potential source of powerful therapy when properly and specifically stimulated. This approach can be used both preventatively and after some injury is realized. For example, a simple foot massage, even by an untrained person, can be great for your feet and brain.

While many problems in the body are the result of either obvious or hidden foot imbalances, some foot problems themselves are secondary to more primary disorders. When this happens, these secondary foot problems can, in turn, cause other problems, another example of a domino effect.

Examples of problems that cause secondary foot dysfunction include structural faults in the spine and pelvis, muscle imbalance, trauma, shoes that don't properly fit, over-supported shoes and those with higher heels, and certain diseases such as diabetes, peripheral vascular disease, neuropathy, inflammation, and arthritis.

Foot problems are perhaps the most common type of structural injury athletes develop. And the most typical complaint about the foot is pain. When pain presents in specific areas of the foot, it most often indicates the source of the problem. For example, pain at the top of the foot may indicate a mid-foot fracture, although there may be other causes of this type of pain.

Many foot problems lead to inactivity. An athlete with a foot injury will often experience a complete cessation of training, unless swimming can be used to maintain fitness. Reductions in training, or forced rest, can make an athlete get out of shape fast; it can also lead to changes in metabolism leading to weight gain, circulatory insufficiency, muscle loss, poor coordination, and other more serious disabilities.

Structurally, improper bike and running shoes can alter how the muscles and joints function, not only in the foot but in leg areas above. Knee movement is the best example of this; with improper footwear, the muscles around the knee and the knee joint may move improperly. When this irregular movement continues, the result is some type of knee injury, usually associated with pain.

## Foot Anatomy Made Simple

In order to truly understand your feet, it's important to be familiar with the basic aspects of the foot's anatomy. This includes the bones, muscles, ligaments, tendons, and other physical aspects. The movements of the foot are also important to be familiar with. A general understanding of what and how things can go wrong in the foot and how to evaluate this leads to a more successful outcome. Pain and pain patterns in feet are important as well.

There's really nothing simple about the human foot. It's one of the most incredible and complex bioengineered parts of our anatomy. It combines power and speed with delicate movement and balance, solid stability with acute sensitivity, and the foot has sufficient endurance to take us almost anywhere we want to go for as long as we live.

The growth of the human foot comes in spurts. During the first ten years of a child's life, foot growth averages about one half-inch a year. Between the ages of ten and twenty, the yearly growth rate slows down considerably, with maturity of growth arriving around age twenty. However, the foot still gets larger with age. This is not true growth but a spreading of the foot due to physical and metabolic changes in the body during one's lifetime. For example, body weight, pregnancy, training, lifestyle, and shoe wear all could influence the foot to naturally expand or not. A foot that naturally expands results in the need for larger shoes through your lifetime; if you don't keep up with foot changes, your shoes may become too tight, contributing to or causing problems. Throughout an adult athlete's life, it's not unusual for the foot to increase two or more sizes during the course of normal activity.

At any stage of development, incorrect posture, poor walking, running and other training habits, and improper footwear can also significantly disturb foot muscle function, joint alignment, and the structure of the bones themselves.

## FOOT-SENSE

We're familiar with our sense of smell, taste, and sight; foot-sense is not as well known but is equally important. For example, if we step on a pebble while barefoot, we react immediately by contracting certain muscles that lift our foot off the pebble. More commonly, we don't have to look to see the position of our foot because we "sense" its location. The same is true with our sense of movement—we don't have to look at each footstep we take in order to walk or run effectively. Foot-sense can also be observed while balancing on one foot. The brain interprets incoming messages from the foot we're balancing on and sends back messages to muscles throughout the body to continuously adjust our posture to keep us from falling. These movements may include tilting the head, moving the arms up and down, or whatever is necessary to keep balanced. Without effective foot-sense, proper body-wide balance could not occur.

The basic anatomy of the foot, like the rest of the body, often has variations in its structures—we're not all exact replicas. But these variations are well adapted for by the muscles. The same is true between the left and right foot. Variations are common, including foot length, which can differ by a whole shoe size or more.

### Bones

At birth, the bones in our feet are undeveloped—there is actually just one bone, with the remainder made up of a softer material called cartilage. By the time we are three years of age, much of the cartilage has become bone, and by age six all twenty-eight bones have taken shape but are still partly composed of cartilage. Even in the adult, some cartilage remains. About a quarter of the body's bones are in the feet. During the developmental stage, interfering with natural foot development can severely impact foot function later in life. For convenience, anatomists divide the foot into three main parts: the forefoot, mid-foot, and hind-foot.

1. The *forefoot* bears about half the body's weight, with the ball of the foot (between the big toe and the rest of the foot) responsible for much of our balance. The four smaller toes are made up of three small bones each, called phalanges. The big toe is called the hallux, and has only two bones (phalanges). Under the big toe (hallux) are two very small, round sesamoid bones within a tendon. The bones of the toes are connected to the longer metatarsal bones that connect to the rest of the foot.

Foot-sense is a vital function for foot stability, to prevent injury, and to recover from an injury. Imbalanced muscles, overuse, disease, and many types of shoes can cause the nervous system to have poor foot-sense, leading to vulnerability to injury and other problems. With poor foot-sense comes a response from the brain to the body's muscles that may not be correct. As a result, the body does not properly compensate for even a minor foot problem, ultimately leading to an injury or worsening of an existing problem.

Because the nerves in the feet significantly affect balance, communicate with the brain, and stimulate foot muscles, encouraging normal foot movement and posture—even for brief periods—can be therapeutic. This is a key benefit of being barefoot—the most natural of all positions for the foot. Improving foot-sense in the feet can be done with almost anyone of any age.

2. The *mid-foot* has five irregularly shaped bones, which, with support from the muscles, form the foot's characteristic arches. It is here that much of the foot's natural ability to absorb shock takes place. The bones that connect to the metatarsals are called the first, second, and third cuneiform bones, and the cuboid bone. Behind these sits the navicular bone.

3. The *hind-foot* contains the talus bone (the ankle), which connects the foot to the two long bones of the leg—the smaller fibula on the outside and the main leg bone, the tibia. The talus bone is also connected to and rests on the calcaneous bone (the heel), the largest bone of the foot, which assists in stability during movement and standing. In the back of the foot, the calcaneous bone is supported by the Achilles tendon.

In some individuals, small extra bones called accessory ossicles may exist throughout the foot. In addition, there may be extra sesamoid bones. When present these extra bones don't inherently pose any particular problem.

### Joints

When two bones come together, they form a joint, which allows smooth movement—flexibility—between the bones. Each bone has softer articular cartilage at its joint end for protection. Joints are surrounded by a cover called the articular capsule, which contains a thick lubricating liquid called synovial fluid. The joints and cartilage cushion the bones and protect them from making direct contact.

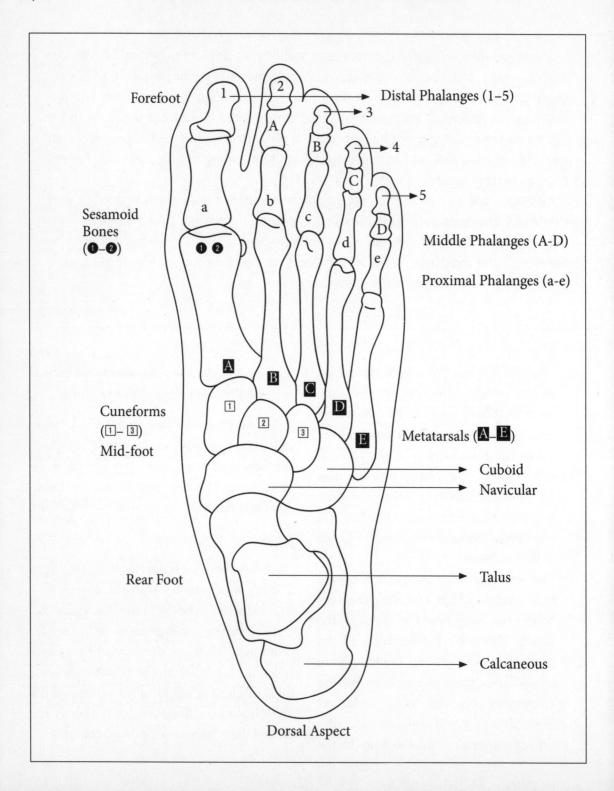

Forefoot

Distal Phalanges (1–5)

Sesamoid
Bones
(❶–❷)

Middle Phalanges (A-D)

Proximal Phalanges (a-e)

Cuneforms
(☐1– ☐3)
Mid-foot

Metatarsals (◼A–◼E)

Cuboid

Navicular

Rear Foot

Talus

Calcaneous

Dorsal Aspect

The foot has some thirty-three joints. Coordination occurs with the help of more than a hundred ligaments, which connect bones to bones, tendons, which connect muscles to bones, and muscles. The bones provide a solid foundation and leverage for muscles to move the body. Perhaps most joint problems are due to muscle problems associated with the joint. For example, muscle imbalance typically causes poor joint movement leading to joint dysfunction and pain. While reading about the muscles below, note that the bones and joints are supported by these muscles.

## Muscles

The foot relies on more than thirty muscles and tendons for motion and stability—not only in the foot itself but indirectly in areas above the foot. The muscles give the foot its shape by holding the bones in position. Without muscle support, the skeleton and all its bones would collapse. Much of the foot support comes from muscles that attach higher up in the leg, with tendons coming down into and attaching to bones of the foot. Many other important muscles are exclusively found within the foot itself.

All the muscles of the foot, ankle, and leg play a vital role in foot movements. Because of the extensive nature of the structure and function of all these muscles, this discussion will be limited to only the most important muscles and muscle groups.

### TIBIALIS POSTERIOR MUSCLE

The tibialis posterior is a long muscle that attaches to the two leg bones—the tibia and fibula—in the middle of the back calf under the large gastrocnemius and soleus muscles (just below the knee). The tibialis posterior muscle runs down the back of the leg around the inside of the ankle (the medial side) and into the bottom of the foot, inserting into different bones. Contracting this muscle allows you to point your foot down (an action called plantar flexion). It also turns the foot inward. The ability to rise on your toes also requires the function of the tibialis posterior muscle.

The tibialis posterior is one of the most important muscles associated with many foot, ankle, and knee problems. It's a key stabilizing muscle for the mid- and hind-foot. When this muscle does not work properly, it can cause a variety of non-specific symptoms, which can be difficult to diagnose.

Because of its importance in supporting the medial arch, abnormal inhibition or "weakness" of this muscle, perhaps its most common problem, causes poor arch support that can lead to excess pronation and other problems. Secondary to tibialis posterior inhibition is often tightness of the gastrocnemius and/or soleus muscles, and sometimes pain in the Achilles tendon. (Recall that abnormal muscle inhibition is a neuromuscular condition similar to a weak muscle.)

### Tibialis Anterior Muscle

The tibialis anterior is also a long muscle and attaches predominantly on the upper half of the tibia on the front of the leg (and slightly to the outside) just below the knee, where it is easily felt as a relatively large mass. It runs downward and becomes a large tendon crossing the ankle, easily visible when lifting the foot. It continues below the ankle and attaches into the first metatarsal bone and the first cuneform bone.

The tibialis anterior muscle raises the foot upward (an action called dorsal flexion) and assists in turning the foot inward. Like the tibialis posterior, when inhibited (weak), it can cause instability of the ankle, and may be responsible for problems in the first metatarsal joint. It may also be a common cause of so-called shin splints, although the posterior tibialis is also commonly involved.

### Peroneus Muscles

The peroneus longus and brevis muscles attach mostly on the fibula on the outside, or lateral side, of the leg, with some parts attached to the tibia. These muscles become a tendon just above the ankle and can be seen just behind the bony end of the fibula (called the lateral malleolus)—the bony protuberance of the outside ankle—where it attaches to the ankle. The longus portion of the peroneus attaches into the cuneform bone and first metatarsal bone, with the brevis attaching to the fifth metatarsal bone.

The peroneus longus and brevis muscles stabilize the outside of the ankle, allowing the outer foot to elevate or evert while the ankle is plantar flexed (foot pointed down). If you try to contract this muscle by pointing your foot down and out, you can easily see and feel it on the outside of the leg.

The peroneus tertius muscle is a much shorter but important muscle that also stabilizes the outside of the ankle. This muscle attaches on the lower portion of the fibula bone on the outside of the ankle and inserts into the fifth metatarsal bone. It allows the outside of the foot to turn upward with the ankle. This muscle is often involved is common ankle sprains, and if it does not heal properly after trauma can help maintain a chronic ankle problem.

### Gastrocnemius and Soleus Muscles

The bulk of calf muscle on the back of the leg is made up of the gastrocnemius and soleus muscles. Together, these two muscles are sometimes referred to as the triceps surae. They attach into the upper leg bones and, in part, above the knee into the back of the thigh-bone, the femur. These muscles are important for rising on our toes during any movement. These two muscles form the Achilles tendon beginning at about the middle of the calf. This tendon runs downward and attaches into the back of the calcaneus bone. Both the muscles and the Achilles tendon provide great support for the foot through stability of the heel.

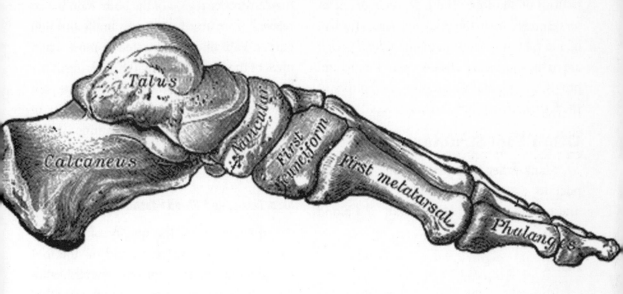

### PLANTAR MUSCLES

There are four layers of muscles on the bottom of the foot consisting of a dozen separate muscles. Overall, these have grabbing actions important for walking, running, foot coordination, and balance. These actions are best observed when barefoot. Wearing shoes can render these and other foot muscles less active and could lead to chronic foot problems. Walking and moving while barefoot improves these and other foot and leg muscle functions.

### Foot Arches

As a means of supporting the weight of the body, for shock absorption and propulsion, and adapting to uneven surfaces and other functions, the bottom of the foot is constructed of a series of arches. Muscles are the key factor in supporting these arches, and maintaining them is vital for normal foot function. Interfering with the normal function of the arches, most often by disturbing the natural action of the muscles that support them, is a common cause of injury and chronic foot problems.

The *medial arch* is one of the two large arches, and is the one familiar to most people. It runs along the inner aspect of the bottom of the foot. A side view (in above drawing) of the bones of the foot (without supporting muscles) clearly shows the magnitude of the medial arch. This arch is maintained by the action of the muscles, especially the tibialis posterior.

The *lateral longitudinal arch* is the second largest arch and runs along the outside of the bottom of the foot. The *transverse or meta-tarsal arches* are in the mid-foot across the ball of the foot and the short *longitudinal arches* are in the hind-foot. The peroneus longus and brevis, and plantar muscles on the bottom of the foot, support these arches.

## Other Foot Structures

Many other structures in the foot support its actions and maintain foot health. These include fascia, nerves, skin, and blood vessels.

### Fascia

Throughout the foot (as throughout the body) are thin fibrous sheaths that have great strength called fascia. This material assists in stabilizing the foot, especially in areas of the joints, and helps bind the tendons helping the muscles in their supporting efforts. The fascia blends with many other soft tissues of the foot and ankle. Important fascia is found on the top of the foot (the dorsal fascia) on the bottom of the foot (the plantar fascia), and around the ankle.

### Nerves

Within the muscles, tendons, ligaments, joints, and other soft tissues of the foot are important nerve endings that sense all movement, pressure, and body position. This information is sent to the central nervous system (spinal cord and brain) so we can respond appropriately to activity of the foot. Next to the spine, the foot has more nerve activity than any other region of the body. Pain is also relayed from the feet to the brain through nerves. Pain fibers are located in most structures of the foot, including the covering of the bones. During injury, the intensity of the pain does not necessarily relate to the severity of injury, as sometimes a relatively minor injury can elicit great pain because of the sensitivity of the foot.

### Skin, Nails, and Blood Vessels

In many ways, the quality of the skin, nails, and blood vessels in and on the foot is a general reflection of our overall health. These areas, like all others within the foot that are not as noticeable, are greatly influenced by diet and nutrition, stress, the brain, our training, and other lifestyle habits.

The skin is obviously important for normal foot function. It protects the structures inside the foot, is an important site for nerve endings, and cushions the foot with the help of a fat pad under the calcaneal (heel) bone.

The skin contains many nerve endings for foot-sense, especially on the bottom of the foot. The skin on the feet is very durable, especially on the sole, and can withstand many more pounds of force compared to the hand and fingers before it is cut open. When the skin is subject to chronic stress, such as excessive wear and tear, calluses develop due to a thickening of the skin.

Calluses are almost always caused by shoes that don't perfectly match the needs of our feet and can be secondary to toe deformities such as a hammertoe or bunion. They typically occur over a bony prominence. A callus that forms on a toe is called a corn. Calluses are usually not painful except certain types that are usually on the bottom of the foot. These may be plantar keratoses, or seed calluses, and are very small. Some calluses put enough pressure on the metatarsal joints to cause pain in the joint. Calluses can usually be differentiated from warts by pinching both sides together—warts are generally tender and calluses are usually not, with the rare exception noted above.

Toenails are adversely affected by trauma, most often by shoes. An ingrown toenail usually occurs in the big toe due to either poor fitting shoes or improper nail trimming, or both. This problem can lead to fungal or bacterial infections.

Another problem found in toenails is the so-called blackened nail. This problem is very common in runners but is found in cyclists and others as well. A blackened toenail is usually due to trauma directly on the nail, which darkens from bruising. The nail may ultimately fall off. A darkened toenail usually means the shoe is too small or otherwise not properly fitting the foot. Some dark toenails are also due to chronic fungal infections.

Blood vessels in the foot are very important to maintain the health of all the structures I've discussed. The arteries bring nutrient-rich blood into the foot, in the form of glucose, fat, protein, vitamins, minerals, and others, including oxygen. The veins carry blood back to the heart and remove carbon dioxide, excess water, and waste products from the foot. Poor blood flow can be due to poor muscle function or abnormally narrowed or closed blood vessels, often seen in early disease conditions. This can cause or aggravate existing foot problems from within. Improper blood flow can also cause skin ulceration, common in diabetics.

## Foot Posture and Movement

When our feet are balanced, our movement, whether walking, running, cycling, or other locomotion, is accomplished most efficiently. This means wear and tear is minimal, as is the energy requirement to keep the feet moving. Any deviation from normal posture and movement causes more wear and tear not only in the foot, but ankle, knee, hip, pelvis, spine, and in other areas. It also causes us to expend more energy on movement—in some cases a significant amount more. Those with a relatively minor foot problem that causes a change in the way they move can waste a significant amount of energy in accomplishing the same task. Even the weight of light sports shoes causes us to expend more energy, with larger and heavier shoes using up even more energy.

Abnormal foot movement can cause a variety of muscles to compensate, adapting in the ankle and knee and resulting in abnormal movement of both joints and related muscles. Foot imbalance can have a negative impact on the knees, hips, pelvis, and spine, and even areas such as the shoulders and into the head. This scenario is a common cause of aches and pains—some serious—above the foot.

### Normal Foot Motions

The foot has a variety of normal movements. The toes can flex, which curls them downward, and extend, bringing them upward. They have slight movement from side to side—seen in spreading the toes and squeezing them together. These actions can make very good exercises for those who need to rehabilitate their foot muscles. If you're unable to squeeze or spread your toes, it may indicate poor muscle function, and only rarely more serious problems.

### Inversion and Eversion

The foot can rotate inward and outward. The inward rotation is called inversion, and results in the sole of the foot turning inward. The muscles that accomplish this are the tibialis posterior and anterior. The outward rotation is called eversion, and the sole of the foot is turned out. The peroneus muscles are important for eversion.

The movement of inversion and eversion takes place in the joints between the talus and calcaneus bones. Pain during these specific movements may indicate a problem with the talus and the muscles that support it, typically the tibialis posterior and sometimes tibialis anterior.

### Gait

The act of moving, such as walking or running, is termed gait. During different types or styles of normal gaits, the stress on the feet can vary; our feet are made to endure this stress. A full phase of a normal walking gait includes the point our heel strikes the ground, through rolling our foot forward, to lifting and pushing off our toes, to swinging our foot forward to strike the ground again. During this normal gait, the foot makes many adaptations. It can effectively adjust to any uneven surface, become rigid enough to propel itself and roll over the big toe, go through various ranges of motion, and effectively absorb shock. This is accomplished by the actions of muscles, with support from ligaments, tendons, fascia, and bones.

A running gait is similar to walking with some exceptions—especially in the heel. Running should not include landing on your heel but rather farther forward such as mid-foot. Runners who land on their heel often do so because of poor foot-sense due to the types of shoes worn. To experience a normal running gait, take off your shoes and run or jog across the room or down the hall. This will usually cause you to land not on your heels but mid-foot (or forefoot), which creates balance in other structures as well.

### Pronation and Supination

During a normal gait, pronation and supination normally occur in the foot. Pronation is very important for shock absorption. During foot strike, the foot goes through many changes—it begins to roll inward, everting slightly, and the arch flattens. This is called pronation. It is a normal action—one that takes place in every step in every healthy foot. The purpose of this is to loosen the foot so it can adapt to the surface, especially on any uneven terrain.

Following pronation, as the foot continues through its gait, supination occurs. This results in the foot turning slightly outward then changing from a flexible foot to becoming rigid so it can propel the foot and push off. During this phase the foot inverts slightly, and the arches get higher, enabling the foot to properly roll over the big toe.

A number of factors can disrupt an athlete's normal gait. The two most common reasons are muscle imbalance and wearing shoes. Sometimes, areas above the foot, such as the pelvis or spine, can abnormally influence foot function. For example, too little or too much rotation of the hip can cause the foot to land in an abnormal position. In addition, injury, pain, and other problems that affect blood flow, cause inflammation, or disturb muscle function in the foot can abnormally alter the gait.

Most shoes change the gait by causing the stride length to become abnormally longer. This causes an abnormal heel strike—hitting the ground farther back on the heel. This is especially a problem during running, as the longer stride places more shock through the foot and into the knee, and occurs despite shoe cushioning or other shoe designs. Barefoot movement of any type does not cause the same stress.

The notion that some people are "pronators" while others are "supinators" is a gross oversimplification that is often presented to an unsuspecting public. That shoe companies make special shoes for one group or the other is an example of marketing hype. We all pronate and supinate. The reason some people *excessively* pronate or supinate is more often from wearing shoes, which cause muscle imbalance. This is especially a problem in children whose feet need to properly develop without shoes.

More importantly, an attempt to "help" a poorly functioning foot with a particular type of shoe or insert is an example of treating symptoms; most cases of foot dysfunction in athletes are due to muscle imbalance. Keeping the foot in a rigid, particular position maintains foot imbalance, not allowing the brain to correct the problem.

Our feet were made for walking, running, hopping, jumping, cycling, and all other natural movements. When we interfere with our natural movement, such as when we wear shoes, problems can arise. Other than in sandals and moccasins, humans evolved barefoot. For millions of years our feet were free. Suddenly, in only the past few hundred years, shoes of many types have restricted our feet, disturbed our gait, and caused untold problems to our feet.

In one sense, the foot is a highly complex structure with intricate functions that scientists are still continuing to unravel and understand. However, the awareness that the foot is a perfectly made natural part of our anatomy and can function just fine on its own will help in our appreciation of this structure and in our ability to prevent and correct most problems we inflict upon it.

## Two Types of Foot Problems

In a very general sense, there are only two broad types of foot problems. The first are those that don't elicit pain or other obvious problems but are silent in their impairment. These are functional foot problems. I have termed these silent foot conditions *asymptomatic foot problems*. The second type includes those that produce pain and obvious disability. I will call these *symptomatic foot problems*. Most foot problems are silent and fall into the first category. These asymptomatic problems are due mostly to relatively minor muscle imbalance. While these problems may come and go without notice, they can also be the cause of the majority of symptomatic foot problems producing pain and disability.

### Asymptomatic Foot Problems

There are a variety of types of asymptomatic foot problems. Most are due to subtle muscle imbalance in the foot, although muscle imbalances in the leg, pelvis, or spine can also contribute. Virtually all athletes have subtle muscle imbalance due to training and competition; this can come from normal wear and tear, but most often it's due to wearing shoes that don't properly match the needs of the foot. Normally, the wear and tear from training and racing, unless it's excessive such as during overtraining, is corrected with recovery; rest allows the body to correct these problems quickly and naturally. And, as noted earlier in this book, a healthy body can correct its own problems quite well.

However, sometimes the body does not correct these problems and they become chronic. This could be due to insufficient recovery but more often is caused by poor shoe fit or over-supported shoes. When this happens, a significant imbalance can occur, leading to symptomatic foot problems. Basically, if you train too hard one day, or longer than expected, you may cause some muscle imbalance that would normally correct itself. But it may not, and this will cause an asymptomatic foot problem. If unresolved—meaning the body or a health-care practitioner does not find and correct the problem—it can become a symptomatic problem. (This same scenario can occur anywhere in the body.)

Muscle imbalance can often arise from a variety of problems, which are often asymptomatic: the trauma associated with overtraining, the repetitive foot stress of cycling or running in shoes not matching the feet, or other stresses.

Muscle imbalance can also be caused by a local problem. A sprained ankle is a common example of a trauma that causes a gross over-stretching of muscles. Other trauma can do the same, such as a blow directly to the muscle in a cycling accident. Even minor trauma, such as regular wear and tear or minor repetitive stress from poor fitting shoes, can sometimes cause muscle inhibition.

Many different types of footwear can cause muscles to become imbalanced. Over-supported shoes, sports shoes that are too soft, and even dress shoes with higher heels or those that don't fit just right are common examples. In addition, supports such as orthotics, braces, arch supports, and other devices can sometimes cause muscle imbalance, especially if the supports don't precisely match the foot or if the support is used too long.

Improper stretching routines can also cause muscle imbalance.

### Symptomatic Foot Problems

Common problems in the foot produce symptoms ranging from pain and localized tenderness, to numbness or tingling, weakness, and reduced range of motion in the form of stiffness or limitation in movement. These symptoms indicate that some aspect of the foot or ankle is not working properly and may even lead to further imbalances. Symptomatic problems are usually obvious and may be due to a variety of causes, including three common ones: chronic muscle inhibition, trauma, and disease (even in athletes).

In addition to symptoms, this type of foot problem is associated with abnormal signs, including calluses, deformities (such as hammertoe), and swollen areas. These signs often indicate a more chronic problem, and sometimes a more serious one.

## Chronic Muscle Imbalance

An asymptomatic muscle imbalance can eventually cause foot pain, injury, or other problems. This is a very common, perhaps the most common, reason for symptomatic foot problems. The pain often comes from a joint that doesn't move properly due to poor muscle function.

Obvious symptomatic foot problems may develop suddenly and others more slowly over a period of time beginning with only the slightest clue. In either case, they may also disappear the same way as many symptomatic foot problems do. This happens because the body may correct them, or the imbalance may be compensated for by other muscles. In some of these cases, the compensation itself—specifically, the muscle involved in compensating—can cause other symptoms. This is part of the domino effect described earlier. It can occur with any group of muscles in the foot, ankle, leg, or above. Sometimes muscle compensation can even shift to the other side of the body. For example, a chronic muscle problem in the right foot may cause the body to shift weight bearing, putting excess weight through the left foot to avoid the stress, with an eventual problem created on the left side.

In the end, it will be the left foot, opposite the side of the primary problem, that produces the symptoms.

Chronic muscle imbalance is associated with some muscles being too tight. Tight calf muscles, tight plantar muscles (the bottom of the foot), or tightness in the front of the leg are common complaints often secondary to primary muscle inhibition ("weakness")—symptoms often described as Achilles tendonitis, plantar fasciitis, or shin splints, respectively.

## Trauma

More serious trauma can cause fracture, serious laceration, or crushing injury. Ankle sprains, for example, are sometimes due to a preexisting foot dysfunction, typically aggravated by improper footwear such as thick-soled sports shoes or high-top sneakers. The most popular shoe in this category is the basketball sneaker. Plain high-top sneakers were popular for many years, but today they have become fancy over-supported, overpriced high-top shoes. Supposedly, the added ankle support, the key feature of this shoe, protects against ankle sprain and other injuries. But studies don't verify this. Actually, these shoes can do just the opposite, as basketball players may have the highest rates of ankle sprains of any sport. When the ankle, or any area of the body, is supported, we run the risk of weakening that area. This is the result of muscles that sense the support and no longer have to

work as much; the result is loss of some of their strength.

Whatever the cause of the trauma, it often results in abnormal muscle imbalance. In a sprained ankle, the trauma damages the muscles along with other important foot structures such as ligaments, tendons, fascia, or even blood vessels. An ankle sprain typically includes damage to the lateral collateral ligaments on the outside of the foot, but at other times different structures may be damaged such as the tendon, local joints or bones, or even nerves. But in almost all cases, muscle imbalance occurs as well, and many of these muscles stay chronically inhibited, slowing recovery time, maintaining pain and often allowing a recurrence of ankle sprain. In fact, the majority of athletes who sprain their ankle will do so again.

If you sprain your ankle, and rule out serious injury, such as fracture, the area should heal relatively fast. Pain that does not diminish or is almost eliminated within a few days or a week of injury may also be associated with muscle inhibition that has not been corrected or compensated for by the body. Many traumatic injuries will recover significantly faster when normal muscle function is restored as quickly as possible.

## Assessing Your Own Feet

Whether you have an asymptomatic foot problem, or one that is giving you symptoms, the first step in correcting the problem is self-assessment.

The first question to ask about a foot problem is how it happened or what caused the problem. If it was trauma—a twisted ankle on a trail run, a bike crash, dropping a weight on it at the gym—that answers one big question. If the problem began soon after you started wearing a new pair of shoes, it may mean the obvious: that those shoes may not properly match your foot. Or perhaps the problem coincided with a new step or modification in your training routine.

If your foot problem feels better with movement, it's generally a good indication that it's a less serious problem. As we move our muscles, they get warmed up and are able to function better. Sometimes an adequate warm-up takes twenty minutes, and some problems may feel better only after this period of time. But don't push yourself if the pain persists.

If a problem worsens during activity, especially after you've had time to warm up, it usually means you should be resting to give the body a chance to heal. It may mean there's a more serious problem, but it could simply be the body needs more recovery time because of muscle inhibition. Pushing yourself in this situation often makes the problem worse and could lead to a chronic, recurring type of problem.

Generally, if your problem feels worse at the end of the day, activity and weight bearing made it worse. Your foot may need more rest. In some cases, you may have accumulated fluid in your foot, ankle, and lower leg. This may be caused by ongoing inflammation, or because you're not able to circulate this fluid back through the veins. The retention of fluid is called edema, and is often associated with a body-wide problem.

Even wearing the wrong kind of non-running shoes throughout the day can make an existing problem worse.

After being off your feet all night, most mechanical problems will feel better because your foot has had time to recover without mechanical stress. Certain problems may not follow this pattern. Plantar pain and the joint pain of arthritis may feel worse as soon as you start walking and gradually feel better after some movement. This may indicate a biochemical component to your problem (sometimes dietary or nutritional), and may be associated with too much calcium being deposited in the area during the night.

The wear pattern on your shoes can depict an accurate picture regarding foot balance. Shoe wear on the back of the heels, along the outside of the shoe, and near the ball of the foot should be similar in both shoes. If it's not, there may be muscle imbalance not allowing normal foot movement.

Another clue that the feet are not balanced is your footprints. If you walk in the sand, dirt, or other area where you can see your footprints, they should show very similar patterns. The same is true for your shoe prints. Look for the prints to be facing slightly outward rather than straight. Prints that are facing straight forward or are pointed outward too much may indicate a muscle imbalance in the pelvis that effects how the feet hit the ground. If you use this assessment, be sure the ground is relatively flat; otherwise you will see a normal deviation in prints.

Finally, most foot problems occur on one side or the other, and rarely are there problems with identical patterns in both feet. When this does happen, it may be simple muscle imbalance but could point to a more serious systemic condition, such as a spinal or circulatory problem, or arthritis.

In many situations, however, general foot discomfort at the end of the day is simply due to wearing shoes not meant for your feet. This becomes obvious when you take your shoes off and move around a bit, only to find significant relief.

Once you have assessed your feet, you will have a better idea of the nature of your foot problem and be better able to decide on what to do next. Often, a foot problem is self-limiting, meaning the body will correct the problem without any other help. The healthier you are, the better and quicker this can happen. If you're allowing your body to fix your feet,

give the process some time. However, if the problem is not beginning to improve in a reasonable period, more help may be needed. An acute foot problem, one involving trauma that does not start to feel better within twenty-four to forty-eight hours, may require some assistance. For more chronic problems, such as the non-traumatic type, one or two weeks should be sufficient time for at least some improvement to be seen. In allowing your body to fix itself, rest may be the key. One of the most powerful therapies, rest can be a double-edged sword if overused. The key with rest is knowing when and when not to use it.

Many athletes have trouble resting when they should. Most foot pain will improve with rest. Rest is the best way for the body to recover from training and competition. Recovery is essential for the body to build up the muscles allowing them to return to normal function. Finding a health-care practitioner for your foot problem may be necessary.

The next chapter takes a closer look at how to fix your feet and how ill-fitting shoes are usually the main culprit.

# PROBLEM AREAS ON THE FOOT

Foot problems are a true epidemic, with certain areas most vulnerable.

## First Metatarsal Jam

Excess pressure and stress through the big toe into the first metatarsal joint behind it is a very common problem. It's almost always due to wearing shoes that are too small. Cyclists are often vulnerable here. This injury involves the bone of the big toe, the phalanx, jamming back into the first metatarsal bone. The first metatarsal joint, between the two bones—the ball of the foot—becomes inflamed and painful. In some situations, when the onset of the problem is very slow, the joint does not elicit pain, but rather the foot adapts by creating another problem elsewhere secondary to the first metatarsal. In a real sense, other parts of the foot are sacrificed to take away some of the stress of the first metatarsal. This is not an uncommon way for the body to adapt when a very important structure, such as the first metatarsal joint, has excessive stress placed upon it. Many ankle, heel, knee, and other problems may be caused by a first metatarsal jam.

This first metatarsal jam can be assessed using two key indicators: the toe itself, and the shoe.

In the toe, pain and swelling in the area of the first metatarsal joint are common. Even a relatively minor jamming of the metatarsal joint over a long period will cause swelling of the joint. This is evident by a slight enlargement of the joint, with a warm feeling to the touch due to inflammation. Sometimes a discolored toenail due to the constant pressure from a shoe that's too tight is obvious. This is especially common in people who wear tight shoes. Even a single long workout or race in shoes that don't fit properly could create a first metatarsal problem complete with blackened toenail. The reason for the toenail's discoloration is tiny hemorrhages underneath the nail, similar to other bruises.

The shoes can also give clues to a first metatarsal jam. Because the foot is wedged forward into the shoe, many toenails can jam into the front of the shoe. Over time, the toenail can bore a hole into the shoe, but more often shoes are discarded before this happens. Even a toenail that is not very long can do this if the shoe is sufficiently tight. This wear pattern can usually be felt inside the shoe. With your fingers, feel inside the shoe in the area where your toenail would rub. You may feel a roughened spot and, in some cases, a layer of material may have worn off the inside of the shoe. This means the shoe is too small—specifically, too short. Keeping the toenail properly trimmed can be helpful, but wearing the proper shoe size is necessary to prevent a return of the problem.

If you have a removable insole, take it out and study it. Look at the wear pattern, especially the indentation made from the toes. Observe any areas compressed by the toes that are not completely on the insert, like they should be. Toes that overlap the top of the insert obviously indicate a too-small shoe.

In a foot that has an atypical shape, or in people with unusual circumstances such as soccer, which requires kicking, other metatarsals can have the same fate. In addition, other traumas can create this problem as well, such as a fall while wearing soft shoes or severely stubbing your toe.

"Turf toe" is basically the same condition. The toe is injured during forced metatarsal movements, such as a push-off injury or other trauma. It usually includes the sesamoid bones under the first metatarsal joint. They may become inflamed, and sometimes fractured. This is evident from local tenderness or pain on the bottom of the foot under the first metatarsal joint.

## Ankle Sprain

Some experts suggest everyone who sprains an ankle have an X-ray, the only way to determine if a fracture is present. But others say this leads to many unnecessary X-rays and expense when other options can help rule out fracture. One issue is clear: Every person with a sprained ankle should be treated as an individual. A professional consensus, known as the "Ottawa Ankle Rules," uses specific questions and examination of key areas to help determine the risk of bone fracture and if an X-ray is necessary.

Immediately after spraining your ankle, a question that should be asked is whether you can bear weight on that foot and ankle, even if it's painful. A second question is whether you can walk four steps, unaided, even with severe pain or a limp, right after your injury. A health professional may also ask you to do this if you go to the emergency room. If you're able to accomplish these tasks, an X-ray may not be recommended because the chances of a fracture are extremely low.

However, despite your ability to bear weight or walk, certain pain patterns may still indicate a potential fracture leading a doctor to X-ray your ankle. The risk of fracture is higher if there is pain in either bone of the inner or outer ankle, along with tenderness in any of the following bone areas:

- The back edge or tip of the lateral (outside) ankle bone
- The back edge or tip of the medial (inside) ankle bone
- The base of the fifth metatarsal (the little toe)
- The navicular bone in the middle of the foot

It should be noted that an X-ray does not always show a fracture if one is present. Some fractures are missed because of technically inadequate X-rays, and even good-quality X-rays may not demonstrate the fracture due to its size, swelling of surrounding tissues, or other reasons.

## Plantar Pain

Pain in the bottom of the foot, generally referred to as plantar pain, can come from a variety of sources. Almost all plantar pain is functional, and therefore X-rays will be negative and the problem can usually be corrected conservatively. If you have plantar pain, first carefully check the skin since a small cut, splinter, piece of glass, wart, or other similar problem can be the cause.

Plantar pain inside the foot, especially in the mid- or hind-foot, frequently comes from tight plantar muscles. This tightness is most often secondary to other muscle inhibition. A "diagnosis" of plantar fasciitis is not indicative of the cause of the problem, and no single remedy for this named condition has proven successful. Two people with the same plantar pain due to tight plantar muscles may have very different causes.

A so-called bone spur may be present in some chronic cases of plantar pain. This is usually associated with long-term plantar muscle tightness. In this case, the tendon of the plantar muscles that attaches to the calcaneus (heel) bone may contain calcium deposits. On an X-ray, this gives the appearance of a pointed "spur" which can give a false impression of a pointed sharp object in your foot. This is another example of the body compensating for a problem: In order to further support the area, the body deposits calcium in the tendon.

Correction of plantar pain usually occurs with improvement of muscle function. In addition to local treatment, chronic problems such as this may require improvements to the body chemistry through better diet and nutrition.

## Ingrown Toenail

An ingrown toenail is a common foot problem. It usually occurs in the big toe due to either poor fitting shoes, improper nail trimming, or both. The area becomes inflamed and painful, and can lead to secondary fungal or bacterial infections.

Conservative treatment is usually effective, including accommodative shoes. Warm foot soaks and proper nail trimming are also very effective. Trimming the nail is best accomplished by cutting it straight across rather than at a curve.

## Stress Fractures

In addition to fractured bones due to trauma, stress fractures are not uncommon in the foot. Stress fractures are usually less severe than other fractures in bones but can still be a significant problem. Most importantly, getting a stress fracture means something is wrong—with training, diet and nutrition, hormones, body mechanics (especially muscle balance), training or racing shoes, and others. Low vitamin D levels are often associated with stress fractures. In many athletes, a combination of factors contributes to a stress fracture.

Pain from a stress fracture typically improves with rest and worsens with activity. There is often some swelling in the area, but sometimes it's not noticeable. The swelling around the bone may prevent a proper diagnosis by X-ray within the first two weeks of injury. Only after some healing has taken place will the X-ray show the problem. In these situations, a bone scan may locate the stress fracture.

Most stress fractures will heal well, more quickly in a healthy athlete, without major therapy. Rest, cooling the site of fracture, cessation of weight-bearing exercise, and hard-soled flat shoes are often sufficient, but each case must be treated individually. Aspirin and other NSAIDs must be avoided as they can delay bone healing.

# CHAPTER 31

# FIXING YOUR FEET STARTS WITH THE RIGHT SHOES

For millions of years, the human foot has been either bare or covered with simple material to protect the bottom of the foot. Sandals were the common covering in warmer climates, with moccasin-type shoes used in colder environments for added warmth. These sparse foot coverings were and are adequate to protect the bottom of the foot from sharp rocks and rough terrain, and didn't interfere with foot function. Foot problems due to being barefoot consisted of the occasional laceration or deep thorn. Today, simple sandals and moccasins are still the most common footwear worldwide.

But with the advent of today's modern shoes came a whole array of foot problems as well as the growth of a new footwear industry that made therapeutic devices and professionals to treat such conditions. The running shoe industry has benefited the most; annual revenues now approach $20 billion.

A 1997 *British Journal of Sports Medicine* paper by Steven Robbins, PhD, described the hazards of deceptive advertising of athletic footwear. Writing about modern athletic shoes, Robbins stated, "Deceptive advertising of protective devices [in shoes] may represent a public health hazard and may have to be eliminated presumably through regulation."

For most of history, shoes were made straight with left and right being identical.

Records show that between the fourteenth century BC in Egypt and the mid-1800s, shoes were essentially produced the same way—by hand. For centuries, shoemakers kept secret the measurements of their clients' feet, to help assure continued business.

In 1845, the rolling machine, followed by the invention of the sewing machine a year later, dramatically changed the shoe industry. By 1860, other more effective shoe-making machines were developed. The next manufacturing breakthrough came in 1875, when Charles Goodyear, Jr., developed a machine that made shoes using a new material called rubber, previously invented by his father.

Today, most shoes are made on machines, but they also require manual assembling. The manufacturing of many shoes, especially athletic shoes produced by big companies, is accomplished in third-world countries because it's very cheap, often a dollar per pair or less.

## How Shoes Can Harm Your Feet

When was the very first time the human foot was injured by a shoe? Probably the first time one was worn. Nothing is more stable, supportive, shock protective, and efficient than bare feet. As soon as a shoe is placed on the foot, there is a loss of mechanical stability and the potential for injury. Perhaps the very first shoe-related injury was a twisted ankle due to surprise instability. Or worse, being overtaken by a lion due to slower run-

ning speed or poor maneuverability in shoes. While most of us don't have to run from wild animals, our shoes can still be dangerous.

Perhaps the first published scientific evidence describing the harm from shoes came in 1954 when researchers Basmajian and Bentzon measured the electrical activity in foot muscles using an electromyographic (EMG) device. This study showed that when shoes were placed on the feet, certain muscles lost significant function. Since that time many other studies have been published in medical journals showing the dangers associated with shoes. These can be easily found in the medical library online, but not easily found in the running magazines.

There are a variety of specific problems associated with wearing shoes. I've broken these subjects down to four general categories: weight bearing, foot-sense and orientation, muscle and bone, and gait.

### Weight Bearing

Our feet support our entire body's weight. Normally, this weight is distributed through specific areas of the feet in order to bear weight most efficiently. During standing, walking, and running, this efficient weight-bearing distribution can significantly reduce the risk of injury. When we wear shoes, our weight distribution can change, often with more weight going through a smaller area of the foot. (An extreme example of this is a woman's high-heeled shoe, especially those with very small pointed heels and small toe box. In this case, all the body's weight is directed into the ground through a very small area—through the heel and the front of the foot.) When we wear a flat shoe or are barefoot, the distribution of weight is over a larger area, although even a flat shoe can interfere with our weight bearing. While sports shoes are not high heels, they also cause weight-bearing distortions.

This example is easily seen with the following experiment. Get your feet wet. Now stand on a flat, dry paper towel. Step off the towel and observe your footprints. Drawing an outline around the print may help you see it better. Next, take a pair of flat shoes that you have worn for a while and observe the area of wear—this will be mostly the back outer corner of your heel and the ball of the foot, and sometimes along the outer edge of the shoe. Now compare the size of your footprint with the area of wear pattern on your shoes. In most cases, your footprint area will be larger, sometimes a lot larger. This is because your contact to the ground is greater when barefoot than in shoes.

The surface area that makes contact with the ground is a significant factor associated with many types of foot problems. If the weight of your body is forced through a smaller area of your foot, (i.e., less surface area), more stress is induced in your foot. Instead, your foot is supposed to disperse the weight-bearing stress through a greater surface area. In addition, with less surface area making contact with the ground, the body has

a lessened ability to maintain proper overall balance.

The flatter and thinner the sole of your shoe, the more your weight bearing is likely to be more natural like a barefoot state. Changing to this type of shoe could have significant benefits for your feet, but you must do this carefully if you're used to thick shoes, those with high heels, or those with a lot of cushioning and support.

## Impact

Our weight-bearing contact with the ground is intimately connected to foot-sense. For many years, sport-shoe manufacturers focused on impact, promoting shoes with shock-absorbing materials to protect us from the impact forces that supposedly caused injury. But after decades of scientific research, experts are unable to demonstrate that our feet are vulnerable to injury from the result of impact, whether from standing, walking, running, or jumping. In fact, what the studies show is that there's *no* difference in injury rates between running on hard surfaces and soft surfaces, or between runners who have heavy or light impact on the ground.

Certainly, excessive impact can injure our feet. And any impact can cause injury when muscle imbalance is present. However, the action of standing, walking, running, and performing other common types of physical activity is quite natural—our feet are made for these activities and the normal impact associated with it. The forces of impact are a natural phenomenon our feet are made to deal with. Actually, our feet use the impact on the ground to decide how much muscle work is needed to run most efficiently. This action is mediated through the nerves and muscles in the feet.

The muscle response to impact also affects comfort. For this reason, all shoes, from the moment you put on a new pair to those that appear too old and worn out, should be completely comfortable. Otherwise, the shoe should not be worn because of the risk of foot damage. Shoe companies may claim that running shoes should be changed every several hundred miles, but comfort is your best guide. So-called worn-out shoes may be just fine as long as they are comfortable and not falling apart.

Still other benefits are obtained from our constant impact on the ground. Bone strength can be improved in those who perform activities that result in harder impact, such as running, especially when compared to activities that have low or almost no impact such as swimming.

### More on Shock Absorption

Shock absorption is another common phrase promoted by running and walking shoe companies. But just because a material has good shock-absorbing ability does not mean it can accomplish this inside a shoe. In fact, shoe materials with good shock absorbency properties are not effective enough to reduce stress in the foot during physical activity. This is because shock absorption in the feet occurs at the same level of intensity whether we wear shoes or not.

The notion that shock and impact are dangerous has led to the idea that we must cushion our feet, especially when walking, jogging, running, or performing other physical activity. Cushioning is a concept most people relate to in terms of comfort and safety. Cushioning can protect your feet against bruising if you should step on a hard object like a sharp stone. However, cushioning can have drawbacks. Shoes that are too cushioned can give our brain the improper perception that the impact is much less than it actually is, which can result in inadequate or improper response by the foot (and rest of the body) to the actual impact. In the course of an easy run in your shoes, this could add up to be a significant cause of injury.

Cushioning is more common in the popular, expensive sports shoes. In a December 1997 issue of the *British Journal of Sports Medicine,* researchers Robbins and Waked wrote that "expensive athletic shoes are deceptively advertised to safeguard well through *cushioning impact* yet account for 123 percent greater injury frequency than the cheapest ones."

### Support

Many shoes have a "support system" built into them. This may be a simple insert or a complex arrangement of built-up stabilizing structures with fancy names. Most of these exist for marketing reasons and not real function. When you support the feet when they don't truly need it, you're asking for trouble. And for most athletes, this need usually does not exist. Some people, however, may need extra support because they have stayed in shoes with too much support for too long, thereby weakening the natural support mechanisms within the foot. For these individuals, their feet don't feel right without the added support. This vicious cycle can be broken by weaning off over-supported shoes and strengthening the muscles of the feet.

Support systems in many shoes contribute to a thicker heel area. When barefoot, our heel and forefoot are about the same level, but most shoes are made so that our heel is higher than the rest of our foot. This unnatural state can ultimately result in reduced muscle function in the gastrocnemius, soleus, and tibialis anterior.

### Foot-Sense and Orientation

Recall the importance of our foot-sense. Within the foot are important nerve endings that sense foot contact with the ground. This information is sent to the brain and spinal cord so we can respond appropriately to activities of the feet, and help regulate all movement and body position. In effect, we orient ourselves—our whole body—as a result of foot-sense.

The primary reason for many common foot injuries is the lack of feedback from the foot despite the same level of shock absorption. This can be the result of increased thickness of the sole, or the types of synthetic materials used in many shoes. In other words, the soles of our feet are not able to properly sense the ground. The relationship between reduced foot-sense and its contribution to injury has been understood in scientific circles for almost forty years.

### K-Sense

Because we are less able to communicate with the ground while wearing shoes, our feet are less able to adapt to the normal impact of regular activity. And it's not just our feet but our whole body. The result is a loss of another type of foot-sense called *kinesthetic sense*, or K-sense. This means our brain is also less aware of our foot position and therefore corresponding body position. Our body cannot adapt properly to normal walking, running, or virtually any movement. K-sense provides us with specific information about our movements, changes in posture, and the mechanical stress on muscles and joints. This problem also can have an adverse effect on our orientation.

An example of K-sense can help us understand how important it can be. Running on a trail requires great K-sense. But everyday activity can be an obstacle course for our feet. If we're walking through a crowded restaurant dinning room to get to our table, we may have to squeeze past chairs, people, other tables, and perhaps even a wet floor to avoid running into these obstructions. We rely on our natural K-sense to do this. And like foot-sense, people (of any age) who have worn thick-soled sports shoes can also have significantly reduced K-sense; with their eyes closed, those with reduced K-sense won't know their exact foot position without looking.

### Gait Effects

Balance is an important component of normal movement, or normal gait. When balance is disturbed due to improper shoes, muscle imbalance and irregular gait can follow. At best, the body will compensate for muscle imbalance with significantly more muscle activity. This can cause the body to use much more energy than normal to accomplish the same movement. In other words, an irregular gait wastes energy.

An irregular gait can also lead to an injury not only in the foot, but the knee, pelvis, low back, or some other areas. Even the shoulders, neck, and head can be affected. Because of the importance of the hip joint during movement, the hips are particularly vulnerable to injury when there is a gait problem.

Abnormal changes in gait are common in master's athletes. These are sometimes attributed to the so-called natural aging process in the feet—the loss of elasticity and arch function resulting in reduced foot function. However, for older athletes who spend sufficient time barefoot, reduction in foot function is not seen to the extent it is in people who spend too much time in shoes.

Runners who wear popular running shoes must contract their *tibialis anterior*— the muscle on the front of the lower leg— more than normal during each step in order to land on their heels. During natural running, with a very flat shoe or when barefoot,

this constant high level of tibialis anterior contraction does not have to take place. This excessive muscle contraction could trigger weakness of the tibialis posterior muscle or other patterns of imbalance. In addition, gastrocnemius and soleus muscle tightness can be a secondary problem, with tightness in the Achilles tendon. In any of these situations, the resulting muscle imbalance can lead to common injuries. The exact area of injury can vary from person to person.

## Buying the Right Shoes

Not all shoes are harmful. The best shoes are those with little or no support, such as moccasins, sandals, flat sneakers, and running shoes with thin and hard rather than soft soles. The correct shoe should feel almost perfect, whether it's a running, cycling, or other sports shoe. This also applies to shoes you may wear much of the day, or even just on special occasions, from casual work shoes to a black-tie affair. The right shoes should wear well, keep their shape over time, tread safely, allow for sufficient foot freedom, minimally distort the foot, if at all, and hold together for years. These characteristics depend on the quality of materials, the manufacturing process, including how the shoe was put together, and how well each shoe matches the structure of your foot. In general, the best shoes are those that are flattest, and ones made specifically for your feet. Unfortunately, most people buy off-the-shelf shoes so it's very important to follow strict guidelines for optimal fit.

Considering that your feet are probably two different sizes, shoe-size numbers (for example size 10 or size 7) have no real meaning, and most companies don't have consistent sizes, which makes finding the optimal shoe a difficult challenge. However, there are a number of things you can do to eliminate common dangers and find the best match for your feet. The most important factor is fit.

## Finding Your Proper Fit

Optimal shoe fit may be difficult for some people, while others have an easy time. While there's a subjective component to shoe fit, other factors are more concrete. You can't predict your size based on previous shoes with specific sizes as shoes between companies can be very different, and even the same shoe in one company can vary in size. This means it's difficult to get the proper fit without actually trying them on and walking in them.

Research from the Battelle Institute shows there are at least thirty-eight factors that influ-ence shoe fit. In addition to length, width, and height, there are many subjective factors, especially those related to feel. This makes most shoes difficult to fit properly. The subjective opinions and attitudes come from both consumer and salesperson, but ultimately you determine if the shoe fits.

### Sizing Your Foot

The majority of people in the Western world probably wear shoes that are too small. Certainly in my practice, where for over thirty years I looked at every patient's shoes and their feet, that was the case. In many situations I would measure the foot and the shoe to show athletes how poorly their shoe fit their foot.

Today's shoe sizes include three popular but different length-sizing systems depending on where the shoes were made. These systems include sizes for shoes made in the United Kingdom (U.K.), which originated in the late 1600s; American (U.S.), originating in the

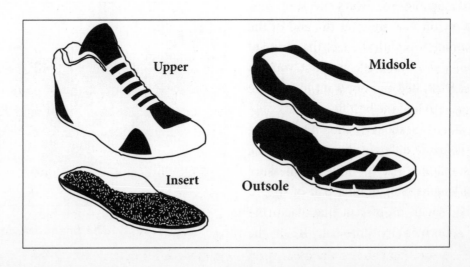

late 1800s; and the Continental or Paris Point metric method, originating in the late 1600s. Other sizing systems also exist. More recently, the Mondo Point system was proposed to replace all other systems. This is based on a simple length and width measurement in millimeters. It would be a great benefit to consumers, but it will probably never be accepted by the shoe industry since it would put all shoe sizes on the same playing field, making marketing—and deception—more difficult.

### Measuring Your Feet

Most adults don't measure their feet when buying new shoes, especially considering that today many shoe purchases are online. As a result, many people squeeze into the same shoe size for years, or even decades. While adult feet stop growing by age twenty, they still get larger through the years—sometimes more than two U.S. sizes. They also get larger within a twenty-four-hour period, typically as the day goes on, returning to "normal" by the next morning, so always measure your feet and try on new shoes at the end of the day. Combine this with the fact that units of measure for shoes are not consistent, you can easily get frustrated and not want to take the time needed to find the best fit.

Consider U.S. shoes. A shoe marked size 10 may be made different than another shoe that's also marked size 10. Both will measure different lengths. Still another pair of size 10 shoes made with a different manufacturing method can measure differently than the

other two size 10s. Actually, it's possible that a shoe marked size 10 could be one of five different sizes. So much for those silver gadgets, called the *Brannock device*, that shoe stores use to measure your feet. In addition, shoes for men, women, and children have different size units—a size 8 men's is much different in length than a size 8 women's.

The three popular size systems don't have much in common either. In the United States, a men's size 10 is the same in Canada, but in the U.K. it's a size 9. The same size in Japan is 27.5, and the continental equivalent size is 43.

In addition to length, width is a very important dimension. The width is measured across the ball of the foot. Add height to the foot and you have volume as another important measurement that is usually neglected. An example of the complexity of shoe fit is with volume, which is best assessed by foot comfort when trying on shoes on a hard floor. By now you may be thinking that this is complicated. It is. But since there's no standard

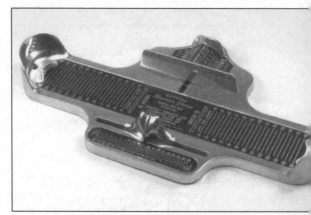

**The brannock device**

for size, none of these numbers should really mean anything to you, with one exception.

### Measuring Devices

One benefit of measuring your feet is keeping track of their *relative* size. This may not relate to shoe size. The Brannock device was introduced in 1927 with the purpose of providing a starting point for shoe fitting, not to dictate the best shoe size. The Brannock device is standardized within itself—they all have the same standard measurements—but these don't precisely match any one kind of shoe size made by any of the companies.

By using either the Brannock device in a shoe store, or doing the measuring yourself as described below, you could, and should, keep track of your foot size just like you would keep track of your weight with a scale, or overall health with a regular blood test. Like most health-related tests, measuring your feet is an important general guide.

Any measurement of your feet should be done in a standing position on a hard floor. Do this at the end of the day. Any meaningful daily size fluctuations must be differentiated from serious health problems, such as edema, certain pathological changes as seen in arthritis, or side effects of drugs.

For an accurate measurement, make a footprint on a piece of paper. Use a damp foot on a paper towel, or draw the outline of your foot with a pencil. Measure the back of the heel to the end of the big toe, in each foot. The purpose would be to see how much your feet

change from year to year, and not relate this to any shoe's size.

## High-tech Shoe "Systems"

For cyclists, skiers, skaters, and those requiring more than just a plain shoe, much of the discussions above still apply, especially the importance of comfort. In the past twenty years, these bike shoes, boots, and other footwear, some with attached mechanical components, have become more specialized. The many different kinds of mechanisms make finding the optimal one more difficult. For example, there are several different pedaling systems available for cyclists, with different ones for road or mountain bikers, triathletes, etc. The different pedal systems provide increased efficiency during pedaling, but the shoe still must fit or foot stress will follow. Finding the shoe and system that best matches your need, like a running shoe, is a matter of trying them on; but this can't be done as easily as trying a few running shoes in the store—it's a more difficult feat since you need to try the whole system on your bike. Once again, comfort is key. Unfortunately, comfort in a shoe can change after thirty minutes of easy riding. Pay particular attention to comfort in the front of the foot, where most wear and tear occurs.

One problem with cycling shoes, boots, and other specialized shoes is that the tighter they are, the more efficient they may be, because there's less energy lost in foot movement. This makes the need for a "perfect fit" even more important. Just don't sacrifice comfort for the notion that a bit more

## 10 STEPS TO A BETTER SHOE FIT

You can get the best fit by following some key points:

1. Never assume you'll take the same size as your previous shoe, even if it's the same type or model.

2. Rely on fit and comfort rather than any particular size.

3. Always plan on spending adequate time when shopping for shoes. Don't rush—if you're short on time, postpone it and set time aside for this important event. You may not find the right shoe in the first store you visit. Most outlets carry only a few of the many shoes on the marketplace.

4. Always try on both shoes. First, try on the size you think would fit best then walk on a hard floor (not carpeted). Even if that size feels fine, try on a half-size larger. If that one feels the same, or even better, try on another half-size larger. Many people don't realize that a larger shoe may actually feel and fit better.

5. Continue trying on larger half-sizes until you find the shoes that are obviously too large. You know especially by the heel—it will start coming off when you walk. Then go back to the previous half-size—more often that's the pair that best matches your feet. There should be at least a half-inch between your longest toe and the front of the shoe for most shoes.

6. Each time you try on a pair of shoes, find a hard surface to walk on rather than the thick soft carpet in shoe stores, where almost any shoe will feel good. If there's

efficiency will make a dramatic difference in performance—it won't. One option over off-the-shelf shoes is to get them custom made, it might be well worth the effort and cost. Just have both feet measured at the end of the day when they may be slightly larger.

Remember, the manufacturer makes new shoes based on trends of style, color, and fancy gimmicks to market the shoe. That's why shoe styles come and go. If you find the shoe that fits perfectly, buy more than one pair. Just be sure to try them all on, since the same shoe may also vary in size.

Some patients I have seen bought larger shoes after discovering their initial problem of a tight fit, only to find that their feet kept getting larger. At some point in time, they ended up with an increase of a whole size or more. I have even seen increases of 2.5 U.S. sizes over a two-year period in adults!

## Weaning Off Bad Shoes

If you feel it's time to make a healthy change for your feet, you may have to go through a "withdrawal" from bad shoes to good. It might be impossible to stop wearing no sturdy floor to walk on, ask if you can walk outside (if you're not allowed, shop elsewhere).

7.  You may also need to try different widths to get the best fit, although many shoes don't come in different widths. The ball of your foot should fit comfortably into the widest part of the shoe without causing the shoe to bulge.

8.  Use comfort as the main criteria. Don't let anyone say you have to break them in before they feel good. The best shoes for you are the ones that feel good right away. While many salespeople are aware of how to find the right shoe size, many are not. Often shoes from mail-order outlets cost less. But be prepared to ship them back if they don't fit just right.

9.  If the difference between your two feet is less than a half-size, fit the larger foot. If you have a significant difference of more than a half-size between your two feet, it may be best to wear two different-size shoes. How you accomplish this is up to you.

10. For sports shoes, many women fit better in men's shoes than in women's. The first rule, though, is that the shoe must fit properly. Some women don't fit into men's shoes, and some stores don't carry or companies don't make men's shoes in sizes that are small enough for many women.

bad shoes one day and start with good ones the next. The reason has to do with the position of your foot, specifically your muscles.

Let's take the case of an athlete wearing thick running shoes for daily training. If he's been wearing this type of shoe for many months or years, his foot muscles, along with tendons and even ligaments, have changed in length to adjust to the shoe. When he suddenly starts wearing a flatter shoe, his muscles, tendons, and ligaments will have to re-adapt. This process may be uncomfortable, and even painful, if he tries to do it all at once.

In making this change, he may feel discomfort right away or it could take a day or two. If his feet have more significant unnatural changes in the joints, such as hammertoe or a bunion, the problem could be worse and take much longer.

For many athletes, these changes need to take place slowly if they're going to make the transition without much discomfort. In many cases, the muscles have become weak and will require a period of strengthening, which could happen during normal movement in good shoes. For some, rehabilitating the feet

## SOCKS

When trying on shoes, wear the socks you would normally wear in them. Socks are not necessary but are mainly for added comfort, especially in avoiding blisters. Like shoes, socks can be too tight, contributing to foot stress. For most situations, socks should be thin and not tight. Thicker socks may require a half-size larger shoe.

Which style of socks you wear—low-cut or above the ankle—and what they're made of—natural fibers (my preference) or synthetics—is up to you. But, like shoes, make sure they fit well; and be careful to avoid the sock interfering with shoe fit.

may be necessary, which can be accomplished by being barefoot. It's not necessary to run barefoot to accomplish this, but just spending time walking and other leisure activities—even just around the house or office—will help balance foot muscles.

For these and other shoe problems, making the change to flat shoes or even being barefoot, as natural as that is, makes your foot feel rather odd and may sometimes be uncomfortable. After all, your feet have been addicted to over-support and have become weak. If you're suddenly without that support you feel, well, naked. This does not mean that flatter shoes or being barefoot is a stressful

state because you don't feel as good; rather your feet have changed because of the kinds of shoes you've worn.

For many people, weaning off bad shoes may take at least one extra measure. First, look at the highest heel height of a current shoe. Compare this to a lower heel or a flat shoe. Your first step in weaning off bad shoes may be to wear a shoe that's about half to three-quarters less in height than the height of the one you currently wear. Try wearing a shoe with this height heel for a few days to make sure your feet don't become painful. If there is pain, you'll require two extra steps and have to wean slower by wearing a shoe whose heel is only one-quarter to half the height of what you're used to wearing before going to one that is half to three-quarters. In some cases, just removing the insert in your current shoe is a good first step to better feet.

Whether you need to take one or two steps in making the transition from bad to good shoes, it may only take a month or two to make the appropriate adaptations to the new foot position. For others, it may take longer. Still others may need assistance from an appropriate healthcare professional. Rely on the feet feeling good for at least a week or two before progressing to the next step. Once you've weaned down to a more flat shoe, you'll wonder how you survived the others.

## Old Shoes

It's been said that old, worn running shoes can cause foot or leg injuries. This may be true if your old shoes were bad to start with. Running shoe companies want people to get rid of their shoes sooner to buy new ones more often. But a good shoe that has a lot of wear may still be good. Properly made running shoes that match your feet could last years depending on your training. Marketing has made many people believe that we have to replace our shoes frequently—every 500 miles or less. This may be true when the shoes are poorly made, but even cheap shoes can last a long time.

A number of factors may cause you to either repair or replace your current shoes. First and foremost, they should remain comfortable. As soon as they cease being comfortable, they need to be repaired or replaced.

Another factor is wear. The two heaviest areas of wear are the heel and under the ball of the foot. If you run properly, there's less wear on the heel. If your shoes wear very unevenly, this could be a problem. For example, if one heel is worn a quarter inch more than the other, this can cause a significant muscle imbalance (which may be the cause of this excess wear to start with). If one heel is worn down much more than the other, repair both heels if possible, or buy new shoes. If the area under the ball of the foot is worn through the sole, sometimes due to an imbalanced gait while running, this is also a reason to repair or replace the shoe.

A common problem in some shoes is the breakdown of the stiffener in the heel area. This is especially troublesome when the heel height is more than about an inch thick. This can create instability in the feet and lead to balance problems.

## Arch Supports, Orthotics, Shoe Lacing, and Other Foot Support

Many shoes have built-in or removable supports, but in addition to these many companies have developed a wide array of foot devices. The first big business for these products, New Balance Arch and Support Company, was founded in Boston in 1906.

Various types of supports are made for the heel, sole, arch, and ankle and include soft and hard materials comprised of cotton, leather, synthetics, plastic, wood, and metal. They come in the form of heel and sole supports, ankle braces, a variety of inserts, and arch supports, including orthotics and others.

In addition to conventional supports, many forms of taping are used in all sports to help support the foot and ankle. In my clinical experience of using conservative treatments for many types of foot problems in athletes, successful outcome does not require any type of support in the vast majority of cases. Successful treatment includes correcting the cause of foot problems such as muscle imbalance. Only on occasion would additional foot support be necessary and almost always for a very short period during which time the foot can heal. In rare situations would support be necessary long term.

Stabilizing or immobilizing the foot or ankle may be necessary in the case of an emergency when the risk of serious damage is suspected and until such time as a proper assessment can be made. These situations, which are very individual, are not detailed in this book.

Unfortunately, the long-term use of foot supports by athletes is very common. Despite the potential risk of further weakening the foot and not treating the cause of the problem, these items are heavily marketed and readily available in many retail outlets and online sites. While these supports come in different sizes and shapes, these are essentially "one size fits all" products since they usually don't specifically match the needs of the individual foot, despite what the manufacturer says.

Some people use these devices for a very short period without success, only to try one type after another with many supports ending up in the drawer unused. If you don't specifically match a particular support to your precise needs, it could lead to long-term worsening of the condition, making proper treatment much more difficult.

In most cases, the use of shoe supports should be considered only after more conservative therapy has been tried without success and before more radical treatment is considered, such as surgery.

### How Supports Can Weaken the Foot

The greatest harm from the use of foot supports is that through their routine use the need for other more appropriate treatments that address the cause of the problem may be overlooked. This is especially true when supports provide temporary symptomatic relief, giving the false impression that the problem is solved.

In some cases, a support will provide symptomatic relief in the area of pain, only to trigger an imbalance or discomfort in another area previously not a problem. For example, you may start using a particular support that provides relief for your foot pain. A week later, your knee may begin to hurt. This can occur due to the initial change made in the structure of your foot by the support, causing other structural changes— sometimes up the leg into the knee, hip, or even lower back.

Supporting a joint when it is not required can actually increase the risk of injury to that joint. This is true not only for the foot and ankle, but also for any joint such as the knee, hip, or those of the low back. The reason is that the added support can reduce muscle function, leading to muscle imbalance. With the additional support, our foot's natural internal support gives way to the external support. In other words, our foot muscles have less reason to work as much since something else (the added support) is doing the job for them. And no support can ever take the place of proper muscle function.

In many cases, a foot support can reduce the ranges of motion in the joints. Reduced ranges of motion can lead to joint and muscle dysfunction, and increase the risk for injuries due to minor twists or turns that normally would not be problematic.

In certain instances, reduced ranges of motion may be necessary to assist in healing, such as after an ankle sprain. However, it's important to remove the support as the body completes the healing process to prevent a continuation of reduced ranges of motion and allow the foot's muscle function to return to normal.

Even when a support is necessary, a softer or semi-rigid support such as leather, rather than a hard or rigid support like hard plastic, may work best for athletes and may even quicken the healing process. This may also apply to the case of a foot fracture, where a semi-rigid rather than a rigid support is usually best. However, these more serious conditions must be treated individually.

### Arch Supports

The notion that our arches always need support is incorrect. They work just fine in their own natural state, as evident from our evolution, where humans have been mostly barefoot. Today, our foot naturally still has a higher arch when not bearing weight, and it flattens out considerably with weight bearing. This is especially true in those who spend a lot of time barefoot and have maintained healthy arch function. Some people confuse this normal flattening with "flat feet" or a pronation problem.

As discussed earlier, the arches of the foot are supported and maintained by muscles. The medial arch is very important, with the tibialis posterior muscle being a key support. Disturbance of muscle function due to shoe problems can lead to muscle imbalance with resulting medial arch dysfunction. In this common situation, addressing the cause of the muscle problem should be the primary treatment rather than using an arch support to take the place of the muscle's normal activity.

Many shoes come with generic supports that can be removed. Some can be easily taken out while others may require a little pulling. These are very general supports that usually don't match the specific needs of your foot. In most cases, you're better off removing as much as possible from the shoe. In addition to allowing your foot to function more freely, the shoe will become thinner and more firm, both healthy attributes. Some of these inserts are meant to cover poor manufacturing work underneath, which can be very rough—in this case it may be uncomfortable to be in this type of shoe without the insert. If the insert is thick, you can replace it with a thinner one.

### Orthotics

The use of an orthotic device should not be a first line of therapy for most foot problems. Orthotics are often prescribed to patients with knee pain. However, many studies have not shown this to be effective. In addition, EMG (electromyographic) studies fail to show any significant differences in the average muscle activity of the tibialis anterior, peroneus longus, and gastrocnemius muscles when orthotics are used.

Placing orthotics in your shoes most often results in the shoe fitting differently, usually too tightly. In this instance, the shoe must either be modified or a different shoe used. Unfortunately, this is not usually done and many people with added support now have worse ill-fitting shoes.

Most orthotics are not custom-made to your foot but to a general model of an average foot. They are often made from hard mate-rials—plastic and sometimes even metal. I could never understand these materials for use in a person without a serious permanent condition as these materials are often used for people who have functional problems. Your foot moves through many ranges of motion during the course of standing, walking, or running. The best material to use is leather since it will move with the foot.

## Heel Lifts

The use of heel lifts has been popular for many years. These are often recommended for plantar fasciitis, Achilles tendon pain, or the so-called short leg syndrome said to contribute to low back and other pains. Just because they may provide some symptomatic relief, however, does not mean they address the cause of the problem.

Heel lifts can make structural changes in the feet, ankle, legs, pelvis, and spine. Yet, studies show that the use of heel lifts can also result in increased impact and increased instability of the foot. The result can be higher weight-bearing stress on the joints in the foot and ankle, and possibly the knees, hips, and pelvis. Like other supports, even if you feel better with lifts, the cause of the problem is usually not addressed.

Heel lifts may provide relief of symptoms in a variety of problems:

- Heel lifts may temporarily improve symp-toms of plantar pain. However, in the pro-cess other areas of the foot and ankle may become physically stressed.

- Some people use heel lifts to attempt to improve low back pain. It's clear that heel lifts can change the posture of the pelvis and low back. However, whether this change makes a real improvement of the problem, no change, or a worsening of the problem is left to chance.

- For those with so-called short leg syn-drome, heel lifts are sometimes recom-mended. However, if the "short leg" is functional, which is almost always the case, and due to muscle imbalance and not a true shortening of one leg compared to the other, heel lifts are not the best remedy since they do not address the problem. For those with a history of a broken bone in the leg or thigh or other causes of a true or *anatomical* short leg, a heel lift may be helpful since one leg is actually shorter. (Although even in these situations, mus-cles should compensate for a short leg, and using a heel lift may interfere with normal compensation.)

- Heel lifts are sometimes used for those with Achilles tendon pain. This is due to the elevated heel reducing the activity of the gastrocnemius muscle, thereby reducing tension in the Achilles tendon. However, in some cases gastrocnemius muscle func-tion is already diminished and one of the causes of the problem.

- The temporary use of heel lifts may be important is certain surgical conditions, such as postoperative management of ruptured Achilles tendon.

### Elastic Support

The popular use of elastic support is different from taping. These supports don't have much effect on foot-sense, presumably because they don't "stick" to the skin like tape and have much less of an effect on the nerves within. Studies have shown that compared to other devices, elastic supports are much less effective in treating various foot and ankle conditions. Like other supports, elastic devices may cause muscle dysfunction if worn for too long.

### Shoe Lacing

Some shoe problems are not due to fit but poor lacing technique. How difficult can it be to tie your shoes? After all, we learned 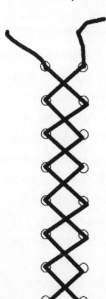 that a long time ago as children. Well, the fact is, many people don't lace their shoes correctly, and sometimes it can make a significant difference in how the shoe fits. In addition, many people don't tie the laces of their casual shoes, making them too loose. This can create instability in the feet.

Sometimes lacing too tight is a sufficient enough stress to cause problems.

Lacing should be snug—not too loose but not tight. There should never be discomfort associated with lacing, or any discomfort under the area of the laces. The most important aspect of lacing is that, after tying your shoes, they should be completely comfortable, and after they've been on for a while, they should be just as comfortable. This should be true for not only the laces but the whole shoe.

There are many different types of lacing used for many different types of shoes by different types of shoe wearers. Using comfort as your guide, you'll always get the best fit. Here are some general tips to lace more effectively:

Always lace from the toes upward, beginning with the holes or eyelets farthest down.

Each set of eyelets you go through with the lace, pull the laces snug, but not tight, so the same amount of tension is evenly distributed through the lace.

Use a crisscross or zigzag pattern—most people and most shoes function best with this approach.

When you finish lacing, all areas of the lace should have the same tension.

Crisscross style of lacing is the most common way to tie shoes in the United States. In Europe, it's more common to use straight lacing, where instead of all the laces going up the shoe in a diagonal pattern, some go from hole to hole straight across.

It's been shown that both the crisscross and European pattern is equally effective. If you find either of these patterns of lacing not comfortable, most likely your shoe does not fit correctly. In addition, the crisscross pattern requires the least amount of lace, so you'll always have sufficient lace for tying. The European style is the second most efficient approach for lace use.

If you have a very irregular foot, you may require any number of different types of lacing, one that matches your particular needs. In this case you may also be wearing special shoes and a specialist should be able to help with lacing. In any situation, don't be afraid to experiment. But always use the comfort factor as the ultimate index.

## Going Shoeless

If you really want to be free, go barefoot. Not that most people will run or bike barefoot, but spending adequate time without shoes is important for physical health. Being barefoot is, in itself, a great therapy—especially if you have a foot problem—because it's the best and quickest way to rehabilitate your feet. It's also one of the best preventive measures to avoid future foot problems.

Without the restriction of shoes, your foot muscles can ultimately return to their natural state of optimal function. In some people, this could take time. For example, if you're used to wearing thick-soled running shoes, being barefoot will be a big transition. But once you experience the freedom of being barefoot, you'll wonder how you got by without it. There are two ways to go barefoot. First, you can spend a certain amount of time walking barefoot, much like a therapeutic exercise. Second, you can incorporate being barefoot

into your lifestyle—just be barefoot as much as possible in all that you do.

Baring your soles may be difficult for some, not just physically but mentally and emotionally, too. After all, we're taught by society that being barefoot is somehow dirty or low class. Yes, when you walk or run barefoot your soles will get dirty. But you'll track less dirt compared to wearing shoes—you'll actually look where you're walking when barefoot and avoid stepping on things you don't think about when wearing shoes. And your feet won't pick up any more germs than your hands or mouth.

For those who need support—not the type in the shoes but mental and emotional support—consider the Dirty Sole Society (www.BareFooters.org), Barefoot Runners (www.BarefootRunner.org), Parents for Barefoot Children (www.Unshod.org/pfbc), and other groups that promote healthy barefoot living. We are not alone.

Physically, making the transition to bare feet will involve toughening up your soles. This sometimes makes people uneasy, but consider that the more time spent barefoot, the less calluses you'll have. Even though your soles may get tougher, you won't notice it except in being able to walk or even exercise barefoot almost anywhere without discomfort. Even though you'll have tougher soles, you'll actually have more sensation in your feet as a result of being barefoot.

Note: The state of being barefoot is referred to as being "unshod"—meaning unshod—while wearing shoes is called "shod."

## Barefoot Therapy

If you still need an excuse to go barefoot, do it for your health. You can even tell people you're undergoing special rehabilitation by order of the doctor. The fact is, being barefoot can help restore normal muscle function in the feet better than any other therapy. It accomplishes this by allowing normal movement and improving foot-sense.

If you're not used to being barefoot, start by walking unshod around your home. It's best without socks, but a thin pair would be acceptable if your feet get cold. Walk on the bare floor, carpeted areas, basement cement, and any surfaces available. Different surfaces will provide different types of stimulation for your bare feet. That's what you're looking for—a variety of stimulation to restore normal foot-sense.

If you have not ventured outdoors after a couple of weeks, take the plunge. This will provide much more foot stimulation because the ground is uneven and not smooth like your indoor surfaces. Walking on grass, dirt, sand, and other natural surfaces will provide great motivation for your feet to improve foot-sense. Even your driveway, sidewalk, and porch can provide additional types of stimulus for your feet. Eventually progress to running short distances.

I'm barefoot indoors at all times, and also spend time outdoors barefoot. I have never sustained cuts or injury other than minor scrapes on occasion, even when running barefoot.

After a couple of more weeks being barefoot, especially with outdoor activity, your foot function should be improving and your feet should feel better. During this period, you should also be wearing shoes that fit properly and better match your feet. This may mean buying new ones and also disposing of the ones that don't fit. Unlike clothing, don't keep your tight-fitting shoes, thinking your feet will someday get smaller. They won't.

Once you've established better foot function through healthy barefoot adaptation, it's important to maintain two habits. First, spend as much time as possible being barefoot throughout the year. Even when the weather is bad, being barefoot indoors virtually all the time can help maintain proper foot function. Second, once you've weaned off bad shoes and restored good foot function, be careful not to return to old bad habits by wearing bad shoes, with the only exception perhaps being the occasional ceremony (although even these situations can be successful with good dress shoes).

There are many exercise programs and types of equipment available to improve foot function, but most won't accomplish any more than the benefits obtained by being barefoot. If your foot problems require more help than barefoot rehabilitation, consider the next most effective home therapy, soft taping.

## Soft Taping

Many different types of taping are used by a lot of therapists for a variety of foot problems. I've tried dozens of techniques through the years with disappointing results. In some cases, these are for emergency purposes, such as following an accident to provide temporary immobilization. In other cases taping is used during an athletic event. At other times it's to provide support during a healing process. Some taping that is too tight, however, can weaken the muscles and ligaments. Instead, you want what I call *soft taping*.

The intention of soft taping is not to directly support the foot or ankle by attempting to physically hold it in place, but to stimulate the sensitive nerves to improve foot-sense, which allows the body to support itself. Soft taping is very light and delicate, using just two pieces of tape.

Recall that foot-sense (along with K-sense) is associated with the feeling of position and movement. The loss of foot-sense can lead to dysfunction and injury, while improving this awareness can restore normal foot function. Soft taping of the lower leg, ankle, and foot improves foot-sense and can be a powerful therapeutic tool for many types of chronic foot problems. These include recurrent sprained ankles, plantar problems, heel problems, and many others including those annoying undiagnosed conditions.

Soft taping is accomplished with two simple steps. It requires one-inch white athletic tape available in most drug stores. Slightly wider or thinner tape is acceptable. Both pieces should be about twelve inches, more for larger and less for smaller bodies. Here are the two steps:

First, place one piece of tape around the lowest part of the leg, just above the two prominent bones on either side of the ankle. This piece should overlap itself by a couple of inches, fit snug but not tight, and should stick to the leg.

Second, attach another piece of tape on to the first, facing downward, and wrap it down the outside and under the mid-foot. Wrap it up the inside of the ankle at the middle of the arch, and attach it to the other side of the first piece. See figure to the right.

If the second piece of tape does not stick well to the first, apply a short, two-inch piece over the attachments to help it stick.

The goal is not to support the foot or ankle, so you should not feel the tape providing any supporting role. It should be comfortable, not tight. At the end of the day when you may have more fluid in your foot and ankle, it should not be tight or uncomfortable. For this reason, in some people it's best to first apply the tape in the early evening.

Leave the tape on for several days. It will gradually begin to peel off—if this occurs sooner, apply new tape. It should not be soaked in a bath but can be wet from a shower and carefully dried. Remove it after a few days and leave it off for a week. If you are spending time barefoot, you should feel improvement in the function of your foot after the first application. If there is no or only very small improvement, tape the foot and ankle again for the same period of time.

In some situations, soft taping may have to be done regularly. This may be the case when bad shoes have been worn for a long time, when you have to wear heavy or over-supported shoes for work, or any footwear that is not comfortable (until you buy new shoes), or as part of a rehabilitation program for a more severe problem such as a stroke or spinal injury.

## Foot Massage

Manual massage may be the oldest hands-on remedy for the feet. While professional massage therapists are now very popular, you can also treat your own feet daily at home, either by yourself or trading massages with others. This foot therapy can improve blood and lymph circulation, reduce muscle tension, improve range of motion in foot joints, and stimulate the communication between the feet and brain to improve foot-sense. Even a five-minute massage for each foot can work wonders. It works best when the foot is completely relaxed, the reason it's best when someone else is doing the work.

The best way to massage the feet is to keep it simple. Start with the feet relaxed, clean, and dry. Place a small amount of organic coconut oil on your hands. The oil is not a necessity but makes the massage easier, and it's good for the skin of the feet (and hands). Begin by slowly and gently rubbing the feet with both hands, all over the foot, ankle, and lower leg. Gently move the foot and toes in all directions, but don't over-stretch anything. Next, use your fingers to massage the muscles, using easy finger pressure in areas of tightness. Some areas will be tender, and

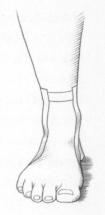

these locations can be massaged more; the foot will feel tender but good if you're applying the right pressure. Continue to work your way up into the leg, where many of the foot muscles originate. This procedure need not be done with hard pressure, and it should not be painful.

As you massage the foot muscles you will often notice small tender areas. These may be tight muscles and may include trigger points—tight, irritated areas in the muscle common in the foot. Trigger points can develop in the muscles from various insults to the body, such as a muscle injury, a sprain, excess activity, and even the stress of bad shoes. When massaging these areas, be firm but avoid causing pain.

The pain of a trigger point is typically felt, or referred to a different area of the body. For example, a trigger point in the calf may cause pain in the heel, while the trigger point itself may not be painful until massaged. A trigger point usually has exquisite tenderness and can be quite uncomfortable. Slow sustained hand or finger pressure and rubbing can help eliminate the trigger point.

## Foot Balancing

Poor foot-sense is a common problem, and the associated imbalance can also affect the knee, hip, pelvis, spine, and areas up into the neck and head. Restoring balance is relatively simple using the three techniques above: being barefoot, soft taping, and massage. Increasing communication between the foot and brain is the goal of this potent therapy.

Many people are unable to balance themselves on one foot for more than a few seconds. This is usually due to poor communication between brain and foot. Try this: with bare feet, stand straight, looking forward with feet close together. Lift one foot by bending and lifting your knee up slightly, and balance yourself on the other foot. You should be able to do this easily for thirty seconds or more. If you can't perform this action, start with attempting to balance on one foot for as long as you can, even if just for a few seconds. Doing this daily can gradually improve the communication between feet and brain. In some individuals, significant imbalances in the foot, especially with certain muscles, may not allow being on one foot for more than a few seconds. Being barefoot, soft taping, and massage may help correct this problem or, in some cases, a healthcare professional may help.

With better balance comes the ability to stay on one foot even longer, and you may be able to perform other actions while on one foot, such as rubbing the foot that's elevated, using a massage as discussed above, combing your hair, or other simple activities. All this will further improve balance by training the feet to communicate better with the brain—and this will help overall balance throughout the body. Make this therapy a regular routine, such as after a shower—

when drying your feet, spend extra time by holding one foot up to include a short massage.

You may note that standing on one foot with over-supported, thick shoes is more difficult due to the restriction of foot-brain communication. However, the more foot-sense you have, the easier this will be as well.

## Other Foot Remedies

In some situations, in addition to the four self-therapies above, certain traditional remedies may be helpful. The two most popular and long-standing home remedies are the use of cold and hot. In addition, rolling tight plantar muscles on a golf ball and strengthening specific muscles that are chronically weak can also be helpful. While these remedies can be very effective, they should not replace those described above, and are best performed in addition. The exception is in situations where rest is necessary or for acute problems where cold may be best.

### Acute Foot Problems

For acute foot problems—recent injuries such as a fall, twisted ankle, or stubbed toe—the traditional RICE remedy of rest, ice (or cold), compression, and elevation can be very effective.

Rest was previously discussed—when your foot needs rest, nothing is better. Rest can prevent further damage following injury and give your body the time and energy it needs to heal.

The use of cold and ice is reviewed below.

Mild compression can help reduce swelling, especially when there are broken blood vessels. Cold compressions should be applied carefully, so as not to further traumatize the area. Even the weight of an ice pack can be enough compression.

Elevation is best done by putting your foot up on your desk, lying on the floor with your foot on the couch, or lying in bed with your foot elevated on pillows. This helps prevent excess fluid from building up in the area of injury and if there are blood vessels broken, helps speed the repair process.

### Cryotherapy

The therapeutic use of cold, cryotherapy, was discussed earlier but will be reviewed here because of its importance for foot problems. Like many therapies, ice can be very helpful when properly applied, but can do harm when used incorrectly. Cooling an area of injury can help reduce inflammation and muscle tightness or spasm, both of which help reduce pain and speed the recovery process.

Ice should never be applied directly to your foot. Instead, use a moist cloth or towel on the skin with the ice applied on top of it. A moist towel helps transfer the cooling benefits, whereas a dry one can partly insulate your skin from the cold. In this way, the cooling effect can reach all areas including, possibly, the bones. The ice can be placed in a plastic bag, with smaller pieces of ice working better than large ice cubes, or you can use a freezer gel pack. Be sure the gel pack is not leaking, as that can be irritating to the skin. In an emergency, a package of frozen peas or other items in your freezer may work just fine.

Applying ice to your foot produces four stages of sensation you can easily feel:

First, the area will become cool, and you will feel this cold effect immediately.

Second, you will feel a prickling or itchy sensation, sometimes described as a burning itch.

Following this you will get an achy feeling—in some cases this can become painful.

The last stage is numbness—the point when you know it's time to immediately remove the ice.

Apply ice until you feel numbness, or for no more than about twenty minutes. When in doubt, remove the ice. The therapeutic effects occur in the early and mid- stage, and risk of ice injury increases in the later stage. You can apply the ice again once the skin temperature has returned to normal, although once every hour or two is sufficient for most situations.

In addition to using cold on the foot, cooling tight muscles in the leg can sometimes help the foot. For example, in cases of heel pain or Achilles pain caused by tight gastrocnemius and soleus muscles, the use of cryotherapy on these leg muscles may be helpful. The other muscle group that commonly becomes tight is the plantar muscles on the bottom of the foot, where ice can also be used.

### Contraindications for Ice

Since the foot is not well endowed with large muscles or fat, the use of ice has the potential to cause harm. Too much ice can literally freeze the skin and small blood vessels, and injure nerves. Essentially, cryotherapy can result in frostbite unless ice is applied with caution.

In many situations, ice is not indicated and should be avoided because it can further injure the foot. Those with rheumatoid arthritis, Raynaud's Syndrome, or any type of paralysis should not use ice. Also avoid ice on areas of reduced sensation. Limit or avoid the use of ice over areas where a large nerve passes close to the skin surface, such as under the ankle bones on the inside and outside of the foot.

A very few number of people have cold allergies and can have adverse reactions to cold. Most people already know the condition exists because of previous adverse reactions to cold, including pain and skin rash. Those with high blood pressure should also be cautious when using ice as it can raise blood pressure.

Care should be taken in using ice boots or other strap-on ice packs because these are often used for too long. They are often used for convenience allowing the person to be active during cryotherapy—itself a contraindication as rest and elevation are often what is required. Do not put these devices on before going to sleep for obvious reasons.

For acute injuries, especially during the first twenty-four hours, certain remedies should be avoided. These include the use of heat in any form, whether a hot bath, heating pad, or heating gel. Heat can aggravate inflammation. An aggressive massage can also create heat and should be avoided. Stretching should not be used for acute problems.

Differentiating between the need for heat or cold is relatively easy—if your foot is hot, cool it; if it's cold, heat it. In general, cooling is the best therapy for acute problems. Cold therapy is easy to use, inexpensive, but often overlooked because of its simplicity.

### Mild Cold Compresses

The benefits of cold need not always come from ice. An excellent alternative is to use a towel soaked in very cold water with excess water rung out. Keep the towel in the refrigerator to keep it very cold. This can have a very good therapeutic effect as well, especially if a five- to ten-minute application is all you require. Don't underestimate the benefits of this approach. It's also safer than the use of ice, which can have side effects.

### Cool Bath

Another method of cooling the foot is a cold bath. This is also a safe and effective form of cyrotherapy, and is often more therapeutic than using ice. A large bucket or small foot tub works well. Place your foot in cold water so it is completely submerged. Add enough ice to prevent the water from getting warm. However, do not fill the tub with ice. Depending on the temperature of the water, you can keep your foot immersed for five to twenty minutes. A deeper bath can also cool the muscles of the leg, which often influence the foot. A deep cold bath that cools the leg muscles is often the best way to improve overall function in the foot and can be more therapeutic than ice placed only on the area of discomfort.

While generally used for acute problems, a cold bath can be very helpful for chronic problems not associated with inflammation. A cold bath can improve muscle balance, especially when you cover the leg up to the knee with cold water. A moderately cold bath can also help recovery from exercise or even a day of wearing bad shoes. In this situation, your feet are tired and hot—even a five-minute cool bath can make your feet feel fresh and alive.

## Blisters

A blister is a vesicle created by the separation of different layers of skin that fills with clear fluid or sometimes blood. A blood blister forms when blood vessels within the blister are broken. Blisters result from a pinch bruise or constant friction, as in the case of poorly fitting shoes. Most blisters occur on the bottoms of the feet and back heel area.

Moist skin produces blisters most easily, with very dry and very wet skin most protective against blister formation. Antiperspirants and powders don't prevent blisters, but acrylic socks may offer additional protection. Rather than look for products and materials that reduce blister incidence, it's best to obtain the best-fitting shoes and socks, which are the best prevention against blisters.

There are two important factors regarding blisters. First, if you get one, it means something is not right and you need to find the cause of the problem. If it's improperly fitted shoes, change them immediately. The second factor is that if you get a non-traumatic blister—such as the common types seen from poor shoe fit—it often precedes an injury. The blister is a sign that you have a significant imbalance. Making the necessary changes immediately can prevent further problems.

If you're new to being barefoot and you get a blister, it may just be that you have not yet adapted by thickening the skin. In this case, more slowly accustom yourself to being barefoot.

Draining the blister with light puncture after a day may result in the best outcome and least discomfort, but be sure the area remains clean and free of chemicals.

Ultrarunners and adventure racers have a novel way of treating blisters. They often use duct tape since the tape adheres to itself and not to the damaged skin area.

## Chronic Foot Problems

A long-term foot problem may be more difficult to treat because the body has been unable to correct it. In some cases, a cold footbath, especially one that includes the whole leg up to the knee, can be very helpful. In other cases, heat may help correct a problem. For some people, certain muscles are too weak and need strengthening. For those who have worn bad shoes for a long period of time, specific soft taping of the foot can help rehabilitate it. Directing therapy at tight muscles may also help, such as in the case of tight plantar muscles.

## Heat

The use of heat therapy, sometimes called thermotherapy or hyperthermia, is one of the oldest home remedies. Warm and hot application can be comforting and emotionally relaxing. Various forms of heating are used from moist hot packs and hot baths to heating pads and hot gels. Moist heat is best as it penetrates better, whereas dry heat can dehydrate the skin.

Heat is generally reserved for more chronic conditions and usually contraindicated in acute problems. Heat dilates the blood vessels within the foot. This allows improved circulation helping to bring in needed nutrients including oxygen and removing unwanted waste products. Heat can also help reduce muscle tightness by relaxing or lengthening muscles. Unfortunately, unlike cold, too much heat can worsen weak muscles since they are already lengthened too much. This is most often the case when heat is applied directly over the muscle.

One benefit of heat applications may be pain reduction. This is especially true with heating gels or creams. This effect is not really therapeutic; rather, the heat stimulation on the skin fools the nervous system, and the brain does not feel as much pain. While this reduces pain, it can eliminate your awareness of a problem with the potential for overuse. Also, be aware that gels and creams often contain toxic chemicals that may enter the body through the skin.

### Contraindications of Heat

When in doubt about using heat, avoid it. You can too easily do more harm than good. Do not use heat when you have an acute injury. Avoid heat on an area that is inflamed, swollen, or bruised. In almost all these situations, the foot will feel warm—an indication to use cold, not hot. Also avoid heat with any skin disorder, diabetes, circulatory problem, or any open wound. As mentioned above, heat can worsen an already abnormally inhibited muscle.

## Strengthening Foot Muscles

Chronic muscle weakness in the foot can be remedied. Even if you have a problem in one foot, it's best to exercise both feet.

Place a small dry towel or your sock flat on the floor. Put your bare foot on top of the sock. By contracting your plantar muscles, attempt to pick up the sock by squeezing your toes with the rest of the muscles on the bottom of the foot, keeping your heel on the floor. If you can do this easily—literally are able to lift the towel or sock—the muscles work fine and there is no need for strengthening exercises. If you cannot perform this task, start with a few seconds of trying to pick up the sock. You should be able to lift the front of your foot off the floor while holding the sock. More than a few seconds may fatigue the muscles, so you can limit the activity to that time frame. Perform this exercise two or three times a day, gradually building up to about one minute for each foot. As it becomes easier, you can switch from sock or towel to a marble or small ball for a better workout.

Once you can easily pick up the sock or marble, begin the next phase of this exercise. This involves lifting the sock or marble and moving it left and right. With your heel planted firmly on the floor, pick up the sock or marble and move it as far to the left as you can, placing it back on the floor. Next, pick up the sock or marble and move it as far to the right as you can, keeping your heel on the floor. Gradually, bring your foot (holding the sock or marble) farther and farther to the left and right each time. Be sure to keep your heel on the floor. You should feel the muscles in your leg as you perform this task. Work up to performing this part of the exercise for about two minutes in each foot, with a few seconds rest between movements. If you feel pain or cramping, slow down; if it continues, there may be more extensive problems in the foot, especially muscle imbalance. In this case, use the four primary therapies discussed above (being barefoot, soft-taping, etc.) for a week or two and try this exercise again.

A third part of these strengthening exercises involves lifting up your foot as far as possible while holding the sock or marble. This strengthens the tibialis anterior muscle more than the previous routine. After picking up the sock or marble, lift your foot straight up, as far up as it will go. Next, bring the sock or marble as far right as possible and place it on the floor. Then do the same to the left. In all movements, raise your foot as high as possible. Over time you'll increase your range of motion as the tibialis anterior strengthens. (For pain or cramping, the same as above applies.)

Once you have strengthened your foot muscles, maintaining strength will occur through normal use, so you generally don't have to continue the exercises. This is especially true if you spend adequate time being barefoot.

## Tight Muscles

In many situations, certain muscles may become too tight. This problem is most often secondary to another muscle being too weak. The most common tightness is in the plantar muscles and calf muscles (gastrocnemius and soleus). These problems are sometimes termed plantar fasciitis or Achilles tendonitis. The names imply inflammation, which is not usually the case, so I prefer not to use these names. Instead, these types of problems should just be referred to as muscle imbalances.

If you have pain on the bottoms of your feet but are able to pick up a towel with your plantar muscles as discussed above, they are probably too tight. Plantar muscles that are too tight can be very painful and are most noticeable when you take your first steps out of bed in the morning—the bottoms of your feet are tight and painful and loosen up as you move around.

The best way to reduce the tightness in the plantar muscles is with a golf ball. It's best to begin this routine later in the day after your foot muscles are more warmed up, otherwise the procedure may be too painful. Place a golf ball on the floor. A thin carpet or bare floor works best. Place your bare foot on top of the golf ball and roll your foot on top of the ball. Apply sufficient weight to feel the tight muscles, but not so much as to cause pain. Roll the ball as far forward as you can and as far back as you can. Be sure to reach the whole width of the foot as well. Perform this task for two to four minutes for each foot. Be aware that relief may only be symptomatic if the primary problem is not addressed.

## Conclusion

It is easy to get seduced by the hype associated with each year's new crop of running shoes. But your most prudent path is to steer clear of the bold, extravagant claims offered by the shoe companies. One of the greatest marathon runners of all time, Abebe Bikila of Ethiopia, who trained barefoot, won the 1960 Olympic marathon running barefoot. Other stories of barefoot runners include South African sensation Zola Budd, a cross-country and middle-distance track athlete who also trained and raced without shoes. This is not to suggest that everyone reading this book throw away their shoes and become natural runners. That too can be just as problematic as wearing the wrong kind of shoes.

You need to experiment with different shoes and styles, while continuing to make adjustments and self-assessments. Don't wait until an injury occurs before making a change. Your feet are quite adaptive. Humans, to a great extent, owe their survival as a species to their feet. Forty thousand years ago, we left Africa by foot and have been moving ever since.

# CHAPTER 32

# THE SUN—
## Vitamin D and Athletic Performance

**D**oes spending more time in the sun improve athletic performance? The ancient Greeks believed athletes should be well bathed by the sun, and their elite athletes trained at the beach and in the nude. The latter might be difficult in today's world, but if your vitamin D levels are too low, the sun can definitely improve your training and racing performance; and in a healthy way. Research indicates that normal vitamin D levels are associated with peak athletic performance. However, a surprising number of athletes have low levels of vitamin D, often because they prevent normal vitamin D production by using sunscreen, avoiding midday sun exposure, and overdressing.

It's important to balance minimizing overexposure to the sun (avoiding sunburn) with obtaining enough sun exposure to allow for sufficient vitamin D production. Normalizing vitamin D levels can improve muscle function, prevent bone problems, help with recovery from training and competition, reduce unexplained muscle pains, and prevent many health problems including many forms of cancer. Normal vitamin D levels may also prevent getting sunburned during long training and racing.

While vitamin D is called a "vitamin," it's really a unique steroid hormone that helps control inflammation and immunity, while improving brain and hormone

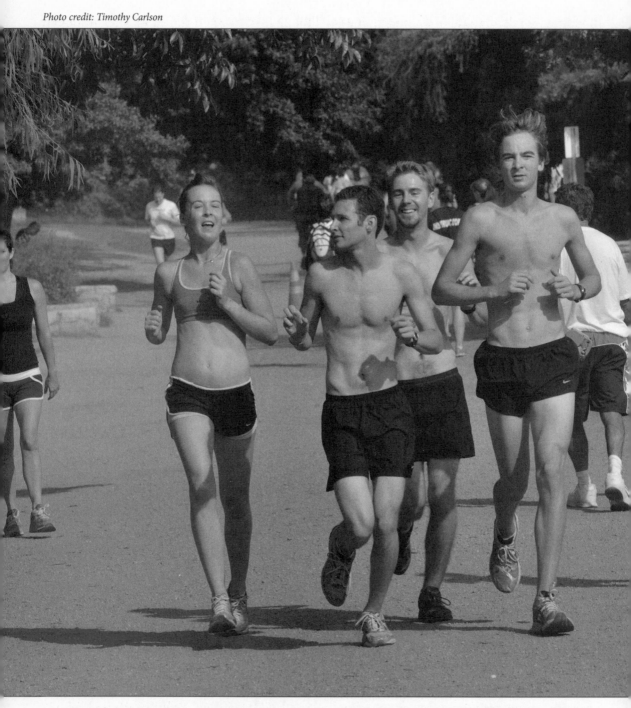

*Balance minimizing overexposure to the sun (avoiding sunburn) with obtaining enough sun exposure to allow for sufficient vitamin D production.*

function, regulating calcium absorption and utilization, and promoting the work of several thousand genes.

For decades, I found low vitamin D levels in athletes I treated. I would then recommend they spend more time in the sun. While this advice resulted in my receiving some nasty letters from dermatologists, current research has shown that the vitamin D–deficit problem is real. A study published in the *International Journal of Sports* revealed that a group of French cyclists, each training sixteen hours a week outdoors, had below-normal levels of vitamin D. Two other current studies measuring large numbers of people in southern Florida and southern Arizona showed significantly high numbers of people were also far below normal levels of vitamin D, despite living in sunny environments.

The key factors associated with an athlete not getting sufficient vitamin D include:

1. Using sunscreen that blocks the vitamin D–producing ultraviolet B (UVB) waves of the sun.
2. Wearing protective clothing, especially materials that block UVB waves.
3. Training early and later in the day, when vitamin D–producing sun exposure is significantly reduced.
4. Darker skin. Even many light-skinned athletes have accumulated enough sun to darken their skin to the point where it reduces their ability to obtain vitamin D from sun exposure. As a result, they need to be in the sun longer to obtain the same amount of D.
5. Proper fat metabolism is necessary for vitamin D production, and those with too high and too low body fat may be unable to release stored vitamin D, which is especially important in winter and early spring when sun exposure produces much less vitamin D.
6. Athletes living at more extreme latitudes, such as northern Europe and Canada, and southern Australia and South America, have significantly less sun exposure throughout the year.

## Testing Your Vitamin D Levels

A simple blood test should be performed as necessary to monitor your vitamin D levels. The lowest levels of vitamin D are in early spring, a good time to test yourself. While different labs can vary in their "normal" ranges, blood levels should be between 50–80 ng/mL (or 125–200 nM/L) year-round, with lower levels in this normal range following winter and higher levels within this range in late summer. How much vitamin D you need from all sources to maintain normal levels is very individual. This is best monitored through taking additional blood tests every few months, adjusting your sun exposure and dietary supplements as needed. Tell your health-care professional to include vitamin D in your next blood test, or get an in-home test kit, which is a very accurate, easy, and relatively inexpensive way to test your vitamin D level. These are available through the Vitamin D Council's Web site (www.VitaminD-Council.org).

Based on recent scientific studies, the currently recommended daily vitamin D levels of 200–400 IU (international units) are grossly inadequate. The average daily need for vitamin D may be as high as 4,000 IU a day in some people.

## Sources of Vitamin D

There are five sources of vitamin D available for athletes. Our primary source comes from the sun, with foods providing small amounts. Fortified foods such as milk and many processed foods are not a good source. Dietary supplements are the most viable option for those requiring more, and artificial light can also be a source of vitamin D for those in colder climates where optimal sun exposure is limited. Let's look more closely at each of these sources.

### Sunshine

It's especially important to obtain adequate vitamin D from sun exposure during the warmer summer months to build stores of vitamin D for the winter. But without sufficient exposure beginning early in the season that brings vitamin D levels in the body to moderate or high levels, the amount of vitamin D stored for winter may be inadequate and additional sources necessary.

How much sun and for how long depends on each athlete's individual needs. For many fair-skinned athletes, exposing arms and legs to sunlight for twenty to thirty minutes—more in northern climates and less as you get closer to the equator during high sun (between the hours of 10 AM and 3 PM) throughout the week without sunscreen may be adequate to start the process of building normal vitamin D levels. In a healthy athlete, this amount of sun can produce 5,000 to 10,000 units of vitamin D—and this amount is healthy, not excessive. Interestingly, we can't overdose on vitamin D from the sun like we can with all other sources, such as from dietary supplements.

As your skin tans, longer periods of sun exposure will be needed to build vitamin D stores for the winter months. That's because those with darker skin will require even more sun exposure throughout the year to obtain the same amount of vitamin D. Those in more northern (and extreme southern) climates may need much more. In general, more exposure may be better as long as you avoid the most important sun stress—sunburn. And as your levels of vitamin D rise and normalize, the risk of sunburn diminishes.

### Food sources

The best vitamin D–containing foods are from animal sources. These include wild salmon, sardines, and tuna, which provide moderate amounts, and egg yolks. Vegetable sources of vitamin D are less adequately utilized by the body, with shiitake mushroom being a modest source.

# AN EXPERT VIEW ON VITAMIN D DEFICIENCY

John Cannell, MD, executive director of the Vitamin D Council (www.VitaminD-Council.org), has extensively researched the topic of vitamin D and athletic performance. He believes that the right amount of vitamin D will make you faster, stronger, improve your balance and timing, etc. How much it will improve your athletic ability depends on how deficient you are to begin with. However, peak athletic performance also depends upon the neuromuscular cells in your body and brain having unfettered access to the steroid hormone, activated vitamin D.

As the lead author of a study entitled "Athletic Performance and Vitamin D" (in the journal *Medicine and Science in Sports and Exercise*), Cannell reviewed reports on the use of sunlamps during the early and mid-1900s in Russia and East Germany to increase vitamin D levels in athletes. They showed this form of artificial ultraviolet irradiation—which increases vitamin D levels—improved athletic function. And these actions caused some to argue that this little known routine provided an unfair advantage during competition. In my earliest days of training and competition in high school and college, there were often news reports about the well-kept secrets that helped former Soviet Union and East German athletes perform better; some claim this was one of their secrets.

In a recent issue of his "Vitamin D Newsletter," Cannell thoroughly described a conversation he once had with a young athletic patient regarding the importance of Vitamin D. Excerpts from that exchange are reproduced here:

"No way, doc," the patient told me. I had just finished telling him about the benefits of vitamin D, explaining that he should take 4,000 IU per day. But he claimed that the U.S. government said he only needed 200 IU per day, not 4,000. He also knew the official Upper Limit was 2,000 IU a day. "What are you trying to do kill me?" I told him his 25(OH)-vitamin D blood test was low, only 13 ng/ml. He had read about that too, in a medical textbook, where it said normal levels are between 10 and 40 ng/ml. "I'm fine doc," adding, "Are you in the vitamin business?" I explained I was not; that the government used outdated values. So I tried a different tact. I brought him copies of recent press articles. "Look," I said, "look at these." Science News called vitamin D the Antibiotic Vitamin. The Independent in England says vitamin D explains why people die from influenza in the winter, and not the summer. U.S. News and World Report says almost everyone needs more. Newsweek says it prevents cancer and helps fight infection. In four different recent reports, United Press International says that it reduces falls in the elderly, many pregnant women are deficient, it reduces stress fractures, and that it helps heal wounds.

He glanced at the articles, showing a little interest in stress fractures. Then he told me what he was really thinking. "Look doc, all this stuff may be important to old guys like you. I'm 22. All I care about are girls and sports. When I get older, maybe I'll think about it. I'm too young to worry about it. I'm in great condition." I couldn't argue. He was in good health and a very good basketball player, playing several hours every day, always on indoor courts.

What could I do to open my patient's eyes? As an African American, his risk of early death was very high, although the risk for blacks doesn't start to dramatically increase until their forties and fifties. Like all young people, he saw himself as forever young. The U.S. government was no help, relying on a ten-year-old report from the Institute of Medicine that is full of misinformation.

I tried to tell him that the 200 IU per day the U.S. government recommends for twenty-year-olds is to prevent bone disease, not to treat low vitamin D levels like his. I pointed out the U.S. government's official current Upper Limit of 2,000 IU/day is the same for a 300-pound adult as it is for a 25-pound toddler. That is, the government says it's safe for a one-year-old, 25-pound child to take 2,000 IU per day but it's not safe for a thirty-year old, 300-pound adult to take 2,000 and one IU a day. I mean, whoever thought up these Upper Limits must have left their thinking caps at home. Nevertheless, nothing worked. My vitamin D–deficient patient was not interested in taking any vitamin D.

What are young men interested in? I remembered that he had told me: "Sex and sports." Two years ago I had researched the medical literature looking for any evidence vitamin D enhanced sexual performance. Absolutely nothing. That would have been nice. Can you imagine the interest?

Then I remembered that several readers had written to ask me if vitamin D could possibly improve their athletic performance. They told me that after taking 2,000 to 5,000 IU per day for several months, they seemed just a little faster, a little stronger, maybe had a little better balance and timing. A pianist had written to tell me she even played a better piano, her fingers moved over the keys more effortlessly! Was vitamin D responsible for these subtle changes or was it a placebo effect? That is, did readers just think their athletic performance improved because they knew vitamin D was a steroid hormone precursor (hormone, from the Greek, meaning "to set in motion")?

The active form of vitamin D is a steroid (actually a seco-steroid) in the same way that testosterone is a steroid and vitamin D is a hormone in the same way that growth hormone is a hormone. Steroid hormones are substances made from cholesterol, which circulate in the body, and work at distant sites by "setting in motion" genetic protein transcription. That is, both vitamin D and testosterone regulate your genome, the stuff of life. While testosterone is a sex steroid hormone, vitamin D is a pleomorphic (multiple function) steroid hormone.

All of a sudden, it didn't seem so silly. Certainly steroids can improve athletic performance although they can be quite dangerous. In addition, few people are deficient in growth hormone or testosterone, so when athletes take sex steroids or growth hormone they are cheating, or doping. The case with vitamin D is quite different because natural vitamin D levels are about 50 ng/ml and, since almost no one has such levels, extra vitamin D is not doping, it's just good treatment. I decided to exhaustively research the medical literature on vitamin D and athletic performance. It took me over a year.

To my surprise, I discovered that there are five totally independent bodies of research that all converge on an inescapable conclusion: vitamin D will improve athletic performance in vitamin D deficient people (and that includes most people). Even more interesting is who published this literature, and when. Are you old enough to remember when the Germans and Russians won every Olympics in the '60s and '70s? Well, it turns out that the most convincing evidence that vitamin D improves athletic performance was published in old German and Russian medical literature.

With the help of my wife and mother-in-law, both of whom are Russian, and with the help of Marc Sorenson, whose book Solar Power is a must-read, I finally was able to look at translations of much of the old Russian and German literature. When one combines that old literature with the modern English language literature on neuromuscular performance, the conclusion is inescapable. The readers who wrote me are right.

If you are vitamin D–deficient, the medical literature indicates that the right amount of vitamin D will make you faster, stronger, improve your balance and timing, etc. How much it will improve your athletic ability depends on how deficient you are to begin with. How good an athlete you will be depends on your innate ability, training, and dedication. However, peak athletic performance also depends upon the neuromuscular cells in your body and brain having unfettered access to the steroid hormone, activated vitamin D. In addition, how much activated vitamin D is available to your brain, muscle, and nerves depends on having ideal levels of vitamin D in your blood—about 50 ng/ml, to be precise.

Why would I write about such a frivolous topic like peak athletic performance when cancer patients all across this land are dying vitamin D deficient? Like many vitamin D advocates, I have been disappointed that the medical profession and the public don't seem to care about vitamin D. Maybe people, like my young basketball player, will care if it makes better athletes.

The medical literature indicates vitamin D levels of about 50 ng/ml are associated with peak athletic performance. Of course, recent studies show such levels are ideal for preventing cancer, diabetes, hypertension, influenza, multiple sclerosis, major depression, cognitive impairments, etc. But who cares about all that disease stuff old people get, we're talking about something really important: speed, balance, reaction time, muscle mass, muscle strength, squats, reps, etc. And guess who's now taking 4,000 IU/day? Yes he is, and he tells me his timing is better, he can jump a little higher, run a little faster, and the ball feels "sweeter," whatever that means.

### Fortified Foods

Foods fortified with vitamin D are *not* a good source for several reasons. First, the levels are very low and quite insignificant when compared to what we get from the sun. Relying on the consumption of vitamin D–fortified foods has clearly failed to prevent abnormal low levels and associated disease and other problems in the population. The synthetic fortification of milk is a common example. Most people would need ten or twelve glasses a day—or more—to consume adequate amounts of vitamin D—something most would not and should not consume. And this form is vitamin D2, which is ergocalciferol, a synthetic form of the type found in plants. In addition, the foods that are fortified are usually unhealthy processed products, such as cereal, margarine, and processed cheese.

### Dietary Supplements

The best dietary supplement is cod liver oil, which provides a concentrated form of natural vitamin D. Cod liver oil is the best type of vitamin D because it contains the vitamin D3 (cholecalciferol) form, which is better utilized by the body than the vitamin D2 form obtained from plants, a common source in other dietary supplements. Vegetarians who won't take animal sources of vitamin D must rely more on the sun. Many supplements of cod liver oil also contain vitamin A, an important nutrient for athletes. However, avoid those that provide you with more than about 5,000 IU of vitamin A a day. High levels of vitamin A can also be toxic (causing such problems as liver stress, loss of bone density, and hair loss), and it can interfere with vitamin D metabolism.

In some individuals who have very low blood levels of vitamin D, even modest amounts of vitamin D supplementation may not normalize blood levels, and much higher doses may be necessary to correct this serious deficiency. In some cases, 50,000 IU a day or more for the first week may be the start of optimal therapy, but this should be done under the guidance of a health-care professional. These doses must be carefully monitored with blood levels to avoid toxicity while assuring levels are returning to normal. These very high doses of vitamin D, both in oral and injectable forms, in doses of 25,000 to 100,000 units, come with a risk of overdose. Vitamin D toxicity can cause significant mineral imbalance, especially of calcium and phosphorus, and fatigue, constipation, forgetfulness, nausea, and vomiting.

## Sun Lights

Tanning or sun beds, "happy lights," and other sources of UVB rays, can increase vitamin D levels. These are readily available for home use and in tanning salons. I don't recommend using them as a replacement for sun exposure but they are helpful for those who may be unable to spend adequate time in the sun. This is especially true in winter months in cold climates, and for those who work indoors all day. With adequate sun exposure in warm weather, cod liver oil supplements, and a tanning bed once a week, even athletes in Canada, northern Europe, and other sun-deficient areas can maintain healthy levels of vitamin D.

## Other Nutrients Associated with the Sun and Vitamin D

Magnesium is an important nutrient to help the body regulate vitamin D. This mineral is often low in athletes. In fact, having done a dietary analysis on almost all athletes I've seen over decades of work, magnesium is one of the more common deficiencies. The best food sources are organically grown vegetables and raw nuts and seeds. These foods will also help you obtain other nutrients needed for better utilization of vitamin D; they include zinc and the vitamins A and K. In the case of vitamin A, however, you'll need egg yolks and other animal foods such as fish since plant foods don't contain vitamin A (they contain large amounts of beta-carotene which the human body can convert to vitamin A but not as efficiently as other animals). Most cod liver oil supplements also contain vitamin A.

As research continues we'll find out more about the nutrients that we need to protect us when spending time in the sun. Various naturally occurring antioxidants from foods, and omega-3 fats, for example, are used by the body in helping to protect us from the possible harm of overexposure, so these nutrients will be needed in adequate amounts especially in sunny seasons. For a long time it's been known that sun exposure reduces the body's folic acid, another reason to consume ten servings of vegetables and fruits each day, which should provide sufficient folic acid.

## Training and Racing in the Sun

Of course, endurance athletes are exposed to significant periods of sun during long training and racing. A common question if you are heading to the Ironman Hawaii is how you can protect yourself from the hot tropic sun, or even during your long Sunday run or bike ride. One observation I made many years ago is that healthy athletes don't burn nearly as much or as fast as those who are less healthy. This may be due to a variety of reasons, as a healthy diet can protect your skin from overexposure to the sun.

Consider these factors:

- Getting roasted by the sun is associated with an inflammatory reaction; the more inflammation, the more severe the burn. But by maintaining a good balance of fats, especially the inclusion of fish oil, you control inflammation and protect yourself better from a long day in the sun.
- A full spectrum of antioxidants—from beta-carotene and lycopene to the vitamin E complex (all eight components) and natural vitamin C—found in the diet can also help protect the skin during sun expo-

sure; in particular, these help control free radical reactions in the skin.

- Because a long day in the sun can significantly reduce the body's folic acid levels, consuming sufficient vegetables and fruits will help offset this, potentially restoring healthy skin.
- Those with normal levels of vitamin D may not burn as fast or as badly as those with low levels.

The body has natural protection from overexposure to the sun. The skin's production of melanin is responsible for this tanning process by providing protection against excess ultraviolet light. It's normal for the skin to redden during very long training or racing, but by day's end, or the next morning, the skin should be back to normal. This does not constitute sunburn, just a sign of high exposure, which should be tolerated by a healthy body. If in doubt about how much burn you have, use cold water immediately after a long period in the sun, which can dramatically speed the healing of the skin. While a cool shower is helpful, getting into cool water, covering all areas of exposure if possible, is ideal.

Even when you're healthy, in long training and racing, certain skin areas will be more vulnerable. The ears, nose, lips, and head are easily burned after training or racing all day in many geographical areas. Proper clothing, including a hat that shades these areas, is very

**Question:** Can you get sufficient sun and vitamin D exposure on overcast days? I just don't like training in the sun all that much and where I live—Cleveland—overcast days seem to be the norm.

**Answer:** Even an overcast, cloudy day can provide you with some exposure to sufficient sunlight to obtain smaller amounts of vitamin D. But on a cloudy day in Cleveland, you might obtain only about half the amount if you're working out midday. The denser the cloud cover, the less vitamin D, and when the air is higher in moisture, such on those humid days, even less. First, establish your vitamin D levels through a blood test; then bring your levels to normal if they're not already there by using cod liver oil if necessary. A follow-up blood test will tell you whether you're successful or not.

important. Even the right length hair can help, especially for the ears and neck. Products such as zinc oxide can also help if necessary. Clothing can also help shade other areas such as shoulders and arms.

Of course, building at least a moderate tan is still a very important way to protect the skin. But if you're racing an ultramarathon in a very sunny location, for example, and know you will burn, using products that rely on zinc oxide may be effective. There are even certified organic versions available.

## Sun Protection Factor—SPF

It should be noted that the SPF—Sun Protection Factor—listed on sunscreen products indicates how much longer you can stay in the sun without burning compared to not having sunscreen. If your skin is unprotected, and burns after thirty minutes, a product with an SPF of 10 would mean you could stay in the sun ten times as long, or five hours. Using that same product a few times during your stay in the sun will not prolong the protection—you would actually need to use a sunscreen with a higher SPF to accomplish this. Sunscreens with an SPF of more than 30 may not offer any additional protection, despite the marketing hype.

Humans have lived in hot, sunny environments for tens of thousands of years. While most athletes spend considerable time outdoors, it's important to not abuse the skin. The concern, however, is that increased sun exposure can cause dry skin, wrinkles, and, the greatest concern, skin cancer. Certainly skin damage and the risk of cancer are possible if time spent in the sun is abused, especially at an early age and when one is not healthy.

Not until the past few decades has the incidence of skin cancer become a growing problem. This period corresponds with the development of sunscreen and other products that attempt to block the sun's rays. Vitamin D is known to prevent many cancers, including skin cancer. William Grant, PhD, who has published many papers on this topic, says that sunscreen is overrated and gives a false sense of security. Other research shows the use of sunscreen can actually increase the risk of malignant melanoma (the most common and deadly form) and other skin cancers. Grant and other researchers describe the problem this way: Most sunscreens block UVB (ultraviolet B waves) very effectively, which is what we make vitamin D from, but sunscreen does not block longer waves that are more dangerous, such as UVA, well. We obtain vitamin D through UVB, and if we block that wave, our sun-stimulated vitamin D production is reduced. And, users of sunscreen often remain in the sun longer because of its artificial comfort. But they are unwittingly exposing their skin to more dangerous UVA and increasing the risk of skin cancer. For this and other reasons, the growing list of research supports the notion that we can prevent a significant number of many types of cancers by spending some time in the sun, without sunscreen—as long as we don't burn.

Some studies show a relationship between sunscreen use and cancer prevention while others have not. Still other studies show sunscreen use can actually increase the risk of malignant melanoma. Unfortunately, sunscreen manufacturers and cosmetic companies spend millions on marketing, using popular scare tactics to convince people to use their products.

For most of my career, I have recommended getting a good tan to protect the skin against excessive sun damage. In fact, tanning provides protection similar to sunscreen, and with protection specifically against the potentially dangerous UVA. A recent issue of *Science* (March 2, 2007) says the same: "A dark natural tan offers unparalleled protection against skin cancer." Not everyone can tan. Extremely fair-skinned people, those with red hair, and those with freckles can burn quite easily, and these individuals must be cautious when outdoors.

My advice has always been the same: Don't put anything on your skin you're not willing to eat! That's because sunscreen, along with so many things people put on their skin, gets absorbed into the body.

# CHAPTER 33

# MEASURING YOUR FITNESS AND HEALTH

**N**o matter where you find yourself on the road to endurance, you will want to keep track of changes affecting your body. Staying vigilant will also help you become more intuitive about your body, allowing you to successfully detect and address signs and symptoms as they gradually develop. You don't want to wait until you develop more obvious problems before realizing there's something wrong.

To help you improve your own self-assessment, I have previously outlined the importance of the MAF Test (see chapter 4) as well as the importance of heart-rate variability, but here are some other general tests, most of which you can easily perform at home. It's important that you record all the test results by keeping track of them in your training diary.

I must emphasize, however, that none of these tests are meant to replace the ones a health-care practitioner may perform. And while each one may be important, they are most accurate when considered as a group, especially in conjunction with other standard diagnostic tests done by a physician. Additionally, the result of one test in isolation may not be as meaningful as seeing the same test results over an extended period of time.

## Body Fat—Measure Your Waist

As I have mentioned earlier, the most simple and practical way to calculate changes in body fat is to periodically measure your waist with a tape measure at the level of the umbilicus, or the belly button. Unfortunately, you can't dictate where fat loss occurs first. Nor can you spot reduce by doing countless sit-ups or crunches. The belly fat won't burn off that way. But as you burn more body fat, you will notice that your clothes are fitting more loosely. People will also tell you that you look thinner, often noticing it first in your face. Since bathroom scale weight is mostly a measure of water, the measurement of fat, which is what most of us need to know, can't be determined accurately on the scale. It's not unusual for an athlete to gain body fat as reflected in a larger waist size, but show no weight gain on the scale.

## Body Temperature

There are at least three ways of using a thermometer to measure your body temperature. One way is to take the temperature under your tongue, a second is taking a rectal temperature, and another method is checking the temperature under your arm (also known as the axillary temperature). The axillary temperature is best taken in the morning. The normal temperature under the arm ranges from 97.8 to 98.2°F (36.5 to 36.7°C). There are times when one or more methods are best, and the results—normal, high, or low—indicate various aspects of body function.

The oral, under the tongue temperature normally is 98.6°F (37°C), with rectal temperatures about 1°F (0.6°C) higher than oral readings. Normal daily variations of perhaps a few tenths may exist, with morning readings being the lowest and late-afternoon temperatures the highest. Nighttime temperatures may also drop slightly, which helps stimulate sleep onset.

### Elevated Temperature

Temperatures above normal may indicate inflammation, infection, or other problems. In the very young and elderly, and in some alcoholics, infections or inflammation may actually lower body temperature. In athletes, an above-normal temperature may indicate training stress or other problems, and the need for rest—a strong indication to cease all training until the problem is found or the temperature returns to normal. The only exception would be immediately after training or competition. Some athletes can have very high rectal temperatures of up to 105°F (41°C) after a hard 5K running race, or following any high intensity activity. This elevation in temperature starts to return to normal levels within minutes of finishing the race. Increases in body temperature reflect the normal compensation by the body. In fact, increases in body temperature parallel oxygen uptake and exercise intensity. Exercise at 50 percent of $VO_2$max can raise temperatures to about 99°F (37.3°C), with intensities of 75 percent elevating temperatures to about 101°F (38.5°C). Even those working in a very physical job, people under emotional stress, and active children may also show slightly elevated temperatures.

## Lowered Temperature

Temperatures below normal may indicate thyroid dysfunction, also called subclinical hypothyroidism. This can occur even when thyroid blood tests are normal. Lowered body temperature can also occur following physical trauma, sometimes called "post-traumatic hypothyroidism." Low thyroid function may also have a close relationship with hypertension.

In addition to low temperature, other signs and symptoms associated with low thyroid function include mental and physical fatigue, weight gain, depression, cold hands and feet, and crying spells. Those who feel good only after exercise stimulation, even a short, easy run or bike ride, may also have a subclinical hypothyroid condition; this stimulation brings body temperature closer to normal.

A common group of drugs can also reduce body temperature. NSAIDs interfere with the balance of fat and can decrease body temperature.

Sometimes low temperatures occur only at certain times of the week or month. This can occur in both men and women, and is associated with changes in hormones. It's best to take your axillary temperature in the morning upon awakening, before getting out of bed. Keep the thermometer under the armpit for a full ten minutes and record the result in your diary. Once you get up and move around, body temperature may rise slightly.

## Blood Pressure

Many people take their own blood pressure using various devices called "sphygs," or sphygmomanometers. But even the best apparatus only provides a general measure of blood pressure. The standard routine is to take the blood pressure in the left arm while sitting with feet on the floor.

The standard numbers, 120/80, relate to the pressures exerted on the walls of the arteries. It is measured as millimeters of mercury (mmHg), with the mercury devices being more accurate than other types (although today's units are usually not mercury-based but electronic/digital). The first number (120 in this example) is the systolic pressure and relates to the pressure in which the heart and vessels contract. The second number (80), the diastolic pressure, shows the pressure at which the heart and vessels relax.

An athlete's blood pressure is always changing, and 120/80 shouldn't be seen as the normal number, with anything above considered abnormal. Nor should we think that lower is better when it comes to blood pressure. Pressures that are too high or too low can be unhealthy, and there's a fairly wide range of normal in most individuals.

## Hypertension

One factor associated with cardiovascular disease is high blood pressure, or hypertension. Athletes are not immune to this problem. It's not only a risk factor for heart disease but overall mortality. Hypertension is generally defined as blood pressures above 140/90. Unfortunately, the intense marketing of hypertension drugs, corresponding with newer definitions of hypertension, have resulted in more people being medicated and even those with normal blood pressure being told they are in a pre-hypertensive state. Indeed, medical journals are now publishing studies that show cardiovascular risk begins with blood pressures as low as 115/75, and that the blood pressure classification of "pre-hypertension" is a systolic pressure between 120–139 and diastolic between 80–89 mmHg.

To make matters worse, most patients are prescribed medication for hypertension without their doctor seeking the underlying cause of the problem. Additionally, most patients are not given appropriate diet and lifestyle guidelines that may reduce their blood pressure to the point where medication may no longer be needed.

Among the problems that may contribute to hypertension is carbohydrate intolerance due to its influence of raising insulin levels. For the Two-Week Test, it's recommended that if your blood pressure is high, you should have it evaluated before, during, and after the Test. That's because for many people, significantly reducing refined carbohydrates and sugars, which reduces insulin levels, will reduce high blood pressure—often dramatically. As a result, if you're taking medication to control blood pressure, your doctor may need to reduce or even eliminate it.

The vast majority of hypertensive patients I initially saw in practice were able to reduce their blood pressure significantly just by strictly avoiding refined carbohydrates and sugars, especially when the aerobic system was improved. Most of these patients were able to eliminate their medication. Other important factors included balancing fats, eating ten servings of vegetables and fruits each day, and controlling stress.

Poor aerobic conditioning can also contribute to hypertension. Those who are inactive and lead a sedentary lifestyle have a significant amount of blood vessels shut down (these are the vessels in the aerobic muscle fibers). These blood vessels remain inactive (they still exist but don't circulate blood) until the aerobic system is better developed, when they start to circulate blood to the newly "turned on" aerobic muscle fibers. Because of increased and improved circulation, aerobic function is an important factor in both prevention and treatment of hypertension. Even one easy aerobic workout can reduce blood pressure for up to twenty-four hours. Anaerobic exercise may not be nearly as effective and can even aggravate high blood pressure through production of the stress hormone cortisol.

Important dietary factors that can prevent or help hypertension include eating sufficient amounts of vegetables and fruits. When certain nutrients are low, such as calcium and vitamins A and C, blood pressure may elevate. Taking these nutrients as a dietary supplement may not provide the same benefits (as most vitamins are synthetic and don't function like those in real food). Basically, by increasing overall fitness and health, blood pressure can be normalized in the majority of people. It's also important to look at the overall picture, as hypertension often means other problems exist. For example, kidney problems and narrowed or "clogged" arteries are commonly associated with hypertension.

## Sodium and BP

A common notion about high blood pressure is that sodium causes it. In some people with existing high blood pressure, excessive sodium intake can magnify the problem. About 30 to 40 percent of those with hypertension are sodium-sensitive. For these individuals, even moderate amounts of sodium can increase their blood pressure further. Obviously, these people should regulate their sodium intake while they are searching for the cause of sodium sensitivity (often an adrenal-associated problem). But salt modification for those who have normal blood pressure is not necessary, as sodium will not raise blood pressure in healthy individuals.

As a necessary nutrient, sodium is essential for all athletes. Overtraining often results in adrenal gland dysfunction causing excess sodium loss, which requires more sodium intake through the diet. An average healthy man of 150 pounds has about 9,000 milligrams of sodium in his body. One-third of this is as part of healthy bones and most of the remaining two-thirds surround the cells throughout the rest of the body, where sodium is a major player in cell regulation. Sodium also helps regulate the acid-alkaline (pH) balance, water balance, the heartbeat and other muscle contractions, sugar metabolism, and even blood-pressure balance.

## Postural Blood Pressure

In addition to using blood pressure to rule out hypertension, measuring the changes in blood pressure in different positions can provide clues about body function. Checking the blood pressure in the lying, sitting, and standing positions can provide additional information. Normally, when you quickly stand up from a lying or sitting position, the systolic blood pressure also rises. This is a normal compensation for the stress of gravity, and if this did not happen, there would be reduced blood flow to the brain. The rise in pressure assures the brain gets the same amount of blood flow as before. From a lying to a standing position, the pressure should increase six to eight millimeters. If this change doesn't take place, it may indicate dysfunction in the adrenal glands or other problems.

Normally, the adrenal glands react to gravitational stress by releasing more norepinephrine hormone, causing a sympathetic reaction. This is, in part, what increases the blood pressure when we stand. No increase or a drop in systolic pressure upon standing is called *postural hypotension* or *orthostatic hypotension*. Sometimes, the drop in blood pressure upon standing results in light-headedness lasting only a few seconds. Though a variety of other factors need to be ruled out, this problem is often the result of a functional adrenal problem.

## Pulse Pressure

Another figure you can obtain from the blood pressure is called pulse pressure. This is not the same as pulse rate. Let's use the example of a blood pressure of 120/80. The pulse pressure is obtained simply by subtracting the diastolic (80) from the systolic (120). In this case, it is 40. The pulse pressure is a general measure of the relaxation of the muscular walls of the arteries. A good, healthy range for athletes is about 30 to 50. The pulse pressure can be calculated in any position, but it's best analyzed sitting. In the standing position there is more stress in the form of gravity, so the pulse pressure will naturally be a little higher. In the lying position, the body is more at rest and the pulse pressure is normally a little lower.

If your pulse pressure is too high, it indicates the arteries aren't relaxing as much as they should. It's like working seven days a week: the body never gets a break. In this situation, the sympathetic nervous system may be too active, and other tests will usually correlate, such as heart-rate variability (HRV). In other situations, it may be that you're taxing your tired adrenals with too much caffeine or overtraining.

You could have a very high pulse pressure and still have a seemingly normal blood pressure. For example, a blood pressure of 130/60 may sound good to most people, but if you figure the pulse pressure is 70, you can see that there may be a problem, indicating that the muscles in your arteries are not relaxing like they should, with increased tension in the cardiovascular system.

What if your blood pressure is consistently around 140/90? Some might say this is hypertension. However, if you look at the pulse pressure, you can see that the body has compensated well with a normal pulse pressure of 50. In this situation, everything may be fine depending on all other health factors.

A low pulse pressure often indicates a slow metabolism with poor circulation. The cells aren't getting enough nutrients, including oxygen. This may be seen in a blood pressure of 100/80 or 90/65. When the circulation is sluggish, the person often complains about feeling sluggish.

The body can compensate for a slightly higher blood pressure if the pulse pressure is normal, and seemingly normal blood pressure may be a problem if the pulse pressure is too high or too low. With age, as your arteries tend to narrow, the normal range of pulse pressure increases. This is also true in athletes.

# Breathing Tests

One of the most important muscles in your body is the diaphragm. This large flat muscle allows us to breathe air in for oxygen and to breathe out to get rid of carbon dioxide. There are two general tests we can use to measure the effectiveness of the diaphragm muscle.

*Breath-Holding Time* is a simple test that measures the general capacity of the diaphragm. It's easy to perform: Take a deep breath and see how long you can hold it. Anyone in good health should be able to hold the breath for at least fifty seconds. If you can't, it may indicate some functional problem.

*Vital Capacity* is a general measure of lung capacity, and a good test for measuring general diaphragm function. Vital capacity can be measured with a handheld spirometer, or with more accurate units that also measure the rate of expired air. The spirometer measures, in cubic centimeters (cc), the amount of air that you can force out of the lungs. This figure can be converted to a percentage of normal capacity, as related to your height. This conversion can be made by your doctor or calculated by the charts that accompany spirometers. You should be at least 85 percent to 110 percent on scale (which goes up to 120 percent). Vital capacity is also related to physiological age: the lower the vital capacity, the older you may be physiologically, and vice versa.

Lowered Breath Holding Time and Vital Capacity usually indicate less than adequate diaphragm muscle function. Most often, it's due to improper breathing (see chapter 25). This is not necessarily related to $VO_2$max, as even athletes with substantial oxygen uptake can have reduced diaphragm function.

## Oral pH

The body has a wide variety of different measurements of pH—reflecting the acid-alkaline balance. The digestive tract has the whole spectrum, beginning with the alkaline oral cavity (pH 7.6), the normally acid stomach (3), an alkaline small intestine (around 8), and a slightly acid colon (around 6.5). A pH of 7 is neutral.

The pH of the saliva, normally around 7.6, is easy to measure at home, while certain health-care practitioners may wish to test the pH of other areas, such as urine, sinuses, or stool. Use pH paper, available in drug and health stores and easily found on the Internet, with a testing range from 5 to 8. Moisten a small strip of pH paper by inserting it into your mouth for at least five seconds. Don't consume any food or drink for about ten minutes before testing. To find the pH, compare your test paper to the color-coded scale on the pH dispenser. A pH of about 7.6 will turn the test paper a dark blue.

Oral pH may be a good general indicator of fat burning. If you have good fat metabolism, pH will be normal. If you need essential fats, the pH will be too low. It's not unusual to see people with fat metabolism problems have an oral pH of 6.0, or even 5.5. If the dietary fats are increased in the proper proportion, the oral pH will eventually rise to its normal 7.6. In addition, too much carbohydrate in the diet can reduce fat burning, and oral pH. Rarely will the oral pH go above 8. If it does, it may be an indication of local infection in the mouth or throat. Diabetics may also have an abnormally high oral pH.

A normal oral pH is also an ideal environment to protect against dental cavities. A bedtime pH above 7 offers this protection, while an acid pH is accompanied by a high incidence of tooth decay. Test children regularly—their oral pH is just slightly higher than adults, around 7.8. Avoid fruit juice, refined carbohydrates, and other acidifying foods to prevent the pH from becoming too acid. (While milk is alkaline, it eventually turns the mouth very acid due to its high content of the sugar lactose.) Many types of toothpaste also lower the oral pH! Check pH after brushing. In adults, a low pH often predisposes you to other tooth and gum problems, including gingivitis.

## Conclusion

The purpose of using any of these tests and measurements is to help ensure that you are not sacrificing health at the expense of fitness. If you feel that your training isn't going as planned, then testing yourself regularly will help you find clues about what might be going wrong. Like any good detective, you need to follow up on these clues. See where they lead. Examine the evidence. It's your body. But if you reach an impasse or need additional information, you should consult a healthcare professional, which is the subject of our final chapter.

# CHAPTER 34

# FINDING A HEALTH-CARE PROFESSIONAL

Sometimes, despite all your good intentions, smart training, and healthy lifestyle, you may need to consult a health-care professional for help with a sports-related injury. When this happens, finding the expert who best matches your particular needs is critical. A variety of doctors, specialists, physical therapists, massage therapists, nutritionists, and others can help successfully treat your injury or improve your health.

In the most favorable scenario, the health-care professional whom you choose should be able to personally relate to your training and competition—better yet if he or she is an athlete. These individuals are on your side; they don't look askew at the endurance sports lifestyle. They understand why you're so serious about and focused on training. (The only real exception to finding the best health-care practitioner, of course, is if you find yourself in an emergency situation, such as being in a bike accident.) If you find the ideal health-

care professional close to home or work, you're lucky. Many athletes I worked with at my clinic would fly in from out of town. Some would stay for several days to receive treatment, go over training and diet, and plan for the upcoming race season.

The first thing to do when seeking a health-care professional is to ask your training partners, those in your running or triathlon club, and even seek local opinions from athletes online. Ask about their success, their experiences, and whether they were treated as a person and not as a condition. In addition, ask how much time the doctor or therapist spent with them during a first visit, and on subsequent visits, and whether the practitioner answered questions and explained what he or she was doing. Also seek out information about philosophical compatibility; you don't want to work with someone who promotes a high carbohydrate diet and anaerobic training throughout the year if that's not your desire.

Before making an appointment, don't be afraid to call their office for information about how this health-care professional practices. This is not unlike a job interview: You want to know about someone before developing a professional relationship. He or she may have a Web site with additional information.

Once you show up for your scheduled appointment, it's important that you provide a significant amount of information about your fitness and health, especially how and when your injury started. This is obtained through the doctor or therapist taking your history, and usually takes a fair amount of time. Some of this can be obtained from extensive questionnaires, much like those used in this book (many of which I developed and used during my years of practice, and which I sent to athletes before their first visit). Furthermore, a dietary analysis is usually necessary to evaluate your nutritional status. I used to ask athletes to keep a food-intake diary for five to seven days.

Observe how the practitioner addressed your needs and concerns. If you have a good feeling about your visit, plan another as necessary. But if you don't feel comfortable, whether or not you can fully articulate why, search for another health professional. It may take some time.

The biggest problem for an injured athlete, especially in our current healthcare system, is that usually he or she will end up seeing a specialist. For example, if you visit an acupuncturist, you'll get acupuncture; visit a surgeon, you may get surgery; visit a dietician, you'll get diet advice. This may not always be the most holistic approach. What if you have both surgical and nutritional needs for the same problem? It's uncommon to find a practitioner who can address all your needs, or who will refer you to another specialist, although these health-care professionals do exist and are worth seeking out. This is why you must actively manage the entire process. It's up to you to find the best health-care practitioners who best match your needs.

## Sports Medicine Practitioners

At one time, sports medicine was made up of two basic types of practitioners—those in mainstream medicine, who were mostly medical doctors and osteopaths, and those in complementary medicine who used so-called alternative therapies. More recently, sports medicine—a general term for all those health-care practitioners who treat athletes—has evolved and transformed itself. Two significant changes have occurred:

Complementary medicine with its many therapies has gained a high level of acceptance. Many of these approaches are used to varying degrees by all types of practitioners, from chiropractors and osteopaths to physical therapists, acupuncturists, and massage therapists. These include biofeedback, diet and nutrition, acupuncture, manipulation (of the cranium, spine, and other joints), homeopathy, and others.

A second change is that many mainstream medical doctors now use one or more of these same alternative or complementary therapies in their practices.

Unfortunately, many practitioners are considered sports medicine therapists simply because many of their patients are athletes, not because they are personally well acquainted with endurance training and racing.

At the risk of sounding too general and leaving out many other types of sports medicine therapies, I'd like to discuss some types of therapies used in sports medicine, beginning with the four general categories of sports medicine practitioners.

The first category consists of practitioners who predominantly provide hands-on care. These include chiropractors, traditional osteopaths, physical therapists, massage therapists, and those employing different manual therapies. Many of these practitioners use forms of manual muscle testing, which can best be described generally as biofeedback.

The second category includes those professionals who deal with lifestyle factors, especially the chemical and mental or emotional aspects of an athlete. These professionals offer dietary and nutritional advice, and dispense other types of non-drug supplements such as dietary supplements, homeopathic remedies, and herbs. With its reliance on imagery and "mental training," sport psychology falls within this category.

The third category includes professionals who incorporate most if not all of the methods mentioned above into one approach, using both hands-on techniques and addressing lifestyle factors such as diet and nutrition, stress management, and herbal and other types of non-drug supplementation. The three predominant groups within this category are Chinese medicine, applied kinesiology, and naturopathy. While many people are not familiar with these professions, most are familiar with some of their individual elements. Chinese medicine was the first holistic approach, using a combination of acupuncture, herbology, manipulation, nutrition and diet, music and color therapy, and other individual techniques. Applied kinesiology employs much of the same and is a Westernized version of Chinese medicine. Naturopathy involves a similar approach with more emphasis on lifestyle factors.

A fourth group are specialists who address more serious conditions. These include surgeons, neurologists, cardiologists, and those who use primarily surgery and medication. They tend to perform emergency care or often use more extreme therapy as a "last resort" approach after other therapies have not succeeded. These will not be discussed here. While their services are sometimes necessary, they treat the minority of sports problems.

There is a fifth group comprised of sports trainers. These individuals work with athletes by providing specific training schedules. While many are former athletes, others are physiologists, athletic trainers, and certified trainers, and they typically don't provide a particular therapy.

## Assessment Procedures

Two main assessment procedures are employed in health care. The first and most common is a symptom-based assessment, in which a specific treatment or remedy is given for a particular condition. In this approach, an athlete who complains of pain on the outside of the thigh down to the knee may be given a diagnosis of iliotibial band syndrome. A number of treatment options are possible for this syndrome, and one or more may be chosen and usually directed at the area of pain.

A second method of assessment is based on a more complete evaluation, which takes into account the athlete's symptoms but includes other tests that consider the whole person. In this situation, the goal of the assessment process is not necessarily to find a name for the condition but to find what is causing it. An athlete with a diagnosis of iliotibial band syndrome might have different sets of problems and causes. An examination is made not only in the area of pain but throughout the body. The practitioner may evaluate the function of the foot and ankle, the pelvis, and other structures, including testing all the muscles that support these areas. The training and racing history is also considered. Treatment is directed at the areas that appear to be the cause of the symptoms, which may not necessarily be the site of pain. In addition, most injuries are also associated with some type of physical dysfunction, such as muscle imbalance. An effective therapy results not only in the elimination of pain but also in the restoration of normal function, which further helps the athlete's overall performance and health.

Unfortunately, many sports medicine approaches have turned into symptom-based treatments in both mainstream and complementary medicine. Consider acupuncture—it was traditionally practiced by assessing the individual's imbalances, regardless of the complaint. Much of this has changed in our fast-pasted Western health-care system, and today acupuncture is more often practiced by treating the symptoms. Other therapies, such as cranial and spinal manipulation and nutrition, have gone the same way. There are many cookbook diets and dietary supplements used for specific conditions: the cholesterol-lowering diet, the weight-loss diet; or mega doses of vitamin C for colds, creatine phosphate for energy, and chromium for fat burning. These cookbook approaches neglect a more thorough assessment since individualized care can be much more effective.

## Complementary Sports Medicine Professionals

Another factor in today's health-care environment sometimes makes it difficult to find a practitioner who is an ideal match. Many use a wide variety of assessment methods, therapies, and lifestyle recommendations not typical of their particular profession, with many using tools that at one time were found only in other disciplines. In the general arena of sports medicine, I've known dentists who used nutrition, podiatrists who treated not just the feet but the whole body, and chiropractors who prescribed drugs. In my own holistic practice, among the activities I was trained for and performed were neurological examinations, sports training, diet and nutrition, manual muscle testing, and various forms of biofeedback.

Because of this, it's now more difficult to find a health-care professional based on his or her title (medical doctor, chiropractor, etc.). And it emphasizes the need to find out what services and products a particular practitioner offers.

It should be noted, however, that while many complementary therapies are still not fully understood, scientific scrutiny of the actual outcomes—how these methods work— have shown significant success. This is one reason for the relatively recent acceptance of these methods by patients and insurance companies. In addition, mainstream medicine has embraced complementary therapies with about half of medical schools and family practice residency programs now including the teaching of some of them.

## Biofeedback

For over thirty years, I have developed and used forms of biofeedback in clinical practice, including training athletes to build endurance, correcting common muscle imbalances, and treating patients with brain and spinal cord injuries. These specific biofeedback approaches include the use of a heart-rate monitor, manual muscle testing and electromyography (EMG) for the assessment and treatment of muscle imbalance, and electroencephalography (EEG) to help stimulate alpha brain waves.

The term biofeedback was coined in the 1960s by scientists who trained human subjects to consciously alter their body function through sensory input to the brain. However, long before mechanical biofeedback techniques emerged, natural biofeedback mechanisms were built into our brains—a key feature in our development, with early humans using it instinctively for survival. For example, sensing uncomfortable temperatures, humans sought ways to adapt through clothing, shelter, and fire; and walking on rough surfaces led to the development of minimal protective footwear.

Because the human brain and body has this built-in capacity for biofeedback, developing various forms that were sensible and useful was relatively easy. This included biofeedback techniques that incorporated equipment, such as heart-rate monitoring, and those that could be done manually where reliance on equipment is not necessary, including EMG- and EEG-type procedures.

While the goal of manual muscle testing is widely varied, there is one common feature among all those professionals using it: Manual muscle testing is an important form of bio-feedback used to help evaluate neuromuscular function, especially in helping to determine muscle imbalance, a common cause of physical injury.

## Chiropractic

While manipulation of the spine has been used as therapy for many centuries, the chiropractic profession, specializing in this technique, dates back only to 1895. Many chiropractors believe that spinal vertebra misalignments, called subluxations, interfere with the normal communication between the brain and body to cause physical, chemical, or mental and emotional imbalances. The chiropractic subluxation refers most often to a spinal joint that is causing problems in the spine or elsewhere in the body. Some chiropractors also address imbalances associated with other joints including the temporomandibular joint and those in the feet, knees, wrists, and others. Chiropractors have successfully treated patients with conditions ranging from back and neck pain to intestinal disorders and allergies. In the United States, chiropractors must receive a doctorate degree (Doctor of Chiropractic, or DC) through a

rigorous education, nearly identical to that of medical or osteopathic school except that it does not include studies in surgery. Many chiropractors are also trained in other complementary disciplines, including diet and nutrition, applied kinesiology, and Chinese medicine, cranial-sacral technique, and others.

Over the past several decades, chiropractic sports medicine and rehabilitation have been emerging fields within complementary medicine. Many professional, collegiate, amateur, and Olympic teams, along with individual athletes, use chiropractic care as a major part of their sports programs.

## Osteopathy

I have studied and used approaches from traditional osteopathy, especially cranial osteopathy. Traditional osteopathy is a manipulative-based therapy using a conservative non-drug approach. There is a stronger focus on the bones of the head and neck and the musculoskeletal system in general. In addition, other therapies are often used by some osteopaths, including acupuncture, diet and nutrition, and biofeedback. Osteopathy was first developed in the 1890s by Andrew Taylor Still, who founded the first college of osteopathic medicine. Still was an American medical doctor and surgeon during the Civil War. He later criticized medicine for overuse of drugs and began using more holistic methods that included diet, prevention, and fitness. By the 1950s the majority of osteopaths were incorporated into mainstream medicine. Today, most osteopaths in the country practice like medical doctors, no longer using their traditional techniques. Their doctor of osteopathy degree (DO) is nearly identical to a medical degree. In many parts of the world, especially Europe, many osteopaths have maintained their traditional roles, often using many complementary approaches.

Cranial osteopathy, developed in 1939 by Dr. William Sutherland, an osteopath, is a subspecialty within osteopathic manipulative medicine. A cranial osteopath focuses particularly on the movements of the cranial bones and their relationships with the spine and sacrum. These cranial-sacral techniques are commonly taught to many health-care professionals. These cranial relationships are described as a dynamic force within the living human body: the "energy" of the central nervous system. In particular, cranial-sacral movement is associated with the circulation of cerebral spinal fluid, which bathes the brain and spinal cord. Osteopaths describe precise movements of all twenty-six cranial bones, which constitute a significant part of the body's self-healing mechanism. Cranial bone movement is associated with the movement of the breathing mechanism; certain bones move specifically with both inhalation and exhalation movement. The amount of movement is in the range of fractions of a millimeter.

Cranial osteopaths believe that any disruption in cranial movement may have an adverse effect on any area of the body, causing imbalances. Problems within the cranial-sacral mechanism can occur as a result of trauma (beginning with birth), daily microtrauma, breathing irregularities, muscular imbalances, and other problems.

Assessment is done by palpation of the cranium, sacrum, and spine; by postural evaluation; by muscle testing; and by other approaches depending on the practitioner. Correction of cranial-sacral problems is accomplished manually by applying gentle pressures at certain points on the cranium and sacrum, often in conjunction with inhalation or exhalation, or through manipulation of certain spinal vertebrae.

## Massage Therapy (Therapeutic Massage)

The profession of massage therapy is comprised of trained, licensed practitioners who perform various types of massage techniques. Massage therapy, also many centuries old, is often used in sports medicine and is frequently recommended by both mainstream and complementary practitioners for athletes who are injured and for prevention purposes. Massage focuses on increasing blood circulation and lymph flow, reducing muscle tension and spasm, improving range of motion, and helping to reduce pain. Foot massage can also stimulate the communication between the feet and brain, helping foot balance and other foot function.

Massage involves soft tissue manipulation of the body's muscles and aids in stress reduction, which can help recovery from training and competition. It can also reduce high cortisol levels to help reduce anxiety, improve the immune system, and help other dysfunction associated with high levels of this stress hormone.

A variety of techniques are used in sports massage, including effleurage, petrissage, and vibration. I have found Swedish massage in particular to be valuable for endurance athletes, especially those with adrenal dysfunction.

Trigger-point massage has also become popular. This approach involves specific finger pressure into myofascial trigger points in muscles and connective tissue to reduce hypersensitivity and muscle spasms. Trigger points may cause restricted and painful movement of muscles, ligaments, and tendons. Pioneered by Dr. Janet Travell in the 1940s, this technique became popular with her treatment of President Kennedy when she was the White House physician. Today, many health-care practitioners perform trigger-point therapy.

## Nutrition and Diet

Various aspects of nutrition and diet are taken into account by so many different health-care professionals that it is difficult to categorize. Many within the field do not consider it part of complementary medicine since nurses and dieticians who work in hospitals and other institutions have been applying a form of basic nutrition therapy for decades as part of mainstream medicine. The differences between mainstream nutrition/diet therapy and the complementary approach are many. Most different is the philosophy of mainstream medicine that associates nutrition with particular deficiency states (i.e., vitamin C prevents scurvy), and that of complementary medicine, which considers the natural foods and nutrients that may improve overall body function, hence endurance. (In doing so, this approach also prevents deficiency.)

Another clear division in the field of diet and nutrition is the recommendation to consume processed foods with fortified synthetic vitamins and other nutrients, versus unprocessed natural foods containing thousands of naturally occurring nutrients.

The same division applies in the arena of dietary supplements. Many sports practitioners recommend high-dose synthetic vitamins much the same way they recommend prescription drugs. Some of these "sports performance" products use synthetic hormones, which can not only reduce the production of your body's own hormones but in some cases are banned in endurance sports. Other products come with the potential of significant health risks. Instead, many other sports practitioners recommend natural products while emphasizing an optimal diet to provide most nutrients.

## Homeopathy

The history of homeopathy begins with its founder, Samuel Hahnemann (1755–1843), a German physician who coined the word *homeopathy* (*homoios* in Greek means "similar"; *pathos* refers to suffering). Hahnemann developed the "law of similars" into a systematic medical art and science. Immunizations, allergy treatment, and other medical approaches are based on this "law," although homeopathy works in a very different way, using extremely low-dose substances to treat patients. In effect, the practitioner seeks to find a substance that, if given in overdose, would produce symptoms similar to those a sick person is experiencing. The most controversial aspect of homeopathy is the dosages. They are produced by a series of dilutions that result in an exceedingly low-dose substance. Homeopaths have observed that the more a medicine has been diluted, the longer it generally acts and the fewer the doses needed to be effective.

More startling is the fact that while homeopaths and scientists agree that solutions diluted beyond 24X or 12C (dilution levels used in homeopathy) may not have any molecules of the original solution, they assert that something remains: the essence of the substance, its resonance, its energy. Many practitioners have difficulty accepting these theories considering their science-based education, while others only look at the end-result success of homeopathic treatments.

Homeopathy evolved in the United States through the work of Hans Gram, a Dutch homeopath who immigrated to the United States in 1825. Today, homeopathy is widespread throughout the world, especially in Europe, Asia, the Far East, Central and South America, Australia, and Russia.

## Naturopathic Medicine

Naturopathy is the holistic practice of natural therapeutics, or natural medicine, which works with a variety of hands-on and lifestyle factors including diet, nutrition, herbal medicine, homeopathy, acupuncture, and physical medicine. In addition to treating a variety of imbalances, the naturopath focuses on functional problems to prevent future illness and injury. These practitioners assess patients through physical examinations, blood and urine tests, nutritional and dietary evaluations, and other methods.

Naturopathy began in the United States in the early 1900s, when many of the natural therapies that had previously existed were joined together into one approach. For unknown reasons, by the mid-1900s, naturopathy rapidly declined as mainstream medicine flourished. Today, the naturopathic physician must obtain an ND degree (naturopathic doctor) from a four-year graduate-level naturopathic college. In the United States, only thirteen states license naturopaths, but with expansion of many complementary practices, naturopathy is once again growing, as other professionals are adopting these approaches, and as the natural therapies movement continues to evolve.

## Chinese Medicine

This approach is one of the oldest known systems of assessment and therapy, dating back five thousand years. Using perhaps the first true holistic approach, traditional Chinese medicine practitioners address every aspect of the patient's life, including physical, chemical, mental and emotional, spiritual, and social facets. Chinese medicine includes four main components: acupuncture, manipulation and massage, herbal and nutritional remedies, and exercise disciplines called *qigong* (the most popular form being *tai chi*).

An important focus in Chinese medicine is assessment, which relies heavily on observation of the person—especially the face, skin, and breath—and on palpation of the radial pulses on the wrist. According to Chinese theory, twelve energy channels, called meridians, contain life's energy (called *chi* or *qi*), the reason why this approach is sometimes called meridian therapy. On each meridian, there are many different points that can be stimulated by manual pressure (acupressure), needles (acupuncture), heat (through the burning of the moxa herb, referred to as moxibustion), and in modern Chinese medicine, electricity (electroacupuncture). Chinese medicine also incorporates therapies such as herbal medicine, music and color therapy, and even psychology.

The basic theory in Chinese medicine is that an imbalance of qi—which consists of yin and yang energy—is the cause of dysfunction, injury, and ultimately disease. The balancing of yin and yang energy is therefore the goal of the practitioner, who may use any or all of the therapeutic tools to accomplish this depending on which is most applicable to the patient's needs based on assessment.

This balance does not stop with the individual but continues into society as a whole. The individual, as well as the surrounding society, is a delicate balance of yin and yang. Yin represents water, quiet, substance, and night; yang represents fire, noise, function, and day. The two are polar opposites and therefore one of them must be present to allow the other to exist; for instance, how can you experience joy if you do not understand sorrow? More interesting is the fact that many ancient Chinese visited their practitioners when they were well, paying the practitioner a retainer to keep them healthy. If they became ill, they stopped paying until wellness returned.

## Kinesiology

Most sports medicine practitioners learn a significant amount about anatomy and biomechanics during their years in training and after. Kinesiology, the study of human movement, is an important part of this learning process.

The study of kinesiology is a common undergraduate and graduate program, with some universities offering PhD programs in this discipline. Students graduating these programs in kinesiology generally work with health-care practitioners in hospitals, on sports teams, and in other arenas to assist in sports training.

Those studying the clinical sciences with a goal of obtaining a doctorate degree in medicine, osteopathy, chiropractic, or other areas often study the same type of kinesiology with more emphasis on neuromuscular function and the use of manual muscle testing as an assessment tool. These individuals are usually healthcare professionals who use complementary medicine, with the name *professional applied kinesiology* (PAK) separating this clinical approach from kinesiology. (It should also be noted that a significant number of people, many of whom don't have college experience in this field, also employ types of kinesiology. These include those in Touch for Health and many other programs that teach lay people certain techniques.)

Many health-care professionals who use various forms of therapy with the name "kinesiology" have evolved in the last fifty years and have incorporated the use of manual muscle testing. Virtually all these different types of kinesiology today—there are dozens—came from applied kinesiology (AK), which was developed in the early 1960s by Dr. George Goodheart, a chiropractor who employed a wide range of complementary approaches, including Chinese medicine, osteopathy and chiropractic, diet and nutrition, and sports medicine. In 1980, he became the first official chiropractor on the U.S. Olympic medical team and in 2001 was on *Time* magazine's list of the Top 100 Alternative Medicine Innovators of the Twenty-first Century.

Much like Chinese medicine, applied kinesiology combines many existing therapies into one system. Applied kinesiology practitioners use manual muscle testing as part of an assessment process that focuses on the physical, chemical, and mental and emotional state. This and other assessment tools help practitioners find the therapies that best match the patient's specific needs. These practitioners theorize that when there is an imbalance in the body, it is usually reflected as a specific muscle imbalance.

There is not a specific academic degree for applied kinesiology; rather, those licensed health-care professionals use manual muscle testing as one of often several complementary medicine procedures. Various professional organizations, such as the International College of Applied Kinesiology, offer postdoctorate courses and certifications in professional applied kinesiology.

## Sport Psychology

In 1956, Roger Bannister became the first runner to break the four-minute barrier in the mile. He later wrote, "Though physiology may indicate respiratory and circulatory limits to muscular effort, psychological and other factors beyond the ken of physiology set the razor's edge of defeat or victory and determine how close an athlete approaches the absolute limits of performance." Sport psychology is not necessarily considered a branch of either complementary or mainstream medicine, but clearly it can be used in conjunction with both approaches. A variety of psychological therapies are often used in sports medicine, including hypnosis, mental imagery, EEG-type biofeedback (neurotherapy), and meditation.

## Conclusion

Forming balanced goals regarding training and racing is a key priority for endurance athletes. All health-care practitioners can play a vital role in helping athletes understand their normal and abnormal physical, chemical, and mental function. By providing objective information about the brain and body, these experts can also help athletes overcome social pressures, media and advertising distortion, and other problems they may encounter.

Millions of athletes, from professionals to recreational enthusiasts, regularly seek help from health-care practitioners. A significant number of these doctors and therapists use many different forms of complementary medicine. Whether the one you visit uses Chinese medicine, biofeedback, applied kinesiology, or some combination of therapies, the two important questions for you to ask are these: Have you completely recovered from your injury or ill health? Has your athletic function improved? In the end, your health is ultimately your own responsibility, and by following the principles outlined in this book, you can have years of sound health and fitness. The lifestyle choice is all that truly matters.

# AFTERWORD

*A living legend in the running and sports science community, Dr. Timothy David Noakes is a South African professor of exercise and sports science at the University of Cape Town. As an endurance athlete, he has run more than 70 marathons and ultramarathons, His running book,* Lore of Running, *now in its fourth edition, remains a classic. In 1996, he was honored by the American College of Sports Medicine for his work in the field of exercise physiology.*

***

I discovered Dr. Phil Maffetone when trying to understand how Mark Allen had been so successful for so long in one of the toughest sporting disciplines on earth, the triathlon. Mark, arguably the finest male triathlete of all time, was quick to acknowledge Dr. Maffetone's contribution.

From Dr. Maffetone, Allen had learned the need to train with circumspection. Years later,

I asked Allen why so few followed Maffetone's proven methods. He replied simply: "Young athletes always think that to be successful, they must do it their own way. They are too proud to listen."

What Allen suggested might be why none had ever come close to matching his own athletic record.

In *The Big Book of Endurance Training and Racing*, Dr. Maffetone shares his lifetime of experience in helping athletes of all abilities to become better. He understands that there is no single magic bullet; that sporting success is achieved by those who control all aspects of their lives. He knows that everything we do each day affects our athletic performance.

For those prepared to listen, there is a wealth of knowledge in Dr. Maffetone's experience. Somewhere out there is the next Mark Allen wondering how to become better. If you read Dr. Maffetone's thoughts, understand them, and put them into practice, you just might be that unique individual.

—**Dr. Timothy David Noakes**

# INDEX